Therapeutic Massage in Athletics

Therapeutic Massage in Athletics

Pat Archer, MS, ATC, LMP

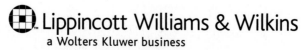

Lippincott Williams & Wilkins
a Wolters Kluwer business

Philadelphia · Baltimore · New York · London
Buenos Aires · Hong Kong · Sydney · Tokyo

Acquisitions Editor: John Goucher
Development Editor: David R. Payne
Marketing Manager: Hilary Henderson
Production Editor: Jennifer P. Ajello
Designer: Risa Clow
Artwork: Dragonfly Media
Photography: Bob Riedlinger
Compositor: Circle Graphics
Printer: Courier Corporation-Westford

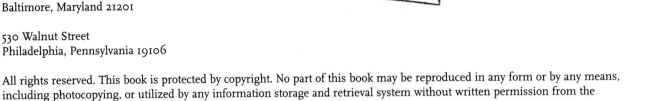

351 West Camden Street
Baltimore, Maryland 21201

530 Walnut Street
Philadelphia, Pennsylvania 19106

Printed in the United States of America

Library of Congress Cataloging-in-Publication Data

Archer, Patricia A.
    Therapeutic massage in athletics / Pat Archer.
        p. ; cm.
    Includes index.
    ISBN-13: 978-0-7817-4269-6
      1. Sports massage. 2. Athletics. 3. Sports physical therapy. 4. Massage. I. Title.
    [DNLM: 1. Massage—methods. 2. Athletic Injuries—therapy. 3. Sports Medicine. WB 537 A672t
2007]
RM721.A73 2007
615.8'22088796—dc22

                              2006005094

The publishers have made every effort to trace the copyright holders for borrowed material. If they have inadvertently overlooked any, they will be pleased to make the necessary arrangements at the first opportunity.

To purchase additional copies of this book, call our customer service department at **(800) 638-3030** or fax orders to **(301) 824-7390**. International customers should call **(301)714-2324**.

Visit Lippincott Williams & Wilkins on the Internet: http://www.LWW.com. Lippincott Williams & Wilkins customer service representatives are available from 8:30 am to 6:00 pm, EST.

08 09 10
3 4 5 6 7 8 9 10

This book is dedicated to the memories of my mother Marian, who was my first inspiration for reading and writing, and my sister Chris, who taught me many lessons in humility, patience, and perseverance.

Preface

This text is based on the knowledge and experience gained through my 30 years working as both a Certified Athletic Trainer (ATC) and a Licensed Massage Therapist. During this time, I have discovered that my experiences as an ATC have made me a better massage therapist; likewise, my massage therapy expertise has helped me become a more thorough and well-rounded athletic trainer. By integrating both of my professions, I have learned to reduce "down time" for the athletes I work with by adding specific massage techniques to standard treatment protocols. To support and encourage other sports health care professionals to develop advanced massage skills, this text outlines the most efficient and effective forms of therapeutic massage for athletics by:

- Providing sound anatomic and physiologic rationale for the inclusion of four specific therapeutic massage techniques.
- Introducing the lymphatic facilitation techniques to therapists who see traumatic edema and inflammation on a regular basis.
- Explaining the differences and similarities among the myriad massage techniques available.
- Outlining the contraindications and precautions for each technique.
- Providing an outline for appropriate and effective integration of these techniques into current sports health care practices.
- Providing examples of stroke combinations for effective therapeutic massage at events and in regular maintenance efforts.
- Providing examples of massage treatment protocols for a variety of common athletic injuries and chronic pain conditions.

ORGANIZATION AND FEATURES

The text is divided into four parts. Part I, Introduction to Therapeutic Massage in Athletics, establishes terminology, discusses the benefits and effects of massage in general, defines basic sports massage, and describes the purpose and use of the basic strokes. Part I also includes information on appropriate massage equipment, supplies, and general body mechanics for therapists when giving massage.

Part II is Anatomy and Physiology for Massage in Athletics. Although an in-depth and thorough knowledge of all human anatomy and physiology is always desirable, this text is not intended to be a detailed anatomy and physiology book. Instead, this text describes only the key anatomic and physiologic concepts that explain and support the use of the specific massage techniques advocated in the book. The basic anatomy and physiology of the cardiovascular and lymphatic systems, muscles, nerves, and the fascial/connective tissue system are included. Rather than go into great detail with each system (something better accomplished by any anatomy and physiology textbook), this text focuses on the key elements that explain how the massage techniques create their desired effects and on the interrelationship of these body systems. Perhaps the most important "new" information in this section is in Chapter 3, which describes the lymphatic system and its role as the primary method of edema removal for the body. Since traumatic edema and inflammation are everyday occurrences in athletics, this in-depth information on how the lymphatic system works and how to stimulate these processes is of vital importance to all sports health care professionals. The final chapter in this section describes the healing process and how this knowledge directs therapeutic choices.

Part III is Therapeutic Massage Techniques for Sports Health Care. I fully acknowledge that one cannot develop sufficient skill in performance of these massage techniques just by reading about them. It is presumed that the students and professionals using this book will do so in the context of a fully outlined course or curriculum that includes hands-on training from a qualified and experienced instructor. The four massage/bodywork techniques described in this text are considered individual specialty techniques by most massage and bodywork professionals.

It is not my intention to write a definitive text on any one of these methods since there are more detailed textbooks and certificate programs available for each of these massage/bodywork styles. Rather, I have distilled and abbreviated some key theories and methodology from each technique and provided detailed guidelines for their use, individually and in combination, to create a therapeutic massage well-suited to a wide array of athletic and clinical environments.

The specific forms of manual therapy advocated in this text are intended to address the body systems that athletes stress the most. They appear to create more immediate and measurable effects on range of motion and tissue flexibility and reduce edema and pain more effectively than many other styles of massage. Since the major objective in sports health care is to keep the athlete performing at his or her highest level on a daily basis, proficiency in each of these techniques is most valuable. Each technique explained in these chapters addresses specific aspects of the common aches and pains associated with athletic endeavors. The neuromuscular techniques are used to address abhorrent muscle tension, the myofascial techniques to address connective tissue restrictions to movement, the lymphatic techniques to reduce pain and swelling, and the deep Swedish/basic sports massage techniques to help the athlete "feel good" and reconnect the injured area to the surrounding strong and healthy body regions. Each chapter begins with a brief history and overview of the theory and purpose of the technique before specific strokes/releases are explained and depicted. The lymphatic techniques in Chapter 7 will be of particular interest because they are new and exciting tools for most sports health care professionals.

In Part IV, Protocols for Massage Used in Athletics, individual techniques from neuromuscular, myofascial, lymphatic, and basic sports massage are combined to form the unique system of therapeutic massage for athletes. Chapters 10 and 11 give examples of event and maintenance massage sequences, and Chapter 13 details massage treatment protocols for several common athletic injuries. Chapter 12 is devoted to assessment guidelines, describing several methods of testing that help therapists distinguish one type of injury from another and how this information is used to direct treatment. Chapter 14 describes other common sports health care modalities and suggests how therapeutic massage might be integrated with them to best serve the athlete.

Some of the key features in the text include the following:

- **Learning objectives** provide clear goals to ensure mastery of the content presented in each chapter.
- **Key terms** are boldfaced at first appearance in each chapter and included in a glossary at the back of the book.
- **Step-by-step procedure boxes** guide the reader through different massage protocols, both visually and with a numbered stroke sequence.
- **From the Field quotes** from athletes, coaches, doctors, sports massage specialists, and physical therapists describe their personal experiences, beliefs, and successful use of therapeutic massage in sports health care settings, which include clinical, high school, collegiate, recreational, and professional athletics.
- **Case studies** provide real-world examples of athletes who have been treated with massage for specific conditions.
- **Bulleted summaries** review essential information and key points in each chapter.
- Approximately 20 short-answer and multiple-choice **review questions** appear at the end of each chapter.

This book is not about teaching readers "my" techniques. Instead, the complex theories and details of each individual therapeutic massage technique have been simplified and are presented in a more generic format that makes it easier to teach and apply to a variety of sports health care settings. This approach leaves plenty of room to teach and use these techniques with your own individual flair and preferences by providing the intellectual scaffolding that helps develop conditional thinking. In other words, therapists, teachers, and students can use the physiologic rationale, general guidelines, and basic stroke applications provided to support and develop their own individual therapeutic skills.

Acknowledgments

I cannot imagine ever trying to write a book without having the support of many, many people, and while I am certain that "thank you" just isn't enough, it is all I have to offer and it is important to say. Many thanks to all at LWW for their guidance and support. Special thanks go to Pete Darcy for "bringing me into the fold" and being such a good cheerleader, to David Payne for being so patient and supportive with me throughout the process (I don't think I made a single deadline, and you simply encouraged me to continue), and to Susan, Nancy, and Christen for your understanding and kind words during my time of deep personal loss. Thanks to all the reviewers for their feedback and suggestions that helped me get to what I was "trying to say" and to all of my colleagues who contributed their "From the Field" quotes—truly some of the brightest stars in the sports health care profession.

A big thank you to Holland McIver for taking care of the glossary. You saved my sanity by handling "the details." Dale Perry, you rocked my world by teaching me all about lymphatic facilitation and helping refine my skills and understanding to this level. It was the need to share this information that made me stop procrastinating and write the book, so thank you.

My undying gratitude goes to Lisa Nelson, LMP, the most extraordinary teacher and learning strategist I have ever known. Without her help, I simply could not have finished. Lisa edited and clarified my words (chopped a lot of the's and that's), checked and rechecked references, kept me organized, positive, and on task for well over a year. She also provided the frequent mental and emotional support I needed when I was feeling negative and unsure of my abilities. I also owe her family, Mark, Kari, Zach, and Tyler, a big load of thanks for allowing her to be away from them for days on end to help me—you're the best.

Finally, I want to thank Heida Brenneke, founder of the Brenneke School of Massage, and my mentor, personal and professional inspiration, and colleague for these past twenty years. You took me under your wing, trusted me, counseled me, challenged me, and gave me the support and encouragement I needed to grow into myself personally and professionally. I simply would not be the person I am today without your love and guidance, and I'm eternally grateful.

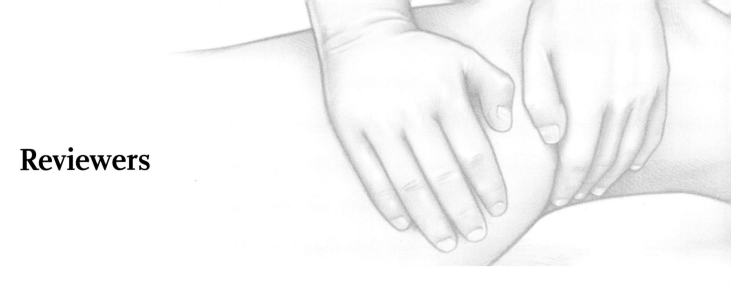

Reviewers

Mitchell L. Cordova, PhD, ATC, FACSM
Associate Professor and Acting Chairperson
Indiana State University
Terre Haute, IN

Lori Dewald, EdD, ATC, CHES
Athletic Training Program Director
University of Minnesota, Duluth
Duluth, MN

Mark Dixon, NCTMB, HHP
Huntington Beach, CA

Cherryanne Gunsch, AAS, PT Asst
PTA/LMT, Still Waters Massage
Fairborn, OH

Bill Holcomb, PhD, ATC
University of Nevada, Las Vegas
Las Vegas, NV

Christopher J. Joyce, PhD, ATC, CSCS
Assistant Professor, Program Director
University of North Florida
Jacksonville, FL

Richard Ray, EdD
Professor and Chair of Kinesiology
Hope College
Holland, MI

Jan Schwartz, BA
Vice President
Cortiva Education
Summit, NJ

Donald Webb
Parkville, MD

Patricia Wilcoxon
Severna Park, MD

Contents

Introduction to Therapeutic Massage in Athletics

Introduction to Massage Therapy

OBJECTIVES

After completing this chapter, the reader will be able to:

- Define the terms *modality* and *technique* as used in therapeutic massage.
- Distinguish a benefit of massage from a physiologic effect, and name four general benefits of therapeutic massage.
- Define and distinguish a structural effect and a systemic effect of massage.
- List five structural effects of massage and explain each.
- Define and give examples of *osteokinematics* and *arthrokinematics*.
- Describe the difference between increased circulation and increased local circulation.
- List the distinctions between the edema removal methods of classic/Swedish and specialized lymphatic techniques.
- List three possible mechanisms to explain how massage reduces pain.
- List nine key steps to good body mechanics for therapists during massage.
- Describe the three general rules of application for all massage techniques.
- Name and define the four therapeutic massage techniques that are the recommended techniques for use in athletics.

Since antiquity, massage has been included as an important element of sports health care. The ancient Greeks and Romans first emphasized the importance of massage for the maintenance of general health and improvement of physical performance. During the European Renaissance, massage, specifically "frictions and rubbing," was considered a standard part of general medical treatment. This is evidenced in the writings of Ambrose Paré, a prominent French surgeon in the sixteenth century. By the late nineteenth century, athletes in the United States and England established "rubdowns" as a regular part of their training and gave this practice a good deal of the credit for championship performances. In our time, massage is included as a part of medical services for the athletes in most international competitions, including championship events for the National Collegiate Athletic Association (NCAA) and national sport federations, as well as most Olympic qualifiers and games.

In one of the earliest athletic training texts, Joseph Dolan defines massage as "the scientific manipulation of the body tissues."[1] He states that the "athletic masseur" has been on the scene since the first football game was played in 1869. The importance of massage at that time is evident in this text because it is the topic of the entire second chapter, whereas modalities such as heat/cold and "electrotherapy" are discussed in only a few paragraphs in Chapter 11. The continued importance of massage is supported by the fact that current textbooks on physical therapy modalities and/or the treatment of athletic injuries include sections on therapeutic massage. In addition, the curriculum guidelines for athletic training programs require that massage be included as a therapeutic modality.

Although massage is acknowledged as an important modality, there is much confusion and disagreement about its practical use and therapeutic benefits.[2–15] The lack of standardized terminology, the many forms of massage claiming to have a set of specific and unique effects, plus the wide range of techniques used in various research projects all make it difficult for sports health care professionals to choose and use any form of massage with confidence. This chapter establishes some standard terminology, describes the benefits and physiologic effects of massage, describes massage supplies and equipment, and introduces the specific massage techniques to be combined as "therapeutic massage in athletics."

Terminology

In sports health care terminology, a **modality** is a therapeutic agent used to effect physical changes. In this text the terms massage and sports massage are referred to as modalities, whereas the specific form of massage/sports massage is considered a technique. In other words, a type of massage that has strokes sharing the same general intentions and methods of application, such as lymph facilitation, is a **technique.**

Benefits and Physiologic Effects of Massage

There is no question that massage is perceived as a beneficial and important modality among sports health care therapists and athletes.[1–15] However, the exact means by which massage creates physiologic changes and how these changes might prevent injury, improve healing, and enhance athletic performance have still not been proved in the minds of many therapists. Many of the original theories on the effects of massage were based on erroneous ideas of human anatomy and physiology, such as the idea that lymph fluid emptied back into the right side of the heart[1] or that lactic acid build-up in muscles caused muscle tension and delayed-onset soreness.[16] As advances in research design and evaluation tools continue, and improvements are made in our understanding of anatomy, physiology, and the mechanisms of injury and healing, the benefits and physiologic effects of massage become clearer.

In the past 50 years, there have been a few extensive literature reviews on the effects of massage,[8,13,15,17,18] and the conclusion of each is that findings are equivocal. Some theories and statements regarding the effects of massage have been supported; others have not. Part of the problem is that many authors and educators continue to reference old research from the 1940s and 1950s. Not only are these stud-

ies insufficient in number to either prove or disprove the theories on massage effects, but the technology of the time makes the accuracy of these studies questionable.[13,17,18] Another issue is that it is extremely difficult to validate the findings of one study with another. This is due to the wide variety of massage techniques used in these studies, as well as the differences in durations of the sessions and in timing of the massages in relation to the activity.

In addition, choices in research design and methods of analysis give a wide range of results. For example, several of the more current research studies are designed to measure immediate changes in range of motion, recovery of muscle strength, and circulation.[13,17,18] Since massage effects tend to be more cumulative than immediate,[3,7,11–13] long-term investigation would be more appropriate and likely to offer more valuable information. However, well-designed studies that investigate long-term massage effects such as improving the range of motion, decreasing the risk of muscle strain, and improving the rate of healing are few and far between. Only research that is carried out over an entire season, or with a full athletic team, and that applies a specific massage technique with well-defined parameters of duration and application can provide validation for some of the claims of the cumulative effects of massage. An adequate number of these types of studies has yet to be designed.

■ BENEFITS OF THERAPEUTIC MASSAGE

In massage textbooks, some authors make a distinction between the terms *indications,* or physiologic effects, and *benefits* of massage. This distinction is related to two different paradigms in health care: the treatment model and the wellness model. The term "indication" implies that a massage technique creates specific and desirable tissue/systemic changes related to an injury or condition. Therefore, massage indications are discussed in the treatment paradigm.[12] The term "benefit" implies that a modality is helpful to overall well-being (wellness), and therefore good, even if no specific injury or dysfunction is present. It supports the concept that it does not matter *how,* or through which physiologic mechanism massage benefits occur, just that they *do* occur. Even if massage is only a placebo, the fact that athletes benefit from its use provides sufficient rationale for its inclusion in certain athletic situations. Most sports health care therapists can recall several examples in which they relied on a placebo such as sugar pills or exaggerated positive reinforcement to help an athlete "feel better."

An athlete's performance can be affected by many *subjective* variables that have nothing to do with body strength, endurance, oxygen consumption, or flexibility. Psychological factors such as mind set, mental toughness, focus, and desire are commonly acknowledged as affecting performance and healing. However, because these psychological factors are highly subjective, it is difficult to quantify and measure the exact effect of these variables on the athlete's performance and healing. The following list of benefits is based on studies of general massage and multiple anecdotal reports from the sports health care field.[3,4,6,8,10,11,13,16,19] Although these studies are not based on the specific combination of massage techniques proposed by this text, nor are they all directed to an athletic population, it is logical to assume that athletes would experience the same benefits as other research populations.

GENERAL BENEFITS OF THERAPEUTIC MASSAGE FOR ATHLETES

- Decreases anxiety, stress, and/or depression[1,3,4,7,8,13,15,19, 21–24]
- Enhances sense of well-being and mental focus[3,7,8,11,20]
- Improves sleep patterns[8,23–25]
- Identifies areas of tension or soreness to be addressed before an injury occurs[2–4,6,10,20]
- Provides *kinesthetic* feedback that helps create a positive state of mind; that is, athletes *feel* muscles relax and joints decompress, leading to a greater sense of ease with movement[3,4,15,20]

Perhaps the most representative study that measures the benefits of massage was done by Field et al.[19] Thirty-two depressed adolescent mothers were divided into a massage group who received ten 30-minute sessions of massage and a control group who received ten 30-minute sessions of relaxation therapy over a 5-week period of time. Both groups reported subjective decreases in anxiety after the first and last sessions, but only the massage group showed a measurable decrease in anxious behavior, in pulse, and in both salivary and urinary cortisol levels. Braverman[8,21,24] gives a good synopsis of several other well-designed studies that collectively demonstrate that massage can lead to less distress and tension, a higher degree of tranquility and vitality, enhanced alertness, and fewer sleep difficulties. It seems logical to believe that an athlete's performance potential and rate of recovery from injury might be positively affected by this decreased anxiety and stress and the enhanced sense of well-being and mental focus. Because regular exercise has been shown to decrease cortisol levels,[8,10,21] this effect may be especially important to athletes whose injury has made it impossible to train at the usual level.

If therapeutic massage is included as a regular part of an athlete's training program, the frequent assessment and reduction of muscle and fascial tensions should help the athlete avoid injury, such as chronic strain syndromes. Although this benefit has yet to be adequately researched, the theory is simple and logical; the more often tissue is thoroughly assessed for restrictions, muscle tension/spasm, and general soreness, the more likely it is that these problems can be found and relieved. However, therapists must be careful *not* to extend this theoretical foundation to conclude that massage *prevents* injury. If that were true, athletes who receive regular massage would never get injured, and we all know that is not the case. One must consider the multitude of variables that increase or decrease the risk of injury; equipment, past injuries, coaching and training methods, and the climate and temperature at the time of the workout, for example. It is impossible to single out any one of these variables as the key factor in prevention of injury.

Other examples of the benefits of therapeutic massage are more related to convenience and the effect on the therapist–athlete relationship. Massage is perhaps the most convenient and flexible therapeutic modality available to sports health care therapists. The therapist's hands are always immediately available, and treatments can be administered in any environment, including an airplane or bus or on the field. In addition, massage provides therapists with the opportunity to demonstrate individual and personalized care to each athlete.

PHYSIOLOGIC EFFECTS: INDICATIONS FOR THERAPEUTIC MASSAGE IN ATHLETICS

Although the subjective benefits of massage are important and helpful to athletes, the specific tissue changes created—the physiologic effects of the massage—determine the true therapeutic value of massage as a treatment modality in sports health care. In most textbooks on therapeutic massage, physiologic effects are described as being direct, indirect, mechanical, or reflexive.[1,7,10,11] This terminology often focuses the discussion on *how* massage creates physiologic changes, which is not always supported by sound research. For example, the reddening and hyperemia in superficial tissues in response to deep massage can be classified as both direct and reflexive. Ultimately, labeling these changes as direct, mechanical, or reflexive is of less importance than recognizing that hyperemia is a physiologic effect of massage and identifying the value of local hyperemia to the athletes. To avoid such a pitfall, this text describes the physiologic effects of therapeutic massage as either **structural effects**—those that create changes in muscle and connective tissue—or **systemic effects**—those created by cellular, circulatory, and/or nervous system changes. In addition, the physiologic effects put forth in this text can be confirmed by research and/or strongly supported by the sheer volume of empirical evidence.

Structural Effects

In athletics, the primary focus of therapeutic massage is the musculoskeletal and myofascial elements of the body. This is because an athlete's physical training places repetitive stress on these tissues. Techniques that create structural changes in muscle tension, joint compression and tension, and connective tissue flexibility are best because these changes can directly affect an athlete's ability to train, perform, and recover from injury. The structural effects of therapeutic massage that are most supported by research and empirical evidence are listed below:

- Improved range of motion[2–8,10,20,26–30]
- Improved general tissue flexibility and muscle relaxation[3–10,20,21,27,28,31–34]
- Reduction of muscle cramps and spasms[2–5,7,10,28,29]
- Relief of myofascial trigger points and neuromuscular tender points[2,3,5,7,25,29–36]
- Reduction of adhesions and enhanced collagen remodeling during healing cycle[3,5–8,10–12,16,20,28,37–39]

IMPROVED RANGE OF MOTION AND TISSUE FLEXIBILITY

Range of motion is a reflection of both osteo- and arthrokinematics. **Osteokinematics** is a measure of the full arc of motion about a joint, for example, flexion/extension and abduction/adduction. Soft tissue flexibility and muscle tension clearly have an impact on the osteokinematics of a joint. **Arthrokinematics** is the normal and necessary joint play that allows free movement of the articular surfaces of the bones within a joint. If you grasp the middle bone segment of one index finger (between the proximal and distal interphalangeal joints) with the thumb and index finger of the other hand and wiggle the bone side to side, you can feel a little bit of the joint play that is arthrokinematics. If joint play is diminished by a tight joint capsule or calcified ligament, for example, the bone ends cannot rotate, slide, or glide through a normal microscopic range of movement, which ultimately decreases the macroscopic range of motion (osteokinematics).

Most of the time a massage therapist should focus on creating structural changes such as stretching and broadening of muscles, tendons, and fascia rather than focusing on increasing a particular range of motion. This is because range of motion is a reflection of both osteo- and arthrokinematics. Improvements in tissue flexibility and muscle relaxation may or may not lead to improved range of motion. However, the perceived value to the athlete of "feeling looser" or "more relaxed" should not be readily dismissed. There is evidence that muscle relaxation and reduced fascial restrictions due to massage allow muscles to contract and lengthen more efficiently, thus improving the length–strength ratio and muscle power.[13,25,35] Furthermore, this sense of tissue flexibility may make a positive impact on an athlete's performance through improved biomechanics.[16] For example, a golfer may improve his or her distance if trigger points and fascial restrictions are reduced. This results in improved trunk and shoulder rotation because the player is more likely to have a full backswing.

REDUCTION OF SPASMS, CRAMPS, AND TRIGGER POINTS

Muscle cramps and spasms are common among athletes, and massage is one of the most effective modalities that a therapist can use to relieve them. A **muscle cramp** is a short-term, temporary muscle dysfunction that usually affects only a single training session or competition. However, **spasms** (sustained tension) are commonly the result of chronic low-grade strains or are functional adaptations to a repeated position or pattern of movement. This often leads to connective tissue restrictions that affect an athlete's performance over an extended period of time. This combination of muscle spasm and connective tissue restriction creates a local ischemia (lack of blood), which leads to tissue hypoxia and stimulation of pain receptors.[15,28,29,35] Furthermore, it has been estimated that the incidence of trigger points as the primary cause of chronic pain can be as high as 74%.[30,35,36] By deactivating trigger points, reducing muscle tension and increasing local hyperemia, massage can decrease pain and diminish hypoxic tissue damage in muscles with these sustained spasms. Chapter 8 outlines a specific method for cramp relief and several neuromuscular release techniques that have proved effective in reducing spasms, trigger points, and tender points.[3,7,26,27,29,35]

ENHANCED COLLAGEN REMODELING

One of the best-documented and most widely accepted structural effects of therapeutic massage is enhanced collagen remodeling. It has been clearly established that repair fibers are first formed in a disorganized fashion and that movement and stress are necessary to establish appropriate fiber alignment, strength, and flexibility (see Chapter 6). Massage administered during the subacute and maturation stages of healing facilitates this process by breaking apart the fibers that are in poor alignment so that movement—passive and active range of motion plus stretching—can be used to establish proper fiber alignment.[15] There is also evidence that some specific massage strokes such as friction stimulate fibroblast activity for improved collagen repair.[38–40] The myofascial techniques described in Chapter 9 are the recommended techniques to reduce adherent connective tissue and break apart poorly aligned fibers.

Systemic Effects of Massage

Substantiating the systemic effects of massage is more difficult than validating the structural effects because the structural changes can be measured through **anthropometric** measurements, palpation, and stop watches and goniometry, whereas complex and/or invasive tools such as Doppler ultrasound, muscle biopsy, radiography, and gas volume/ratio analysis are necessary to measure many of the systemic changes. Current research shows strongest support for the following systemic effects:

- Enhanced *local* circulation, that is, venous flow and superficial hyperemia[1,3,4,6–8,10–12,15,17,20,41]
- Decreased traumatic edema[2,5,7,8,10–13,29,42–44]
- Decreased pain[3,5–8,10–12,14–16,18,21,28–30,35,36,40,45–47]

ENHANCED LOCAL CIRCULATION

One of the most commonly claimed and widely accepted physiologic effects of massage is increased circulation.[1,3,4,6,7,10–12,20] Without agreement on what constitutes increased circulation, such as which particular cardiovascular process should be measured to indicate this increase, a comparison of results among different studies often creates more confusion than clarity. For example, in a 1949 study by Wakim et al., it was demonstrated that massage increased peripheral blood flow by 50%.[13] However, a 1952 study showed that massage had no effect on blood flow. Subsequent studies over the 1970s and 1980s have results at both ends of this spectrum as well,[8,13,17] and two separate studies in the mid-1990s by Tiidus[17] concluded that several different forms of massage had no effect on blood flow in either the quadriceps or forearm muscles.

Current research does show that massage improves local venous flow, which in turn creates a momentary decrease in capillary pressure that empties capillary beds.[8,13] This could be viewed as increased circulation, although there is no unequivocal evidence of reflexive arterial filling in response.[8,13] In addition, an increase in superficial circulation (skin) with massage is well supported[8,41]; however, this effect may be more appropriately viewed as hyperemia than increased circulation.[41] Because of this contradictory information regarding massage and increased circulation, other claimed physiologic effects such as improved nutrition–waste exchange and improved lactic acid removal must also be questioned because they are derived from the supposition that massage increases circulation.[3,6,8,11,15,18,21] Furthermore, if the goal is to increase circulation, then it can be argued that exercise is the best modality for athletes. This may not be true for a massage therapist working with more sedentary or completely immobilized patients. In these patients, the possible improvement in circulation derived from massage and passive movement could be of vital importance.[7,11]

This text suggests that sports health care therapists focus less on *increasing overall* circulation and more on creating the proven effects of improved venous flow and hyperemia. These two physiologic effects are well substantiated[8,13,21] and have distinct therapeutic value to athletes. **Hyperemia**, indicated by external reddening of the tissue, is strictly defined as more blood in a specific area. This is most likely due to a local vasodilation rather than increased circulation. This vasodilation may be due to an increase in heat, to an increase in histamine release, or to parasympathetic stimulation (Box 1-1).[8,13,15]

REDUCTION OF EDEMA

Because traumatic edema and low-grade inflammation are common in the athletic population, any modality that stim-

BOX 1-1 NET PHYSIOLOGIC EFFECTS OF THERAPEUTIC MASSAGE

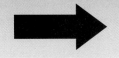

↓ Pain
↑ Range of motion
↑ Force production
↓ Effusion/edema

↑ **Function and performance potential**

ulates edema removal must be considered valuable. Massage strokes that move blood through the superficial veins create a momentary negative pressure in the capillaries, which then improves fluid movement out of that tissue region. This may help reduce edema; however, it is somewhat limited because it addresses only fluid that has already been reabsorbed into the capillaries. Edema is extra fluid in the interstitial spaces.

Although general massage does move interstitial fluid, it simply shifts fluid from an injured area to an area with intact blood and lymphatic vessels. A good analogy for how this may help to reduce edema is to imagine a baseball field after a hard rain. A puddle of water often forms in the batter's box because the ground has been fully saturated and no longer absorbs the water. Coaches and groundskeepers all know that sweeping the water out of the batter's box into surrounding "dry ground" dissipates the puddle. This is exactly what a massage therapist is doing with general massage: moving the fluid to dry ground for better reabsorption. These general massage methods of edema reduction are somewhat effective,[2,5,7,8,10-13,29] but they do not stimulate the lymphatic system—the body's natural edema removal system.

In contrast to general massage, lymphatic facilitation techniques directly improve the function of the lymphatic system to enhance *edema uptake*. The manual lymphatic techniques have been well researched, and their effectiveness at edema removal has been proved beyond reasonable doubt (see Chapters 3 and 7). Therefore, sports health care therapists can use both general massage and lymphatic massage techniques to reduce traumatic edema.[42-44] Theoretically, improving the rate of edema removal could also improve an injured athlete's rate of return to activity.

REDUCED PAIN

Although our understanding of the mechanisms of pain is still incomplete, massage has been recognized as an effective pain-reducing modality since the beginning of athletic endeavors.[3,5-8,10-12,14-16,18,45,46] The most obvious mechanism for pain reduction with massage is through the gate control theory, which is thoroughly discussed in Chapter 4. In addition to gate control, massage can reduce pain by improving tissue flexibility and reducing muscle spasms and trigger points, which indirectly decreases nociceptor stimulation.[15,28-30,35,36] In a similar manner, when swelling is reduced, pain is also reduced because the chemical and pressure stimulus to nociceptors is decreased. Furthermore, several good research articles confirm the effectiveness of massage for pain relief in both delayed onsets muscle soreness and postsurgical pain.[15,45,47] Ultimately, because pain is based on an individual's perception, the psychological benefits of therapeutic massage cannot be ignored as a mechanism of pain reduction.[21,40]

When the benefits and physiologic effects of massage are viewed together with the anecdotal evidence, it presents a strong case for the regular use of therapeutic massage in athletics. This is not to say that massage should be a substitute for any of the therapeutic modalities currently used in sports health care, but it is considered an important ancillary technique that may be the modality of choice in certain situations.

Guidelines for Selecting Massage Equipment and Supplies

The proper equipment and supplies must be used for massage to be effective and comfortable for both the athlete and the therapist. The athlete must be in a stable, fully supported position that allows easy access by the therapist to the area being massaged, and the therapist must be able to use proper body mechanics (described later in chapter) in application of the strokes to protect him/herself from strain. An equipment line that has proved its durability and reliability is usually a wiser investment than the less expensive items that may need replacement in 2 to 3 years, especially if there are budget constraints.

The minimum equipment/supplies required for therapeutic massage in a sports health care program is an adjustable-height massage table and an emollient designed specifically for massage. The variety of equipment, supplies, and the manufacturer selected is largely a personal choice based on budget, individual preferences, and the intended therapeutic environment. There are many reputable massage equipment and supply companies to choose from, but there are some newcomers to the market with equipment look-alikes that may not have gone through the same intense product testing as those of older and larger companies. Therefore, it is suggested that equipment and supplies be purchased from companies and suppliers that have been in business for several years, so there is a product history that can be investigated. The proximity of the company to your facility or institution may also be a consideration to minimize shipping costs and to allow occasional personal visits by the manufacturer's representative. The following guidelines are offered to help therapists make informed decisions regarding the best equipment and supplies for use in their particular athletic environments.

■ THE MASSAGE SURFACE

Any flat and padded surface might be considered an adequate surface for massage in the short term; however, a table, chair, or cushion system that is specifically designed

A male tennis player has been in rehabilitation for 4 weeks with a mild plus rotator cuff strain and has just returned to light practice. His first workout calls for general running and footwork drills, plus ground stroke volleys for 5 minutes each to forehand and backhand. After this warm-up, he is to do 10 no-spin serves at half his normal power and pace before attempting full service strokes. At the end of the 10-minute ground strokes, he comes to the massage therapist with some anxiety about trying the serves because he is beginning to feel some tension around the shoulder and up through his neck. The therapist has the athlete sit in a massage chair and performs a 15-minute upper body basic sports massage routine that includes assessment and release of tender points in all rotator cuff muscles, the trapezius, and pectoralis major. In the last 5 minutes of the massage, the therapist uses lymphatic facilitation to clear the neck, terminus, and axilla before returning the athlete to practice. The athlete talks to his coach, and they agree that he should try just a few serving strokes without striking a ball to determine whether he is ready to perform an actual serve. After four strokes with no pain, the athlete begins the regular service stroke and completes the full workout without any further pain or tension. After the athlete has showered, the therapist reevaluates the same muscles for tender points and performs a 10-minute general upper body basic sports massage before the athletic trainer ices his shoulder and sends him home. Pre- and post-practice massage is continued throughout the first week of his return to full workouts, then tapers to twice per week before changing to an as-needed schedule. His recovery and return to full competition are uneventful after this.

for massage ensures that the work is safely and effectively performed over the long term. The risk of injury to therapist and/or athlete is greatly reduced by choosing a high-quality surface with a few key features that have been demonstrated to work well in sports health care clinics and at competition sites.

The Massage Table

The most versatile and stable surface for therapeutic massage is a table designed specifically for massage. The standard physical therapy and treatment tables found in most clinics generally *do not* make good massage surfaces because they do not have adjustable-height legs and have minimal padding. When choosing a massage table, look for the following[2,7,12]:

- Adjustable-height legs with secure, easy to adjust locking mechanisms.
- A detachable and fold-down face cradle that can be adjusted for height and tilt angle. Make sure that the base for the face cradle is sturdy and that the adjusting mechanism is quiet and easy to use.
- A minimum of 2 inches of foam padding for both the table and face cradle.
- A strong middle cross-piece and hinge where the table folds.
- A strong material for the carrying case with a shoulder strap.
- A table of appropriate weight based on its function. Weight for portable tables should be in the 5- to 15-pound range. Heavier tables are good for setting up and taking down in the training room or clinic, but are difficult for travel.

If the table is to be used in the clinic only, all of the above features except weight and carrying case are still important. Because multiple users are common in clinics, consider an electrically powered table for quick and easy height adjustments, if possible. Another very nice, but nonessential, feature for a massage table is an arm-rest shelf that is situated underneath the face cradle. It may be a separate attachment or a permanent part of the table that folds down.

The Massage Chair

Another option for therapeutic sports massage is the massage chair, or field chair (Fig. 1-1). This type of chair allows the therapist to work on the athlete while he or she is seated with chest, arms, and head supported by the chair. These chairs are lighter and smaller than massage tables, making them well suited for travel and for massaging in small, confined areas. A disadvantage of the massage chair is that the only truly comfortable and well-supported position for the athlete is leaning forward with chest and face on the pads. This limits access to the lower extremity muscles, and the variety of massage techniques that can be applied while in a seated position makes the massage chair less versatile and desirable than a table. Massage chairs are generally best suited for event massage with upper body athletes like tennis players and golfers, who are less likely to need extensive work in their legs at the event. Massage chairs are not

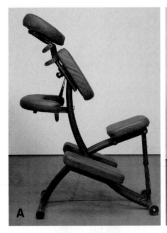
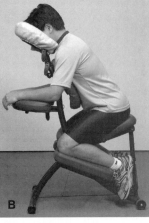

FIGURE 1-1 **Massage chair.** **(A)** Notice the two angle adjustments for the face cradle, plus separate height adjustments for the face cradle, chest pad, arm shelf, and seat. **(B)** The athlete is properly positioned on a massage chair.

recommended for regular use in the clinical setting or for event massage with athletes likely to need lower body focus such as tri-athletes and those who do marathons. Massage chairs should have features such as the following[2,7,12]:

- Multi-plane adjustable face cradle
- Adjustable-height legs and chest pads
- Adjustable-height and adjustable-angle seat
- Quick and easy set-up and breakdown
- Carrying case with shoulder strap

Bolsters, Draping, and Cushion Systems

Standard bolsters and draping are required in classic massage, but optional in sports massage. Many therapists prefer not to use bolsters in event massage because the athletes are usually flexible enough in the ankle to lie flat when in prone, and accommodate a flat supine position without undue strain on the low back. In addition, bolsters

are another surface/item that must be cleaned between each athlete, and they tend to get very dirty at outdoor events. However, bolsters are recommended when massage is given in a clinical setting.

Because athletes are generally clothed during sports massage, draping for modesty is not an issue. However, some therapists like to drape, generally with a towel, for other reasons such as keeping the athlete warm, wiping sweat and dirt off the athlete before massage, and removing the emollient from the skin at the end of the massage. In pre-event massage, this rubbing with a towel to remove emollient becomes part of the massage plan to invigorate the athlete (Fig. 1-2).

Massage cushion systems are an extremely lightweight, portable, and versatile method of support for therapeutic massage. These specifically designed cushions can turn any smooth, flat surface into a suitable massage table, or they can be adapted for use with the athlete in a seated position leaning forward in a chair into the folded cushions on a table, bench, or flat surface of suitable height. These cushion systems are contoured and shaped to support the spine in a neutral position when lying prone and to avoid compression of the soft tissues such as the stomach or breasts. A good system has chest and abdominal sections that separate to allow the therapist to adjust the support according to the length of the athlete's torso, to create an extremely stable position for an athlete in need of side-lying work, or to position a specific body part as needed for access to deeper muscle groups. Also, simply lying down on the cushions after a long bus or airplane ride can position the athlete in such a manner that tight and cramped muscles are encouraged to let go[2] (Fig. 1-3).

If a full cushion system is not used, it is advisable to select several different sizes and shapes of individual cushions to support different body parts during the massage. A standard set of individual pillows or bolster should include both a full round cylinder (4- to 6-inch circumference depending on the size of athletes seen on a regular basis) and a "half-round" cylinder. These bolsters are generally

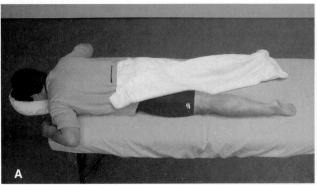
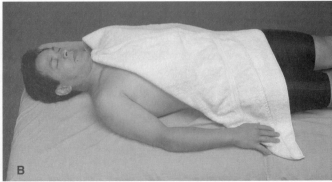

FIGURE 1-2 **Optional draping.** **(A)** Towel draping for lower body. **(B)** Towel draping for upper body.

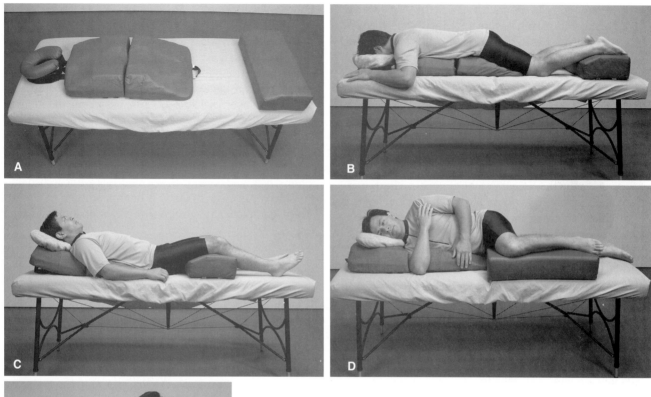

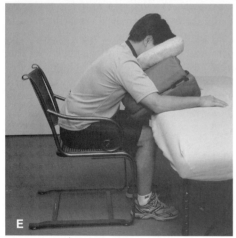

FIGURE 1-3 Full-body cushion systems. These systems offer good support for the athlete in a variety of positions on any available flat surface of an appropriate height. **(A)** Cushions can be separated and adjusted in several ways. **(B)** Prone position of athlete. **(C)** Supine position. **(D)** Side-lying position. **(E)** The cushions can also be adopted for massage of the neck, back, and arm from a seated position if a massage chair is unavailable.

placed under the athlete's ankles when in a prone position, under the knees when supine, and under the top leg (with the bottom leg straight) when in the side-lying position.

■ MASSAGE EMOLLIENTS

Many of the therapeutic massage techniques described in this text are done without an emollient, but some of the techniques require that the hands glide or slide over the surface of the tissue while still engaging the tissue in a slight stretch. In these cases, an oil, lotion, gel, or cream specifically designed for massage should be used rather than non-massage lotions, balms, and creams. These non-massage emollients are generally a poor choice for several reasons. First, the absorbency rate of these substances is highly variable, making it difficult to apply consistent and predictable pressure, glide, and stretch to the tissue. In addition, analgesic balms or creams can cause problems for the athlete and the therapist because the repeated stroking of massage can create too much heat and counterirritation. Moreover, the therapist and/or athlete may develop serious skin irritations from continued exposure to these counterirritants and analgesics. Following are some characteristic differences among massage emollients[2]:

- *The slide–stretch ratio:* The viscosity and absorbency of an emollient make it more or less slippery on the tissue, and the amount of tissue stretch achieved is in an inverse ratio to the slide. In other words, the more slide, the less stretch, and vice versa. Therefore, the slide–stretch ratio can be high on slide or high on stretch. In general, the optimal situation is to have a balanced slide–stretch ratio.

- *Stains:* Most massage emollients in use today do not stain clothing and treatment linens as much as those of the past. However, the residue from some types of emollient is much more easily removed than others. Naturally, this is one of the points for therapists to consider in selecting their preferred emollient.
- *Spilling:* Again, the viscosity of the emollient determines whether it easily stays put in the therapist's hand or on the athlete's body part when applied. Less dripping and spilling occurs with the higher viscosity emollients, which also tends to decrease the amount of staining that might occur to clothing or treatment linens.
- *Storage and spoilage:* Emollients used in the athletic environment should not require special storage and should have a shelf life of at least 6 months. The type of container for a particular emollient plays an important role in how easily it can be stored and how well it resists contamination. All of the emollients can be purchased in bulk, and the bulk containers are generally equal in ease of storage and retardation of spoilage to the smaller containers.
- *Daily dispensers:* The style of the daily use dispensers makes a difference in how easily that particular emollient is used in the treatment clinic. Because many therapists commonly use one dispenser in the clinic, pump-top jars with a wide, stable base that do not have to be picked up for dispensing and do not tip over easily are generally the best choice.

From the Field

"We've been using some form of massage in our program for many years now and have found it to be an important addition. The athletes with nagging pain and problems from past injuries seem to benefit most from the massage, and our track athletes and coaches really believe in the value of a good warm-up massage at events."

Bob Grams, ATC

**Head Athletic Trainer
Seattle Pacific University**

Oils

The slide–stretch ratio for oils is very high on the slide side, allowing the therapist's hands to easily glide over the surface of the skin throughout the entire massage session. However, the tissue cannot be engaged and stretched on anything but a superficial level. Because of spilling, the squeeze bottles for massage oils are easily contaminated and difficult to handle. Simply said, they can quickly become a sticky, greasy, unsanitary mess. Oils also tend to run a higher risk of staining clothes and linens and go rancid faster than most lotions, gels, and creams. In addition, oils are absorbed into the skin very slowly, so that it is not uncommon to hear an athlete complain about feeling too greasy or slippery after a massage when oils are used.[2]

Lotions

Lotions are more viscous and absorbent than oil, increasing the ability of the therapist to stretch the tissue during massage. However, the higher absorbency rate of lotion can be a problem because as the skin soaks up the lotion the slide factor is decreased over the course of the massage. The therapist may have to re-apply the lotion several times during the massage to maintain the proper slide–stretch ratio for the tissue. Lotions have a slightly lower risk of staining clothes and linens than oils, and they have a little longer shelf life if stored properly at an average room temperature.[2]

Gels

Gels have a medium viscosity and absorbency. The slide–stretch ratio is similar to that of oils at the beginning of the massage, meaning that gels can be a little slick. As the massage continues, however, the slide–stretch ratio quickly shifts toward more stretch, making the gel emollient act more like a lotion. This variability in the slide–stretch ratio requires that therapists practice frequently with the gels to determine the proper amount to apply in different situations and on different athletes. The staining and storage quality of massage gel are better than oil and similar to that of lotion.[2]

Creams

Among the four types of emollients, massage creams have the highest viscosity and moderate, consistent absorbency rates. Therefore, massage creams have the most balanced slide–stretch ratio throughout the massage, and very little spillage as the emollient is applied. Staining and rancidity are rarely issues with high-quality massage creams. However, some creams come in a large tub or jar that is quickly

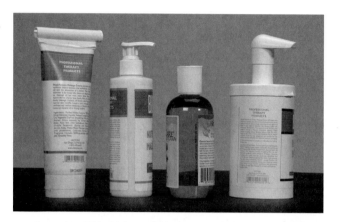

FIGURE 1-4 Therapists may choose from a variety of different emollients.

and easily contaminated in addition to being difficult to handle at events. To avoid this potential problem, look for creams that come in a refillable squeeze tube or pump-top jar for the best hygiene and handling[2] (Fig. 1-4).

Some massage oils, lotions, creams, and gels may contain herbal analgesic additives that have lesser counterirritant properties than analgesic balms commonly used in athletics. You may choose a plain emollient or one with additional analgesic properties as suited to the needs of the athlete. An emollient with mild analgesic qualities may be good when an athlete has some preexisting muscle soreness or a mild chronic strain in superficial muscles. However, other athletes may not like any kind of scented emollients, regardless of whether it is a mild herbal additive or a stronger menthol-based analgesic (Table 1-1).

Application Guidelines for All Massage

Within the modality of massage, there are many forms of soft tissue manipulation that are classified and named as specific techniques, such as Swedish massage, shiatsu,

foot reflexology, neuromuscular technique, and others. In this text, the specific massage techniques that are easily integrated into common sports health care procedures and that best address the pathophysiology of athletic injury are named and outlined later in this chapter. Regardless of which specific theory or combination of techniques the therapist uses, there are a few common guidelines for introducing touch, safely and effectively engaging the tissue, organizing the sequence of strokes or maneuvers, and reducing the risk of chronic strain to the therapist.

■ PROPER BODY MECHANICS

To avoid chronic strain syndromes, therapists must focus a good deal of attention on their overall body mechanics and specific stroke applications. The use of proper body mechanics ensures that the desired effects on the tissue are achieved, and the risk of injury to the therapist is greatly reduced. The first key to good body mechanics is to make sure that the massage table is adjusted to the proper height. Figure 1-5 shows a simple method of estimating the proper working height for all therapists. However, only through trial and error can therapists find the best table height for their individual body type.

The therapist's posture, stance, use of weight and strength, and careful attention to joint and full body alignment all play important roles in making the massage safe and effective for both therapist and athlete[2-4,7,12] (Fig. 1-6). The general goal is to maintain a balanced, relaxed stance and to use the larger muscles of the legs and torso to lean into the tissue for added depth rather than pushing with the hands and elbows. A *stride stance* is generally preferred over parallel-foot stance because it allows the therapist to lean into the tissue and shift weight forward or backward without moving the feet and losing pressure in the stroke. In a stride stance, the center of gravity is easily centered between the forward and back foot, but most of the therapist's weight is on the back foot to push forward into the tissue. This stance also helps the therapist maintain a neutral wrist position and push from behind the stroke.

TABLE 1-1	Comparison of Emollients		
	Oils	**Lotions and Gels**	**Creams**
Slide–stretch ratio	High slide	Moderate slide Moderate stretch	Moderate slide Good stretch
Staining	High	Moderate	Low
Spilling	High	Moderate	Low
Storage/spoilage	Poor	Average	Average

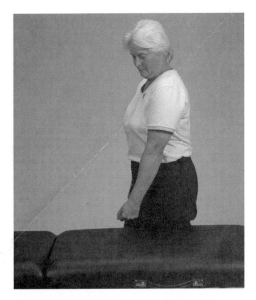

FIGURE 1-5 Estimating proper table height. To estimate the appropriate working height of your table, take an easy stride stance at the side of the table and extend your arms slightly (hands in line with your chin). Your closed fists should clear the table surface by 2 to 3 inches.

Another key to good body mechanics is for the therapist to *square the hips, shoulders, and feet* toward the hands and tissue being worked. This helps the therapist avoid twisting and bending during the massage and therefore decreases back stress. In addition, the squared position works with the stride stance to ensure that the pressure of deep strokes is applied more by leaning into the tissue than by pushing with the hands. Therapists should also concentrate on keeping a posture of *head up, chest open, and shoulders down* to reduce tension in the neck, chest, and back. This position could also be described as keeping a straight spine with the hips directly under the shoulders and using bent knees to move the hands through the tissue. Using *relaxed hands and neutral wrists* (little or no flexion/extension, radial/ulnar deviation) and allowing the arms to hang naturally are also important mechanics to reduce the therapist's risk of developing chronic strain syndromes such as tendonitis and/or carpal tunnel syndrome.[2-4] Deep breathing on the part of the therapist during massage helps keep the neck and chest open and relaxed and serves as a gentle reminder to the athlete that he or she too can relax and let go of muscle tension during the session. Following is a summary of good body mechanics:

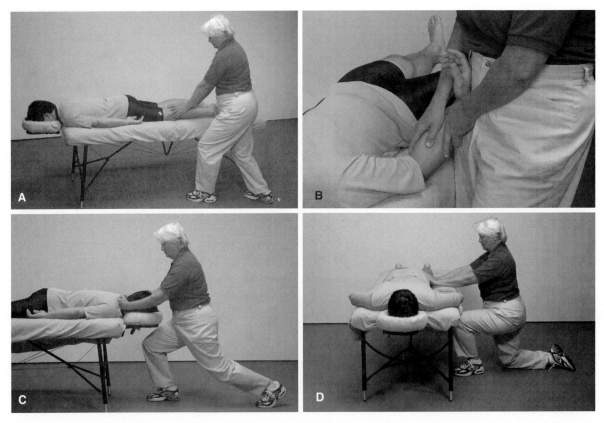

FIGURE 1-6 Good body mechanics. (A) The head and chest are up with arms extended, a stride stance is used with both knees slightly flexed, the hips are aligned with the shoulders, and the shoulders and hips are square to the therapist's hands. **(B)** Note that the hips and shoulders are still squared and that a stride stance is still used to accomplish this. **(C)** A long stride is necessary for deep work in the upper trapezius. **(D)** Kneeling at the side of the table to work over the lateral thigh helps to keep the wrists neutral.

- Use a stride stance.
- Keep the head up and shoulders down and back (chest open).
- Keep hips directly under the shoulders and knees bent.
- Square hips, shoulders, and feet to the tissue being worked.
- Let the arms hang naturally with elbows close to the side of your body.
- Lean into the tissue; use your body weight.
- Keep the hands soft, relaxed, and contoured to the body/tissue area.
- Use a neutral wrist position as often as possible, especially with deep strokes.
- Breathe deeply and regularly.

In addition to these general body mechanics, each individual massage technique and each stroke has its own specific mechanics that ensure maximum effectiveness with minimum stress to the therapist. These stroke-specific mechanics are addressed later in this chapter with the individual technique and stroke descriptions.

Figures 1-7 and 1-8 illustrate improper poor body mechanics and technique.

■ GENERAL RULES OF APPLICATION

In addition to good body mechanics, some basic concepts of safe and effective soft tissue manipulation apply to all therapeutic massage techniques. First, it is important to *work superficial tissue before deep tissue*. This may sound simplistic because it is obvious that massage is applied through the outside and most superficial surface, the skin. The rule simply reminds therapists that the objective is to assess and address the superficial tissues before attempting to access the deeper muscles, ligaments, and tendons in a general body region. In other words, one must introduce touch and outline the area to be worked with superficial massage strokes before increasing the pressure to affect the muscles and deep fascia. This can be of great psychological importance to the athlete, communicating a caring attitude by demonstrating the therapist's mindfulness of any fear or pain the athlete might be experiencing. This superficial-to-deep concept is also applied in making recommendations for specific stroke sequences within a massage technique. For example, massage in a particular muscle group or body region begins with strokes that are light and intended to affect mostly skin and superficial fascia (effleurage). Strokes that require deep pressure or are directed at a small focal point of tissue (friction and trigger point) are not added to the massage of that muscle group until the middle or later half of the massage.

Second, it is best to *work general to specific*. Just as an athlete goes through a warm-up period before intense practice or competition, the tissue needs to be prepared for more intense work. Therefore, long and/or broad massage strokes that cover an entire muscle group or body region should precede focused work on a specific area of tenderness or adhesion. For example, the entire back or limb should be stroked and kneaded before addressing a specific muscle group in that region, and the entire muscle group should be addressed before a specific muscle attachment. When time is a constraint, the general work may be limited to just a small area of surrounding tissue before focusing on the tight or tender point, but the general to specific guideline still applies. Again, the general sequence of strokes common to each particular massage technique is based in part on following this principle.

Third, objective *assessment and findings should guide the massage*. Each athlete has a different medical history, psychological make-up, tissue type, and stress points based on the individual's biomechanics. All these variables give the therapist a changing picture of an athlete's needs each day. Although it is common and important to have a "standard" back or leg massage routine, therapists must fully assess the status of that particular athlete on each particular day, even when no injury is present, to determine what structures need a little extra work, need to be avoided, or need to be treated with a different modality. When there is no specific injury, a good deal of the assessment may occur during the massage rather than being a separate process. In other words, after a few quick questions about how the athlete is feeling and whether he or she is aware of any problem areas, the therapist begins the massage in the body regions and muscle groups stressed by the athlete's particular sport. As the massage progresses, the therapist feels areas of tension, spasm, tenderness, adhesions, and/or fibrous bands, which indicate the need for a specific stroke or technique (ie, myofascial) to reduce adhesions and neuromuscular to decrease tension. Therapists often shift the focus of the massage based on these findings and spend more time in a particular area, or they change the technique or stroke being used. (Box 1-2)

BOX 1-2 SUMMARY OF MASSAGE APPLICATION GUIDELINES

- Work superficial tissue before deep tissue.
- Work general, large areas before specific points within a body area.
- Let objective assessment and findings guide the massage, even when there is no specific injury.

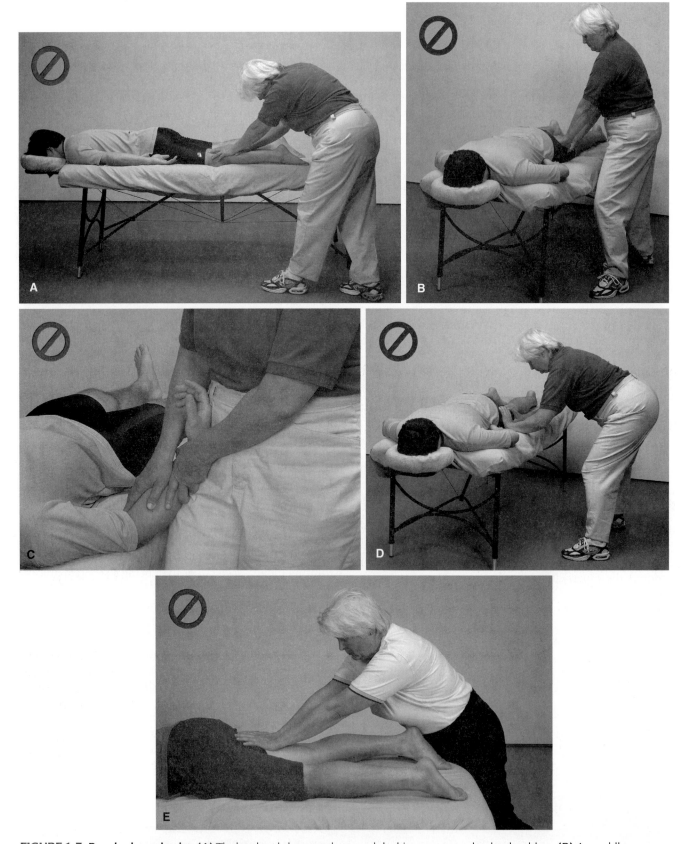

FIGURE 1-7 Poor body mechanics. (A) The head and chest are down and the hips are not under the shoulders. **(B)** A straddle stance with toes pointed out makes it difficult to transfer weight into your hands. **(C)** When the hips are not squared to the hands, the low back and neck of the therapist are strained. **(D)** If therapists attempt to work over the lateral thigh without kneeling or using a deep stride the back, quadriceps, and wrists are under great strain. **(E)** When hips get stuck at the corner of the table, knees lock, the pressure of the stroke is diminished, and the back is strained.

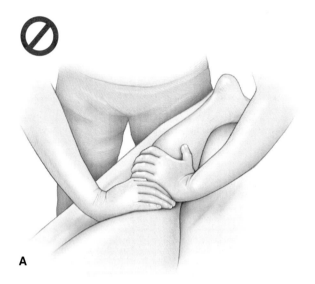

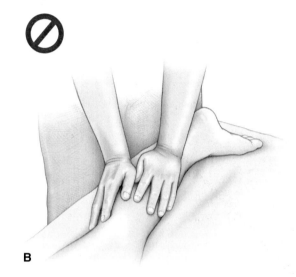

FIGURE 1-8 Stress to the wrists. (A) Avoid putting this lateral pressure on your wrists by not applying effleurage with the hands positioned across the vertical line of the stroke. **(B)** Avoid this hyperextension stress to the wrists by keeping your weight behind your hands in all gliding strokes.

When a specific injury is present, a thorough assessment is necessary to determine massage indications and contraindications as well as to determine the need for referral and/or the inclusion of other treatment modalities. Guidelines for assessment of common athletic injuries are outlined in Chapter 12.

Massage Techniques Most Beneficial to Athletes

The modality of massage can be defined very simply as the patterned and purposeful manipulation of soft tissue with therapeutic intention. However, a seemingly endless number of specialized techniques and forms of massage exist, and not all of them are appropriate or effective techniques for sports health care (Appendix A). The therapeutic massage advocated in this text is a combination of specific techniques that address the unique musculoskeletal, fascial, and circulatory stresses placed on athletes during training and competition. All therapeutic massage is guided by the therapist's knowledge of anatomy, physiology, the healing cycle, principles of athletic conditioning, the purpose and use of other treatment modalities, and the principles of injury rehabilitation. Of the many styles of massage and bodywork available, the therapeutic massage most useful for a sports health care therapist is a system of work that combines four specific massage techniques: basic sports massage, myofascial techniques, neuromuscular release, and lymphatic facilitation. One or all of these techniques can be used to help athletes maintain their normal training routine, to prepare for and recover from events and competitions, and can be used in the treatment and rehabilitation of specific injuries (Table 1-2).

■ BASIC SPORTS MASSAGE

Basic sports massage is a combination of deep Swedish massage and a few strokes specific to sports massage, such as rhythmic compression, pin-and-stretch, and active releases. The deep Swedish strokes are applied with greater depth and specificity and at a more vigorous pace than traditional massage when used in basic sports massage.

■ MYOFASCIAL TECHNIQUES

Myofascial techniques consist of any method used to stretch, broaden, and soften fascia and other connective tissue elements. These techniques can be used to address large connective tissue/fascial zones, a specific anatomic site, or a specific tissue lesion/tear/adhesion. Myofascial techniques focus on achieving the structural effects of therapeutic massage and, in doing so, may reduce local ischemia.

■ NEUROMUSCULAR RELEASE

Neuromuscular release methods include any technique that is directed at reducing abnormal muscle tension. These techniques may be based on normal muscle physiology and proprioception, or site-specific pathologies within the musculoskeletal system. Neuromuscular release techniques are more specifically directed toward the structural effects of

TABLE 1-2	Summary of Therapeutic Massage Benefits and Effects			
Benefits	**BSM**	**MR**	**NMR**	**LF**
↓ Anxiety/stress/depression	X			
Enhance sense of well-being/mental focus	X			
Identify and relieve areas of stress/tension	X	X	X	
Provide positive kinesthetic feedback	X	X	X	
Structural Physiologic Effects				
↓ Adhesions and fascial restrictions		X		
↑ Tissue flexibility and muscle relaxation		X	X	
↑ Range of motion		X	X	X
Relieve cramps and trigger points			X	
Enhance collagen remodeling		X		
Systemic Physiologic Effects				
Enhance local circulation (hyperemia and venous flow)	X			X
↓ Traumatic edema				X
↓ Pain	X	X	X	X

BSM, basic sports massage; **LF**, lymphatic facilitation; **MR**, myofascial release; **NMR**, neuromuscular release.

massage. However, improved local blood flow, a systemic effect, may occur when abnormal muscle tension is reduced.

LYMPHATIC FACILITATION

Lymphatic facilitation is a unique style of massage specifically directed at reducing traumatic edema. The lymphatic facilitation strokes and sequences described in this text are adaptations of the manual lymph drainage techniques used to treat lymphedema. These techniques are directed toward creating systemic changes, specifically increased edema uptake and lymph flow. The lymphatic facilitation techniques provide sports health care therapists with a unique and highly desirable set of complementary skills for treatment and rehabilitation of athletic injuries.

The following chapters provide therapists with comprehensive descriptions of the physiologic rationale for use, the intentions and purpose, benefits and effects, and the indications and contraindication for each of these four therapeutic massage techniques. Therapists who fully understand these principles and spend enough time to master the manual skills set forth in this text should be considered as true sports massage specialists.

SUMMARY

- Massage is considered a therapeutic *modality,* whereas the specific style or type of massage is referred to as a *technique.*
- Four specific therapeutic massage techniques are beneficial and efficiently used in athletic environments: basic sports massage, lymphatic facilitation, neuromuscular release, and myofascial techniques.
- Therapeutic massage provides several *benefits* to athletes, such as decreased anxiety, improved mental focus, and early identification of tight and/or tender areas that are difficult to quantify and measure.
- The physiologic effects of massage can be divided into two categories: structural and systemic. There is more good research to support the structural effects of massage than the systemic effects.

- Therapists must use equipment and supplies specifically designed for massage to achieve maximum therapeutic value and to avoid injury to self.
- Massage emollients have different qualities, and some care must be used to select the proper emollient for each situation.

- Proper body mechanics for all massage includes using a stride stance with the hips, feet, and shoulders square to the tissue being worked; keeping the head-chest up and the shoulders down; and using relaxed hands with neutral wrists.

Review Questions

SHORT ANSWERS

1. Name five key features to look for when choosing a massage table.
   a.
   b.
   c.
   d.
   e.

2. Name three key features to look for when choosing a massage chair.
   a.
   b.
   c.

3. Name at least two advantages that using a full-body cushion system offers for massage.

_____

_____

_____

4. Label each of these statements as being true for: O (oils), L/G (lotions/gels), or C (creams).
   a. ____ has the highest slide ratio.
   b. ____ provides moderate slide and good stretch.
   c. ____ begins with high stretch and changes to low.
   d. ____ has the lowest risk of spilling.
   e. ____ provides the lowest amount of tissue stretch.

MULTIPLE CHOICE

5. Three keys to good body mechanics are:
   a. Straight back, knees bent, hips square to the stroke
   b. Straight arms, bent back, straight knees
   c. Toes forward, head down, elbows bent
   d. Knees bent, toes out, chest closed

6. The general guidelines for application of massage include: determine the focus of the massage via a thorough evaluation, and which one of the following:
   a. Begin with the back and always use an emollient.
   b. Work from superficial to deep and general to specific.
   c. Work specific ligaments first, then do full muscle massage.
   d. Begin all massage with effleurage, and finish with tapotement.

7. Which of these is considered a benefit of massage?
   a. increased circulation
   b. decreased edema
   c. improved mental focus
   d. improved collagen alignment

8. Normal joint play between the two bones of a joint is the definition of _____
   a. flexibility.
   b. arthrokinematics.
   c. osteokinematics.
   d. range of motion.

9. Increased flexibility, decreased adhesions, and improved range of motion are all examples of _____ of massage.
   a. the benefits
   b. systemic effects
   c. reflexive effects
   d. structural physiologic effects

10. Any massage technique that stretches or broadens connective tissue is classified as a _____ technique.
    a. basic sports massage
    b. myofascial
    c. neuromuscular
    d. lymphatic

11. The term most closely associated with the physiologic effect of increased local circulation is _____
    a. edema.
    b. hematoma.
    c. ischemia.
    d. hyperemia.

12. Which style of therapeutic massage has the primary intention of decreasing muscle tension?

a. Basic sports massage
b. Myofascial
c. Neuromuscular
d. Lymphatic facilitation

13. Which of the following is considered a systemic physiologic effect of massage?
    a. Decreased pain
    b. Improved flexibility
    c. Decreased fibrotic adhesions
    d. Improved collagen alignment

14. Which of the following is a proven effect of massage on circulation?
    a. Improved nutrient waste exchange
    b. Improved lactic acid uptake
    c. Improved venous flow
    d. Enhanced arterial flow and cardiac output

15. Which therapeutic massage technique is best at reducing traumatic edema?
    a. Basic sports massage
    b. Myofascial
    c. Lymphatic facilitation
    d. Neuromuscular

16. What physiologic process seems to be the primary method for massage to reduce pain?
    a. Massage increases the level of dopamine.
    b. Certain strokes stimulate histamine release.
    c. It improves lactic acid removal.
    d. The gate control theory.

REFERENCES

1. Dolan JP. Treatment and Prevention of Athletic Injuries. Danville, IL: The Interstate Printers and Publishers, 1955.
2. Archer PA. Massage for Sports Health Care. Champaign, IL: Human Kinetics, 1999.
3. Benjamin PJ, Lamp SP. Understanding Sports Massage, 2nd ed. Champaign, IL: Human Kinetics, 2005.
4. King RK. Performance Massage: Muscle Care for Physically Active People. Champaign, IL: Human Kinetics, 1992.
5. Archer PA. Three clinical sports massage approaches for treating injured athletes. Athletic Therapy Today 2001;6(3):14–20.
6. Cash M. Sport and Remedial Massage Therapy. London: Ebury Press, 1996.
7. Fritz S. Mosby's Fundamentals of Therapeutic Massage, 2nd ed. St. Louis: CV Mosby, 2000.
8. Braverman DL, Schulman RA. Massage techniques in rehabilitation medicine. Physical Medicine and Rehabilitation Clinics of North America 1999;10(3):631–648.
9. Verhoef MJ, Page SA. Physician's perspectives on massage therapy. Canadian Family Physician 1998;44:1018–1020,1023–1024.
10. Prentice WE. Therapeutic Modalities for Physical Therapists, 2nd ed. New York: McGraw-Hill, 2002.
11. Salvo SG. Massage Therapy: Principles and Practice, 2nd ed. St. Louis: Saunders/Elsevier, 2003.
12. Tappan FM, Benjamin PJ. Healing Massage Techniques: Classic, Holistic, and Emerging Methods, 3rd ed. Stamford, CT: Appleton & Lange, 1998.
13. Cafarelli E, Flint F. The role of massage in preparation for and recovery from exercise. Sports Medicine 1992;14(1):1–9.
14. Dryden T, Baskwill A, Preyde M. Massage therapy for the orthopaedic patient: A review. Orthopaedic Nursing 2004;23(5):327–332.
15. Pornratshanee W, Hume PA, Kolt GS. The mechanisms of massage and effects on performance, muscle recovery, and injury prevention. Sports Medicine 2005;35(3):235–256.
16. Meagher J, Boughton P. Sports massage. Garden City, NY: Dolphin Books Doubleday & Co, 1980.
17. Tiidus PM. Manual massage and recovery of muscle function following exercise: A literature review. Journal of Orthopaedic and Sports Physical Therapy 1997;25(2):107–112.
18. Boone T, Cooper R, Thompson WR. A physiologic evaluation of the sports massage. Athletic Training 991;.25(Spring):51–54.
19. Field T et al. Massage reduces anxiety in child and adolescent psychiatric patients. J Am Acad Child Adolesc Psychiatry, 1992;31:1:125–131.
20. Kuprian W. Physical Therapy for Sports. Philadelphia: WB Saunders, 1982.
21. Field T. Massage therapy. In: Davis CM. ed. Complementary Therapies in Rehabilitation. Thorofare, NJ: SLACK, Inc, 1997.
22. Field T et al. Children with asthma have improved pulmonary functions after massage therapy. J Pediatr 1998;132:854–858.
23. Hernandez-Reif M, Ironson G et al. Breast cancer patients have improved immune and neuroendocrine functions following massage therapy. Journal of Psychosomatic Research 2004;57:45–52.
24. Sunshine W, Field TM et al. Fibromyalgia benefits form massage therapy and transcutaneous electrical stimulation. J Clin Rheumatol 1996;2:18–22.
25. McLeod I, Mistry D, Archer P et al. Massage therapy utilization and application in the treatment of myofascial trigger points. Advanced Track Seminar June 2005; NATA Annual Meeting.
26. Crosman LJ, Chateauvert SR, Weisberg J. The effects of massage to the hamstring muscle group on range of motion. Journal of Orthopaedic and Sports Physical Therapy 1984;168–172.
27. Gazzillo LM, Middlemas DA. Therapeutic massage techniques for three common injuries. Athletic Therapy Today 2001;6(3):5–9.
28. Juhan D. Job's Body: A Handbook for Bodywork, expanded ed. Barrytown: Station Hill, 1992.
29. Chaitow L, DeLany JW. Clinical Application of Neuromuscular Techniques, vol. 1: The Upper Body. Edinburgh: Churchill Livingstone, 2000.
30. Lucas KR, Polus BI, Rich PA. Latent myofascial trigger points: Their effects on muscle activation and movement efficiency. Journal of Bodywork and Movement Therapies 2004;8:160–166.
31. Morelli M, Seaborne D, Sullivan S. Changes in H-reflex amplitude during massage of triceps surae in healthy subjects. Journal of Orthopaedic and Sports Physical Therapy 1990;12(2):55–59.
32. Morelli M, Seaborne D, Sullivan S. H-reflex modulation during manual muscle massage of human triceps surae. Arch Phys Med Rehabil 1991;72:915–919.
33. Morelli M, Chapman C, Sullivan S. Do Cutaneous receptors contribute to the changes in the amplitude of the H-reflex during massage? Electromyogr Clin Neurophysiol 1999;39:441–447.
34. Sullivan S, Williams L, Seaborne D et al. Effects of massage on alpha motoneuron excitability. Phys Ther 1991;71(8):555–560.
35. Simons DG, Travell JG, Simons LS. Myofascial Pain and Dysfunction: The Trigger Point Manual, 2nd ed. vol. 1: Upper Half of the Body. Philadelphia: Lippincott Williams & Wilkins, 1999.
36. Gerwin R. A study of 96 subjects examined both for fibromyalgia and myofascial pain. Journal of Musculoskeletal Pain 1995;3:121.
37. Cyriax JH, Cyriax PJ. Illustrated Manual of Orthopedic Medicine, 2nd ed. Boston: Butterworth & Heinemann, 1993.
38. Cook JL et al. Overuse tendinosis, not tendonitis; Part 2: Applying the new approach to patellar tendinopathy. The Physician and Sports Medicine 2000;28:31.

39. Gehlsen GM, Ganion LR, Helfst R. Fibroblast responses to variations in soft tissue mobilization pressure. Medical Science and Sports Exercise 1999;31:531–535.

40. Guthrie RA, Martin RH. Effect of pressure applied to the upper thoracic (placebo) versus lumbar areas (osteopathic manipulative treatment) for inhibition of lumbar myalgia during labor. Journal of the American Osteopathic Association 1982;82:247–251.

41. Hinds T, McEwan I et al. Effects of massage on limb and skin blood flow after quadriceps exercise. Medicine and Science in Sports and Exercise 2004;36(8):1308–1313.

42. Casley-Smith JR. Modern Treatment of Lymphoedema. Adelaide, Australia: Henry Thomas Laboratory, Lymphoedema Association of Australia, 1994.

43. Foldi E, Foldi M. Textbook of Foldi School. Austria: self published, English translation by Heida Brenneke, 1999.

44. Kolb P, Denegar C. Traumat letic Training 1983:Winter:

45. Forchuk C, Baruth P et al for women with lymph 27(1):25–33.

46. Cherkin DC, Sherman K tiveness, safety, and co spinal manipulation f 2003;138(11):898–906.

47. Smith LL, Keating MN, Ho of athletic massage on delayed onset musc tine kinase, and neutrophil count: A preliminary report. nal of Orthopaedic and Sports Physical Therapy 1994;19(2): 93–99.

2 Sports Massage

OBJECTIVES

After completing this chapter, the reader will be able to:

- Define sports massage and name three categories of this style of massage.
- List three differences between classic massage and sports massage.
- Name and define the three subcategories of event massage.
- Define maintenance massage and name the primary massage techniques used in this category.
- Define treatment massage and identify the technique that is unique to this category.
- Define the five general categories of classic/Swedish massage strokes, and describe the intention/purpose of each.
- Describe proper stroke mechanics and specific cautions for each of the classic massage strokes.
- List four specific contraindications for all basic sports massage strokes, and explain why they are contraindicated.
- Describe three types of friction strokes that are generally applied with an emollient, and two types that are applied without an emollient.
- Describe the purpose and proper stroke mechanics for rhythmic compressions and active assistive techniques.
- Describe the cautions and contraindications for rhythmic compression and active assistive release.

Therapeutic massage in athletics, often referred to as sports massage, is broadly defined as the scientific and intuitive application of massage, movement, and stretching to physically active individuals. The techniques used in the sports massage modality are not exclusive to athletics. Instead, the specific combination of techniques advocated here—basic sports massage and myofascial, neuromuscular, and lymphatic techniques—distinguishes sports massage as a unique system of massage for a specialized population.

Just as there is a difference in coaching during practice and during a game, the type of massage given to an athlete varies according to the setting, timing, sport, status of the tissue, and the athlete's medical history. A massage performed on an athlete just before the beginning of a competition has different goals and uses different techniques from those of massage used in treating a sprained ankle. Several variables must be considered to determine the best combination of massage techniques and strokes to be used in each individual massage situation. Therapists must consider:

- *Timing:* Whether the massage is to be provided before, after, or between activities and how close it is to the start and/or finish of the activity will direct the choice of techniques and duration of the massage for the therapist.
- *Setting:* Massage may be given at the site of the activity among all the hustle and bustle of the event or in a quiet and private treatment clinic. The location affects the choice of equipment, strokes, and duration of the massage.

- *Common stress areas:* The biomechanics and common training practices of a particular sport create common stress areas in the athletes. Knowing these common areas helps the therapist make decisions about which muscle groups need more prolonged and specific massage and which can receive abbreviated, general massage.
- *The training and competition schedule:* This information helps determine the frequency of massage and affects the specific goals of the massage, that is, scheduling massage on light training days and waiting until the noncompetitive season to make postural corrections.
- *Other treatments/modalities/exercises:* The effectiveness of the massage can be enhanced or diminished by other modalities. Therefore, some consideration must be given to whether the massage should be administered before or after different treatments.

Categories of Sports Massage

Sports massage has been divided into different categories by several authors.[1–5] In 1982, Werner Kuprian[2] identified four categories of athletic massage: training, preparatory, intermediary, and warm-down. All of Kuprian's categories describe massage administered before, during, or after the activity, which is a rather limiting view of both the modality of massage and the sports massage technique. In a more recent text, Benjamin and Lamp[3] break down sports massage into five major applications: recovery, remedial, rehabilitation, maintenance, and event. These categories give a more complete view of the common uses of therapeutic massage in athletics. However, the distinctions among remedial, rehabilitation, and maintenance massage are small and may not be as helpful to the therapist as a broader classification system.

This text describes only three categories of sports massage:

1. Event
2. Maintenance
3. Treatment

■ EVENT MASSAGE

Event massage is designed to help the athlete prepare for and recover from physical exertion. It is administered on the day of activity and generally at the site of the activity. Event massage is fast-paced and of short duration, usually lasting only 10 to 15 minutes. Therefore, it is generally done only on the large muscles of either the upper or lower body, whichever is more stressed by the activity. There are three subcategories of event massage that are based mostly on the timing of the massage:

- Pre-event
- Inter-event (massage given between bouts of exercise or competition that occur on the same day, such as track, tennis, or swim meets)
- Post-event

The primary massage techniques used in all of the event massage categories are the basic sports massage techniques detailed in this chapter. In Chapter 10, the goals, stroke combinations, and sequences for event massage are fully detailed.

■ MAINTENANCE MASSAGE

Maintenance massage is more of a full-body massage that is generally administered to athletes in a clinical setting rather than at the site of competition. The intention of maintenance massage is to minimize the negative effects of exercise and keep the athlete training and competing at his or her highest level by *maintaining* tissue flexibility and muscle relaxation. As previously theorized, regular massage can identify and reduce areas of tensions and/or tenderness before the athlete's performance is impacted and therefore decrease the risk of some injuries. This explains why this category of massage can also be called preventive. A maintenance massage is tailored to the specific needs of that athlete by thoroughly addressing the muscles under most stress—depending on his or her sport—and administering general massage to the rest of the body when time allows.

In maintenance massage, therapists combine the basic sports massage techniques with more specific myofascial and neuromuscular techniques to achieve the goals of tissue maintenance and injury prevention. For example, a maintenance massage for a sprinter would likely begin with the hips and legs and focus specific myofascial and neuromuscular techniques on these muscle groups and fascial lines for 45 minutes and then finish with basic sports massage to the upper body. Maintenance massage is the focus of Chapter 11.

■ TREATMENT MASSAGE

When the athlete has suffered an acute injury or when the chronic strain of activity has accumulated to the point at which training and/or performance capacity are diminished, the massage is classified as treatment massage. Like the maintenance classification, treatment massage is generally administered in the clinic, but this massage is more focused and limited to the injured joint or muscle and the surrounding tissue. The primary intention of treatment massage is to enhance the healing process and to help an athlete return to full activity more quickly. The principles and methods of treatment massage are detailed in Chapter 13.

Treatment massage is individually designed according to the type of injury, stage of healing, severity of injury, and the other modalities being used by the therapist. All of the basic sports massage, myofascial, and neuromuscular techniques are used in the treatment massage, and the lymphatic facilitation techniques are added. The addition of lymphatic facilitation to current treatment protocols provides sports health care therapists with a new, unique, and simple method of addressing traumatic edema that has a wealth of supporting research.

What Is Basic Sports Massage?

Perhaps the most basic and common massage technique practiced in this country is the Swedish or classic style of massage. This form has been developed, described, and refined over the past two centuries by several prominent figures such as Pehr Ling, Dr. Johann Mezger, Albert Hoffa, and Dr. James Mennell.[6–9] A Swedish/classic massage is an integration of gentle movement and light stretching with five styles of massage strokes: effleurage, pétrissage, friction, tapotement, and vibration/jostling. An emollient is always used with classic massage to create a relaxing slow rhythm, flow, and connection between strokes and/or body regions during the massage. These characteristics support the primary intentions of Swedish massage, which are to reduce stress and anxiety, improve relaxation and general tissue flexibility, create a sense of well-being, and reconnect the body, mind, and spirit of the patient.[6–12]

In contrast to classic massage, basic sports massage is a deeper, more invigorating, and more anatomically specific massage that combines the standard Swedish massage strokes with a few new strokes, specifically rhythmic compressions and active assistive release (Table 2-1). The pace of basic sports massage is much faster than the classic style of work, and use of an emollient is optional rather than mandatory because sports massage therapists often need to work through the clothing of an athlete. Most notably, basic sports massage is focused on the specific muscle groups, fascial zones, and/or areas of stress created in the athlete by his or her sport activity rather than being a full body massage like the classic technique.

Basic Sports Massage Strokes

The five classic Swedish massage strokes, effleurage, pétrissage, friction, tapotement, and vibration/jostling, form the foundation for basic sports massage. However, when used in basic sports massage, these classic strokes

TABLE 2-1	A Comparison of Swedish/Classic Massage to Basic Sports Massage					
	Intention	Emollient	Duration	Focus	Pace	Client Status
Swedish/classic massage	Soothe and sedate	Always	1–1.5 hours	Full body	Slow and rhythmic	No clothing
Basic sports massage	Invigorate	Optional	10–20 minutes	Major muscle groups: upper or lower body	Fast and vigorous	Light clothing

are modified to make them deeper and more specific. These modified strokes are used in the same general sequence as in classic massage—that is, pétrissage before friction—and may be preceded or followed by the new basic sports massage.

■ EFFLEURAGE

Effleurage is any stroke in which the hands glide or slide over the superficial tissue. This implies that a lubricant is always used. Application of the emollient is accomplished with a light effleurage stroke before increasing the depth to the therapeutic level. In deep effleurage, the full surface of the therapist's hand is pressed firmly into the tissue and pushed in a linear direction along the surface of the body area. The hands can be moved together as one unit in an alternating hand-underhand stroke, or fists and forearms can be used for added depth in large muscle areas such as the back and posterior leg. Deep effleurage creates a ridge of tissue in front of the hands as they glide together up the body region. It is important that the ridge of tissue be pushed distal to proximal or toward the heart when working in the extremities to avoid undue stress on the one-way valves in the superficial veins.

Stroke Mechanics

To maintain the neutral wrist position, good stroke mechanics require the therapist to push the tissue with his or her body weight *behind the hands* rather than directly over the hands (Fig. 2-1). In a good effleurage stroke, the hands of the therapist are firm without being stiff and slightly rounded to conform to the contours of the body. The tissue is engaged by the full hand, that is, in the palm and finger pads. A common mistake in stroke mechanics for effleurage is to either hyperextend the fingers so that the pressure of the stroke is coming only from the fingers or to push the tissue with the heel of the hand only (Fig. 2-2). Remember that depth is always created by leaning in with body weight rather than pushing with hand and arm strength.

Compared with classic effleurage, the deep effleurage used in basic sports massage is applied with a shorter stroke and at a more vigorous pace. For example, the classic effleurage for the posterior leg is a full-length stroke from heel to hip, and generally, a minimum of three strokes are applied. In basic sports massage, one full-length stroke is followed by three to five strokes from knee to buttocks, then three to five strokes from heel to knee, and finally one or two full-length strokes. Of course, the depth and vigorous pace of deep effleurage should be established gradually with slower and more superficial strokes in the beginning.

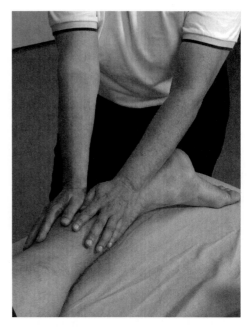

FIGURE 2-1 Correct hand position for effleurage. Pressure is evenly distributed over palms and fingers.

Purpose and Effects

Effleurage strokes create more systemic than structural effects. Even though deep effleurage does create a slight superficial stretch, it is more effective at moving blood through the superficial veins and out of local capillary beds.[6–9,13,14] Effleurage is generally used as a beginning stroke for each body part because it is superficial, and gives the athlete kinesthetic awareness of the full length and suppleness of the body part being massaged. It also assists both therapist and athlete in general assessment of the tissue.

Effleurage strokes can be used in any category of sports massage, but consideration must be given to the requirement of an emollient. There may be some event massage situations in which the therapist might choose to avoid the use of an emollient. For example, using an emollient in a pre-event massage for a marathoner when there is high temperature and humidity may make it difficult for the athlete to dissipate heat if the lubricant is not completely removed after the massage. In the maintenance and treatment categories, the massage must be planned, so that dry work, such as myofascial release, is done before the emollient is applied for effleurage. The tissue cannot be slick with emollient if the deep tissue is to be engaged, stretched, and broadened.

Cautions and Contraindications

Deep effleurage should not be used in an area immediately over or distal to an area of edema or a severe hematoma. Because circulation is impaired in bruised and edematous

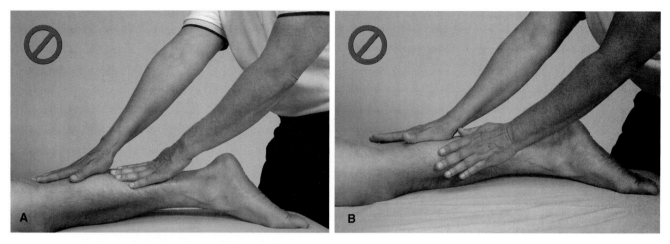

FIGURE 2-2 Incorrect hand positions for effleurage. (A) Flat fingers without pressure in the palms. **(B)** Pressure only in the palms.

tissue, pushing more fluid into the area with deep effleurage may dislodge a blood clot or increase the edema. In addition, any direct pressure over the area could disrupt the formation of fragile granulation tissue and disrupt the healing process. Only the lymph facilitation techniques described later are light enough to use in and around acute swelling or a hematoma. None of the basic sports massage strokes should be applied directly over the following:

- Inflamed or edematous tissue
- Varicose veins
- Open wounds or rashes associated with skin diseases
- Cysts, tumors, or hematomas

■ PÉTRISSAGE

In pétrissage, the superficial tissues are separated from the underlying surfaces by using one or both hands to grasp, lift, and squeeze a large segment of tissue. Three standard forms of pétrissage are applied with an emollient: two-handed, one-handed, and bilateral, but all use the same basic stroke mechanics. In a two-handed application of pétrissage, the hands are positioned side by side across the muscle; then an alternate squeeze and lift motion, such as left hand–right hand–left hand, is applied with the fingers and palms while the hands are pushed (sliding) over the tissue in a figure-8 pattern (Fig. 2-3A). Note that the tissue in between the hands is the focus of the work. The alternating circles of two-handed pétrissage must be applied in an overlapping pattern to effectively loosen and soften the tissue. When working over a smaller area such as the forearm, a one-handed pétrissage that uses the same squeezing and lifting motion is just as effective as a two-handed pétrissage. The hand slides through the tissue in a circular line (Fig. 2-3B),

which usually parallels the long bones. In bilateral pétrissage, hands are placed on opposite sides of the muscle group and slide through the muscle group with an alternate grasping motion (Fig. 2-3C). When these styles of pétrissage are included in sports massage, they are applied at a more vigorous pace with less emphasis on slow and smooth transitions between muscle groups. Theoretically, when massaging the extremities, pétrissage strokes should begin at the proximal end of the extremity to loosen muscles and connective tissue to decrease resistance to fluid flow. This concept is similar to the idea of taking the cork out of a bottle before pouring. However, the need for beginning at the proximal end of a limb has not been substantiated by research at this time.

Another form of this stroke, called **compressive pétrissage**, is also applied with an emollient, but rather than lifting the superficial tissue the hands press the tissue away from the underlying structures. There are two forms of compressive pétrissage: (1) lift and press, also called fulling,[7] and (2) kneading. In the lift and press form of compressive pétrissage, both hands are used to lift the muscle mass up away from the bone, then the palms of both hands press the tissue down and away from the bone (Fig. 2-4A & B). In the kneading form of pétrissage, the hands are positioned on opposite sides of the muscle mass, and then pressed together pushing the superficial layer of tissue up between the palms of the hands (Fig. 2-4C). Therapists with small hands may prefer compressive pétrissage to the standard form of the stroke when working with heavily muscled athletes.

Pétrissage can also be effectively applied without an emollient and over clothing. In a dry pétrissage application, the therapist is "walking" the hands through the muscle by grasping and releasing the tissue without sliding. The dry pétrissage technique is most effective (softens and loosens a larger section of tissue) when both hands are used simultaneously to grasp and release the tissue. Once the tissue is

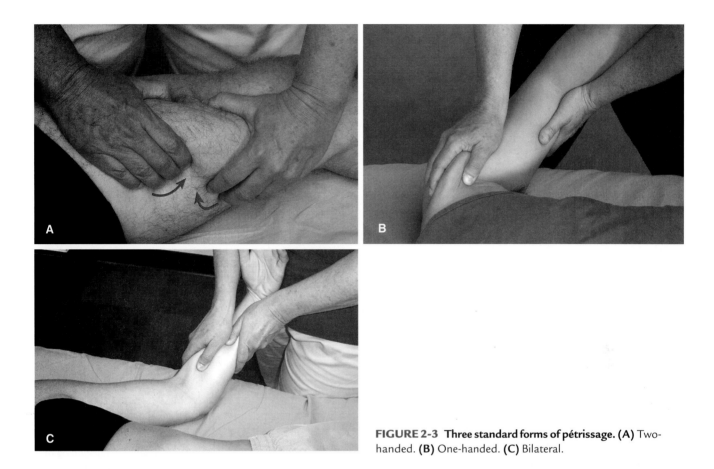

FIGURE 2-3 **Three standard forms of pétrissage. (A)** Two-handed. **(B)** One-handed. **(C)** Bilateral.

lifted away, a brief twist or pull of the tissue before release may increase this effect.

Stroke Mechanics

For pétrissage to be effective, the full hand must be in contact with the tissue. The curved thumb and heel of the hand are used for stabilization while the fingers scoop the tissue toward the thumb. This scoop-and-squeeze action is used to lift the superficial tissue away from underlying layers for a gentle stretch and loosening. To avoid undue stress on the thumbs and wrists, therapists must focus much attention on keeping the hands soft and contoured with equal amounts of tissue under the palms and fingers. The lift and squeeze is created by curling the fingers under the tissue to engage it with the pads of the fingers and thumb as depicted in the Figure 2-3, rather than pressing flat straight fingers into the tissue (Fig. 2-5). The flat finger squeezing motion puts all the stress of the stroke into the small muscles in the palm of the hand (lumbricals) and often feels "pinchy" to the athlete. Another part of the "soft hand" mechanics is to focus on keeping the web space between the thumb and index finger in a "J" shape rather than extending the thumb to an "L" shape. Open-

ing the thumb to an L or wider causes major stress in the extensor tendons of the thumb and wrist and should be avoided.

Purpose and Effects

The pétrissage strokes are used mostly for their structural effects. The superficial stretch created by lifting the tissue combined with the squeezing action of the hands loosens and softens the tissue. Because the hands don't slide, dry pétrissage is more effective than the standard pétrissage strokes in creating this loosening in the deeper tissues. Pétrissage may have an indirect effect on fluid movement by decreasing the restriction of tissue around blood vessels to allow easier local flow.

As the loosening and softening process occurs with pétrissage, the area is being prepared for deeper work, and the tissue is being assessed for restrictions. Pétrissage strokes are also believed to improve skin and muscle tone. This toning effect may be the result of stimulating the muscle proprioceptors with alternating increase and decrease in tension and length from the lift, squeeze, and release action of the stroke. Although there is no research on this effect of pétrissage, the anecdotal evidence clearly supports the

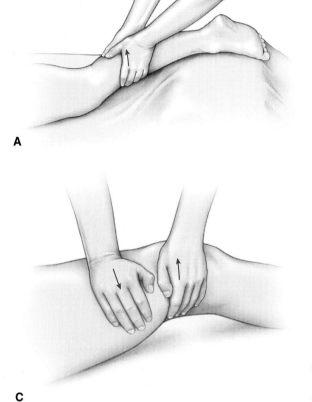

A

B

C

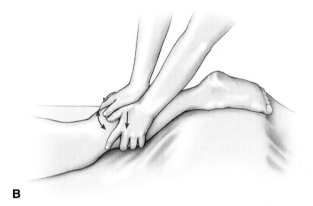

FIGURE 2-4 Two forms of compressive pétrissage. (A) Beginning of lift and press, or fulling. **(B)** Finish of lift and press/fulling. **(C)** Kneading style of compressive pétrissage.

hypothesis. To stimulate this toning effect, pétrissage must be performed at a brisk pace and moderate depth. A slow-paced pétrissage with more slide than lift will have a minimal effect on loosening and no toning effect, but it will be effective at improving muscle relaxation.

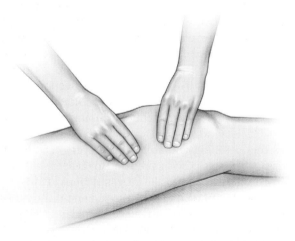

FIGURE 2-5 Incorrect stroke mechanics for pétrissage. The hand is stiff with the fingers and thumbs extended instead of curled. Pétrissage done in this fashion feels "pinchy" to the athlete and creates undo stress to the hands of the therapist.

Cautions and Contraindications

Pétrissage strokes are used in all categories of sports massage, but a slower pace must be used in post-event massage to avoid stimulating a cramp. In addition, the same considerations must be given to the use of pétrissage strokes that require an emollient as is given to effleurage use in pre-event situations.

▪ FRICTION

The general definition of friction is any stroke that applies compression and stretch to the tissue. The elbow, fist, palm, heel of hand, thumb, or braced fingers may be used to perform friction strokes, and the direction of the stretch may be across the muscle fibers, linear, or a combination of these. In all styles of friction, the tissue is pressed firmly into the underlying surfaces, and then the superficial layers are pushed over the underlying surface to a point of resistance/restriction for stretch and release. Friction strokes are designed to address the connective tissue elements of the musculoskeletal system, and different strokes are used to address the different elements. For example, broad friction strokes with fists or full hands are best for

A 33-year-old man has been an elite cyclist for many years at the ultra distances. He had a history of idiopathic chronic low back pain, which finally resulted in a L-5/S-1 diskectomy at age 30. He was living with constant low-grade pain in his low back that limited his ability to train to compete. In early 2003, he set his sights on winning a state championship race in the following year, so he found an experienced therapist and began regular massage. In his initial visits, the therapist noted that his lumbar and sacral motions were decreased, with spinal extension being the most limited and painful. There was also a significant difference in muscle mass between his right and left legs in both thigh and calf. His abdominal muscles and hamstrings were weak, and the iliopsoas and quadriceps were tight and dominant. His weekly massage session included trigger-point releasing in the iliopsoas, gluteus medius and minimus, piriformis, adductor magnus, pectineus, and quadratus lumborum, plus lots of spine extension movements and stretches for the quadriceps, psoas, and piriformis. He also did the recommended stretches on his own and began a core stability strength program. He continued to work out and compete throughout the 2003 season even though his low back pain came and went according to the intensity of his workouts and competition schedule. Between races, his massage session continued to focus on trigger-point and myofascial releases. However, he sometimes felt sore for a day or two after these sessions, so if he had a race coming up the therapist shifted to a more general massage with lots of pétrissage and gliding frictions. Gradually, the frequency, intensity, and duration of his pain diminished, and he achieved his goal of winning the 2004 State Champion jersey. He feels more in control of his symptoms than ever before and has every intention of holding his title in the upcoming year.

large fascial planes like the lumbosacral aponeurosis and iliotibial band, whereas thumbs or braced fingers can be used for the smaller and more specific work in areas such as the myofascial divisions between muscle groups and musculotendinous junctions.

Friction strokes can be applied with or without an emollient with the understanding that the slide–stretch ratio of the emollient changes the effective depth of the stroke. Effective friction strokes that use an emollient are broadening, linear, and reverse-J. Broadening friction is applied as a straight cross-fiber stroke (Fig. 2-6A). using hands or fists to engage the tissue in a light stretch. In the reverse-J stroke, also called circular friction, therapists use thumbs or loose fists to engage the tissue in an upside-down J pattern that both lengthens and broadens short segments of the tissue as the hands slide through the full muscle (Fig. 2-6B and C). Figure 2-6D depicts simple linear friction with loose fist gliding with pressure through the paraspinal muscles.

When no emollient is used, the stretching and broadening effects of friction are enhanced. One common non-emollient friction is a stationary form of broadening friction. This site-specific friction is an effective way to address one specific site, such as the common tendon of origin on the hamstrings and the origin of the long head of the triceps (Fig. 2-7). A specialized form of friction that adds passive movement to the linear techniques, called pin-and-stretch friction, is another common friction stroke used in basic sports massage. Pin-and-stretch, also called soft tissue release,[15] is applied without an emollient. First, the therapist positions the body part in a neutral or shortened position so that the tissue is soft, then presses with moderate depth and scoops the tissue into a taut/stretched position. Once the tissue is "pinned" in this manner, the body part is slowly lengthened to intensify the stretch (Fig. 2-8).

Stroke Mechanics

Because friction strokes require moderate to deep pressure into the tissue, proper stroke mechanics must be used to avoid injury to the therapist while still ensuring that the strokes are effective and comfortable to the athlete. First, the effectiveness of each friction stroke depends on how the compression and tension are applied to engage the tissue. It is the stretch part of the stroke that is necessary to achieve the desired effects. Therefore, the depth of the compression must not restrict the movement of the superficial layer of tissue. The best way to achieve this is to scoop under the tissue (see Fig. 2-6B), which creates a fold of tissue in front of the hands or thumbs, rather than to press straight down, which creates more of a dent or hole in the tissue. The second consideration in good friction mechanics is to use proper alignment of the therapist's hands, wrists, thumbs, and fingers. Wrists should be maintained in neutral during fist friction (see Fig. 2-6), and thumbs must be held close to the index finger to be in alignment with the radius, as in Figure 2-6B, rather than using the lateral edges of the thumbs (Fig. 2-9A), and fingers should be squeezed together to form one single unit as depicted in Figure 2-7A. When thumbs and fingers are used in friction strokes, the therapist must focus the pressure on the pads of the thumb/finger by keeping slight flexion at the

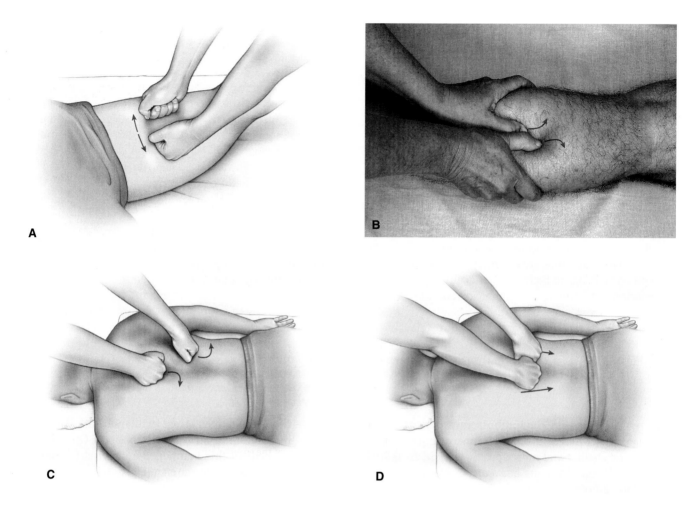

FIGURE 2-6 Friction strokes that require an emollient. (A) General broadening across hamstrings. **(B)** Reverse-J with thumbs. **(C)** Reverse-J with fists. **(D)** Linear.

distal joint rather than hyperextending and pressing into the tissue with the volar surface of that joint (Fig. 2-9A). Finally, body weight not hand and arm strength, should be used to create depth in all friction strokes.

Purpose and Effects

In sports massage, the friction strokes play a primary role in creating the desired structural effects of the massage. Friction strokes are the best type of massage strokes for stretching and broadening of muscles, reducing fascial restrictions, and enhanced collagen remodeling. The stretching and broadening actions of friction help athletes maintain general flexibility and full pain-free range of motion. The stretching and pressure of the strokes are believed to cause a histamine release from the mast cells, which creates a local hyperemia that enhances local fluid movement. When the tissue feels fibrous and/or adhered during pétrissage, friction is a good follow-up stroke through that area.

Cautions and Contraindications

The friction strokes described above can all be used in every categories of sports massage and should be used after the tissue has been softened a little by the pétrissage strokes. Therapists should be cautious about how rapidly they add depth to the strokes and should slow the pace of application in post-event and treatment categories of sports massage to avoid pain and possible stimulation of a muscle cramp. In cases of hypothermia, vigorous friction rubs are contraindicated in the extremities because it may force cold and acidic blood toward the heart, leading to a shock response.[16] In this case, all massage is contraindicated, and appropriate first aid measures become the priority.

▮JOSTLING

The jostling strokes included in basic sports massage are more vigorous forms of shaking that move larger masses

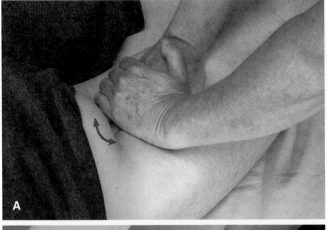

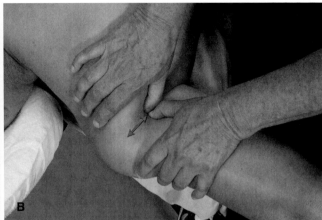

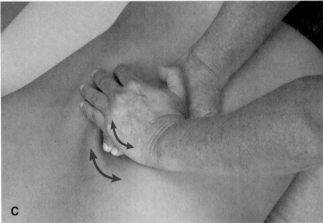

FIGURE 2-7 **Site-specific friction. (A)** Braced fingers over the origin of hamstrings. **(B)** Braced thumbs over the origin of the long head of the triceps (tendon). **(C)** Braced fingers in the paraspinals.

of tissue than the style of vibrations common to classic massage. In two of the most common forms of jostling, the therapist maintains a stationary hand position. To jostle a large muscle group such as the quadriceps or hamstrings, the hands are pressed under the edges of the muscle mass to lift it away from the bone. Then the entire muscle group is shaken side to side (Fig. 2-10A).

This technique can be expanded to full limb jostling that rocks the entire torso, leg or arm back and forth (Fig. 2-10B). The third form of jostling is a traveling stroke in which one or both hands are used to engage the tissue, shaking as they are pulled through the length of the muscle (Fig. 2-10C).

Stroke Mechanics

There are no specific stroke mechanics to be aware of for the jostling strokes other than the general body mechanics for all massage. However, therapists are reminded that it is the *rhythmic* movement of the muscle or body part that creates the desired effect, and the *speed* of the jostling must be adjusted according to the size of the therapist, muscle group, and/or category of massage.

Purpose and Effects

All the jostling strokes stimulate the mechanoreceptors in the muscles, providing kinesthetic feedback to help identify and release subconscious tension or holding. This effect is often described as reduced muscle guarding,

FIGURE 2-8 **Pin-and-stretch friction stroke in the triceps.**

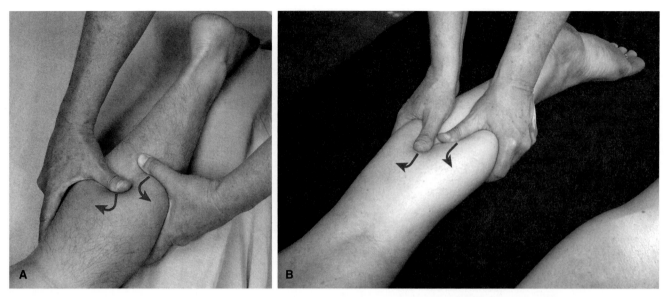

FIGURE 2-9 Two examples of poor stroke mechanics with friction strokes. (A) Thumbs are hyperextended so the tissue is incorrectly engaged with the interphalangeal joint. **(B)** Lateral stress is being placed on the thumbs because they are not in alignment with the radius.

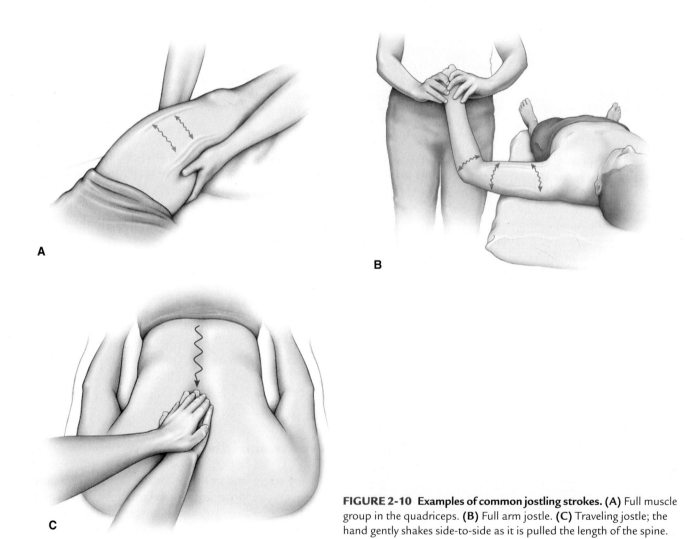

FIGURE 2-10 Examples of common jostling strokes. (A) Full muscle group in the quadriceps. **(B)** Full arm jostle. **(C)** Traveling jostle; the hand gently shakes side-to-side as it is pulled the length of the spine.

which should improve overall muscle relaxation without the sedating effect of classic vibration techniques. Jostling also loosens superficial tissue; probably more through the reduced muscle tension than through direct stretching or broadening. Jostling can be invigorating when applied at a brisk pace or relaxing when a slower pace is used. In the event category of sports massage, jostling is often used as a beginning stroke for each new body part and as a transition stroke between large muscle groups and other strokes. In pre-event massage, vigorous jostling is also a good choice of stroke for the end of the massage to leave the athlete feeling invigorated.

Cautions and Contraindications

With a history of dislocation, vigorous full-limb jostling in that extremity must be avoided. However, the large muscle groups in the limb may be jostled with a slower, less vigorous pace. In post-event massage, avoid vigorous jostling to reduce the risk of stimulating a cramp. As with the friction strokes, vigorous jostling is specifically contraindicated in cases of hypothermia, and appropriate first aid must be administered.

■ TAPOTEMENT

Tapotement is a percussive stroke in which the therapist alternately strikes the tissue with an open hand, loose fist, or fingertips (Fig. 2-11). The most common varieties of tapotement are:

- Spatting—using the palm of the hand
- Drumming—using a loose fist
- Hacking—using the ulnar border of the hand
- Pincement—using the thumbs and fingers to pick up the tissue in a rapid but gentle pinching movement
- Cupping—using a cupped palm of the hand so that the outer borders of the hand make contact with the tissue while the palm does not

Stroke Mechanics

Regardless of which surface of the hand is used by the therapist, the fingers and wrists should be relaxed and soft. The hands should rise only 3 to 4 inches from the tissue before dropping back down to the tissue to decrease the likelihood of being overly exuberant and causing tissue damage. Therapists must use knee flexion rather than trunk flexion to maintain this safe height relationship without causing

tightening of the hands, wrists, and back and to avoid strain.

Purpose and Effects

The pace of application and the type of tapotement used can change the effect of the stroke on the tissue. The consistently observed tissue changes associated with tapotement are a slight reddening of the area, muscle toning or relaxation, and an overall sense of invigoration for the athlete. The alternate striking action of tapotement is believed to stimulate a histamine release that causes the hyperemia, and the reflex muscle response of toning or relaxation is theorized to occur in response to stimulation of the stretch reflex. The results of tapotement, whether it tones or relaxes the muscles, are based on the choice of location, depth, rhythm, and duration of the application.[3,6–8,13] In cases of disuse muscle atrophy (after coming out of a brace or cast), pincement and/or tapping used in combination with brisk pétrissage can help the muscle regain its normal tone. If tapotement is applied in the large muscle groups like the gluteal muscles and hamstrings with moderate depth and pace for a period of several minutes, it can also have the opposite effect; muscle relaxation. Cupping tapotement has been used effectively to reduce congestion in the lungs. Therapists must use specific patient positioning and a prescribed pattern of cupping over the back and chest to achieve this effect, so cupping is not a recommended tapotement for basic sports massage. In athletics, tapotement is generally used for its invigorating and toning effect and mostly in the pre-event category of basic sports massage.

Cautions and Contraindications

Heavy tapotement strokes such as beating and hacking should be used only in thick or heavily muscled body areas, and no tapotement strokes should be applied over joints or floating ribs. Athletes with asthma should not get tapotement over the sternal and/or pectoral regions because anecdotal evidence suggests that it may stimulate an attack. Tapotement is generally too vigorous for post-event massage and should be specifically avoided in muscles that have experienced cramps during the activity. In cases of neurologically based atrophy (paralysis), the deep tapotement techniques of beating and hacking are contraindicated, because the protective reflex contraction of the muscles and the normal pain response are most likely compromised. In cases of paralysis or other degenerative neuromuscular conditions, only the pincement and tapping styles of tapotement are recommended, and even these should be used with great caution to avoid severe tissue damage.

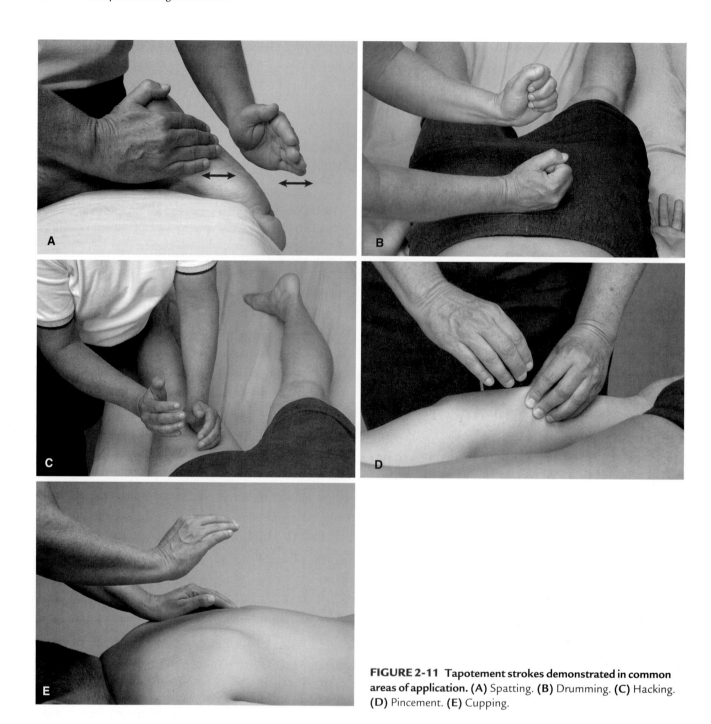

FIGURE 2-11 Tapotement strokes demonstrated in common areas of application. (A) Spatting. **(B)** Drumming. **(C)** Hacking. **(D)** Pincement. **(E)** Cupping.

■ RHYTHMIC COMPRESSION

In rhythmic compression, the therapist uses one or both hands in a loose fist or open palm position to apply a rhythmic press and release of the muscle belly directly into the underlying bone. The direction and depth of the stroke are designed to create a squeezing action on both sides of the tissue between the bone and the therapist's hands.[1,3–6,9] Rhythmic compression strokes do not use emollients and are easily applied over clothing, which can be an advantage in the event category of sports massage.

Stroke Mechanics

The loose-fist method of application for rhythmic compression is recommended over the open-palm method because the therapist can keep a neutral wrist and apply deeper pressure when working in larger muscle groups. A good loose fist is formed by gently squeezing the thumb next to the index finger, and the finger pads into the heel of the hand. This position creates a firm flat surface across the fist and prevents hyperflexion stress to the therapist's hands. When possible, double fists should be used to cover more tissue

From the Field

I am well aware of the importance, no the necessity, of regular massage from a qualified and experience sports massage specialist. I have relied on massage to keep the aches and pains of my training schedule under control and to help resolve the many minor injuries that have occurred over the years. I've realized that there is a direct correlation between when I break down and how long it's been since my last massage. Any time I'm training for a big competition I make sure I'm booked for a weekly massage a month or two in advance.

Kent Murdoch

Competitive Cross Country Skier
2001 and 2003 Masters National Champion

area, and the fists should be held close together to press into the tissue as one unit (Fig. 2-12).

In some smaller muscle groups or bony areas such as the anterior compartment of the leg, chest, forearm, and brachium, open palm(s) or the heel of one hand may be all that is needed to create the desired tissue compression (Fig. 2-13). It is essential that the therapist compresses the tissue directly into the bone without pushing the tissue mass off to one side, creating a shearing force that may lead to mild damage. To avoid this shearing action, let the arms hang slightly in front of the body holding the upper arms close to the chest. In this position, the therapist can look down and see that the fists/hands are aligned with the chin, as depicted in Figures 2-12 and 2-13. From this position, the tissue is compressed straight down into the bone until resistance is felt. At this point of tissue resistance, release the pressure allowing the tissue to rebound/expand slightly, then press again in the same general location, with each stroke slightly overlapping the previous one. When the pressure is released, the hands should remain in contact with the tissue, but at a more moderate depth that allows the rebound. It generally requires a minimum of three rhythmic compressions into the same tissue area before the desired effects of softening and hyperemia occur. However, the true gauge for the therapist is to notice a palpable softening of the tissue before moving to the next zone of the muscle. Gradually, the entire muscle mass has been covered with this alternating press–release action. The final point on stroke mechanics relates to overall body mechanics. The compression of the tissue should be established by

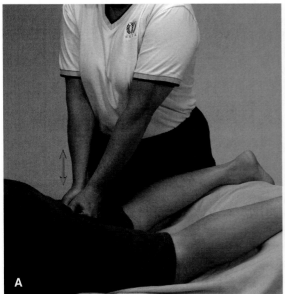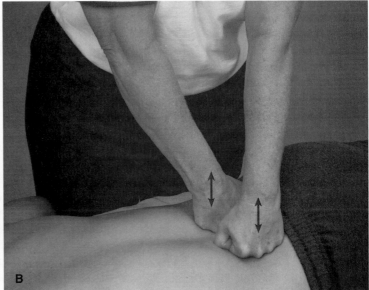

FIGURE 2-12 A double-fist hand position is preferred for most rhythmic compression in large muscle groups. (A) Hamstrings. **(B)** Paraspinals.

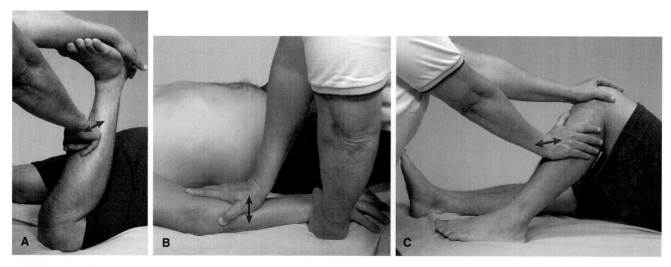

FIGURE 2-13 Alternate hand positions for rhythmic compressions. (A) Single loose fist over the anterior compartment. **(B)** Single palm for smaller muscles like those in the forearm. **(C)** Heel of hand in the anterior compartment.

the therapist leaning into the tissue with his or her body weight rather than pumping with hands and elbows only. Not only is this pumping action stressful to the therapist, it is less effective especially in thick tissue areas.

A common variation of the rhythmic compression technique is to lightly grasp and lift the tissue before compressing. This form of rhythmic compression is similar to the lift–press style of compressive pétrissage. However, because compressive pétrissage is applied with an emollient and rhythmic compressions are not, the intentions and effects of these strokes are different—compressive pétrissage stretches tissue *away* from the bone, whereas rhythmic compression squeezes tissue *into* the bone. The grasp and lift can be done with one hand before the other presses the tissue into the bone (Fig. 2-14), or both hands can lift before pressing down with the palms in larger muscles such as the hamstrings or gastrocnemius. This "lift–compress" variation is most useful in body areas where both the muscle and the underlying bone are rounded, such as the brachium and upper gastrocnemius. The lifting of the muscle mass before the compression helps to stabilize it and keeps the force of the stroke pushing the tissue into the underlying bone rather than creating a shearing force that rolls the muscle off to the side.

Purpose and Effects

A brisk pace is necessary to stimulate the release of histamine from the mast cells, which creates a deep hyperemia and gives the muscle a softer feel. The hyperemia effect of rhythmic compression is particularly helpful to athletes in pre-event massage because it keeps blood in the muscles about to be stressed by the activity. In addition, because this stroke is done without lubricant, it can be used in place of effleurage and can be used for general assessment to locate tight and tender regions in the muscles. The softening effect of rhythmic compression is important in post-event and maintenance massage both to prepare the tissue for deeper work and to return the muscle to its normal flexibility.

Cautions and Contraindications

Because the rhythmic compression strokes apply such deep pressure into the tissue, they should not be applied over any joint or bone projections. Ideally, the strokes are applied only in the muscle belly, and caution is used over the fascial divisions of that area. The pace and depth of rhythmic compressions must be moderated for post-event massage to avoid creating pain and/or muscle cramps in the fatigued and sore muscles of the athlete. Use of these strokes is not recommended in most treatment massage plans, especially during the acute and sub-acute phases.

ACTIVE ASSISTIVE TECHNIQUES

Active assistive techniques are specialized forms of broad friction that are often considered too deep and specific for use in classic Swedish massage. First introduced to most massage therapists by Benny Vaughn, ATC, LMT, CSCS, active assistive release is also known today as active release technique, active myofascial release, osteokinematics, soft tissue release, and muscle release techniques. The many names given to the techniques do not change the method of application or the primary effects of the strokes. These

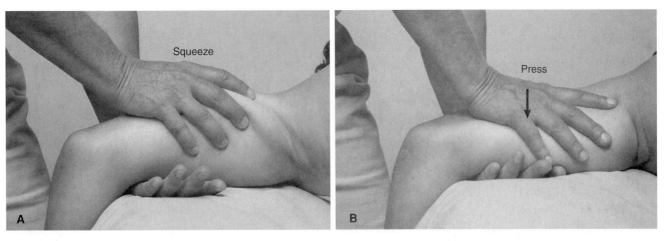

FIGURE 2-14 **Examples of the lift–compress style of rhythmic compressions. (A)** Start of one-handed lift–compress rhythmic compressions. **(B)** Finish of lift–compress.

techniques combine a friction stroke with an active muscle contraction by the athlete to create either a broadening or lengthening effect.[1,3] Active assistive techniques may be applied with or without and emollient.

Stroke Mechanics

In active assistive broadening, the therapist positions the body part so that the muscle is in a neutral or lengthened position and positions his or her hands (loose fists or the heel of the hands) at either the proximal or distal end of the muscle belly. The therapist instructs the athlete to slowly and actively shorten the muscle (concentric contraction) while the therapist simultaneously applies a down-and-out pressure to stroke across the normal muscle fiber direction to intensify the broadening action of the contraction. This process is repeated in the next segment of muscle until the full length of the muscle has been broadened, which may require three or four contractions. Depending on the fiber arrangement of the muscle being worked, the broadening action may require that hands stroke straight out as depicted in the standard broadening friction in Figure 2-15 or that they fan out from a pivot point as depicted later in Chapter 11, Figure 11-13. This fanning-out motion is particularly useful in muscles with an oblique fiber direction such as the quadriceps.

In active assistive lengthening, the therapist positions the body part so that the muscle is in a short position, and positions the hands (loose fists or the heel of the hands) at the distal end of the muscle belly. The therapist instructs the athlete to slowly and actively lengthen the muscle (eccentric contraction) while simultaneously applying a linear friction stroke parallel to the normal muscle fiber

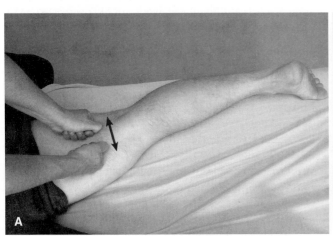
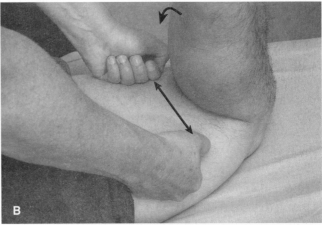

FIGURE 2-15 **Active assistive broadening. (A)** Start of broadening across hamstrings. **(B)** Finish position for active assistive broadening.

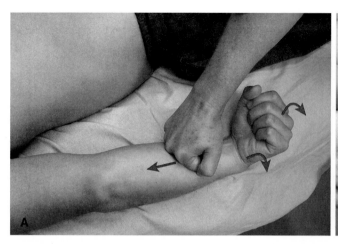
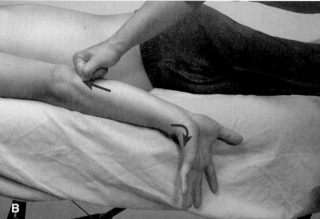

FIGURE 2-16 Active assistive lengthening. (A) Start of lengthening in wrist/finger flexors. **(B)** Finish position for active assistive lengthening.

direction to intensify the lengthening action of the motion (Fig. 2-16). Most muscles require more than one contraction for the stroke to be completed over the entire muscle.

The intensity and depth of the tissue broadening and lengthening are increased when the active assistive strokes are applied without an emollient. In the dry applications, the therapist first engages the tissue in either a broadening or lengthening stretch and maintains that stretch throughout the athlete's contraction. Because the therapist does not stroke through the tissue, only a small segment of muscle can be worked at a time. Therefore, several contractions are required to cover the full length of the muscle.

Purpose and Effects

Active assistive techniques are used to achieve structural effects of sports massage. Because the full muscle is actively engaged during a contraction, the connective tissue releases may occur at a much deeper level in the muscle and in areas not directly under the hands of the therapist. As the muscle fibers naturally broaden and lengthen during the contraction, the pressure of the friction stroke intensifies these movements to release any restriction between the fibers. These techniques are particularly useful when thick and matted scar tissue is deeply embedded in muscle tissue. The active assistive techniques also cause a reflexive reduction of muscle tension, presumably by stimulating the muscle spindle and Golgi tendon organ with intensified lengthening and tension input.

Cautions and Contraindications

Because of the intensity of these strokes, they should not be used in treatment of an acute muscle strain until the

maturation stage of healing. Although the active assistive techniques can be used in all three categories of sports massage, the dry applications may be too intense for event massage.

■ STRETCHING AND RANGE OF MOTION

It is appropriate and necessary for therapists to incorporate stretching and passive range of motions into sports massage. Generally, the range of motions should be applied before stretching, and both should be added to the end of the massage after all of the soft tissue strokes for that body region have been completed. Static or gradual stretches are the most common form of stretching for event work, while facilitated stretching techniques such as Proprioceptive Neuromuscular Facilitation (PNF) and Post-Isometric Relaxation (PIR) (Chapter 9) are more appropriately used in the maintenance and treatment categories and should be applied with caution in post-event work to decrease the risk of stimulating a muscle cramp.

When stretches are incorporated in basic sports massage, the intention is to return muscles to their normal length after reducing muscle tension and/or connective tissue restrictions *not* to affect a long-term improvement in muscle length. This is particularly true in event massage, where the primary intentions are to loosen and soften the tissue and give the athlete the kinesthetic feedback of easy pain-free range of motion and stretch. Even when facilitated stretching is used in maintenance and treatment massage, the goal is simply to return the muscle to its normal status of full extensibility and rebound. When that is accomplished, range of motion and stretch are likely to improve as well. However, if the muscle tension and connective tissue elements all are healthy, months of regular stretching are often required for an athlete to achieve and maintain any

TABLE 2-2	Purpose/Effects of Basic Sports Massage Strokes
Purpose/Effect	**Strokes That Best Produce the Effect**
Assessment and preparation for deep work	Effleurage Pétrissage Rhythmic compression
Improve local circulation (venous flow)	Effleurage Linear friction
Create hyperemia	Rhythmic compression Frictions Active assistive release
Stretch and broaden	Frictions Active assistive release Stretching (static or facilitated)
Reduce muscle tension/muscle relaxation	Pétrissage Jostling Prolonged tapotement
Improve muscle tone[a]	Pétrissage (rapid) Tapotement

[a]Theoretic/supported by anecdotal evidence.
Modified from Massage for Sports Health Care. Champaign, IL: Human Kinetics, 1997. © Patricia Archer.

significant increase in a specific range of motion or stretch. Table 2-2 shows the best strokes to use for an athlete's particular purpose.

All three categories of therapeutic massage in athletics include a few of these basic sports massage strokes in the massage sequences and protocols. However, the other therapeutic massage techniques must be used in addition to basic sports massage to formulate appropriate maintenance and treatment massage protocols. Basic sports massage is best suited to the event and maintenance massage categories of therapeutic massage because the basic strokes are designed to create mostly structural changes, in an abbreviated time frame.

SUMMARY

- There are three categories of basic sports massage: event, maintenance, and treatment.
- Event massage is designed to help athletes prepare for and recover from physical exertion. It is subdivided into pre-event, inter-event, and post-event. Basic sports massage strokes are used in event massage.
- Maintenance massage is regular massage given in a clinical environment that is intended to minimize the normal aches and pains associated with rigorous physical training. Basic sports massage, myofascial, and neuromuscular techniques are used in maintenance massage.
- Treatment massage is administered when a specific injury has occurred, with the intention of facilitating the healing process and safely returning the athlete to activity as soon as possible. Lymphatic facilitation is added to the other three therapeutic massage techniques to encompass treatment massage.
- Basic sports massage differs from classic/Swedish massage because it is brief and focused on specific muscle groups or body areas rather than being full body, is applied with a rapid pace that is not intended to soothe or sedate the athlete, may or may not use an emollient, and is often applied over clothing.
- In addition to standard effleurage, pétrissage, friction, vibration, tapotement, and stretching, basic sports massage uses two unique strokes: (1) rhythmic compressions and (2) active assistive release.
- The basic sports massage strokes can be used in all three categories of event massage. However, tapotement and contract–relax stretching may not be the best choices for post-event massage because of the increased risk of muscle cramping.

Review Questions

SHORT ANSWERS

1. Define basic sports massage.

2. Name the five stroke categories from Swedish/classic massage that are also used in basic sports massage.
   a.
   b.
   c.
   d.
   e.

3. Name the five contraindications for all basic sports massage.
   a.
   b.
   c.
   d.
   e.

MULTIPLE CHOICE

4. The two types of compressive pétrissage are:
   a. Active assistive and two-handed
   b. Kneading and lift-press
   c. Alternating and bilateral
   d. Pushing and pulling

5. Which of these strokes are used to assess and prepare the tissue for deeper strokes?
   a. Friction and jostling
   b. Pétrissage and friction
   c. Effleurage and pétrissage
   d. Active assistive release

6. What strokes are best at creating the structural effects of stretching and broadening tissue?
   a. Effleurage
   b. Pétrissage
   c. Jostling
   d. Friction

7. Softening muscles and creating a deep hyperemia are the intentions of _____ strokes.
   a. Rhythmic compression
   b. Pétrissage
   c. Jostling
   d. Tapotement

8. Which hand position should be used to apply rhythmic compression in the heavily muscled areas such as hamstrings and quadriceps?
   a. Single open palm
   b. Single fist

   c. Double fist
   d. Braced flat fingers

9. Which of these general friction strokes must be applied with an emollient?
   a. Stationary braced thumb
   b. Single fist
   c. Braced fingers
   d. Linear

10. What type of movement/contraction do athletes perform during active assistive broadening?
    a. Isometric
    b. Eccentric
    c. Concentric
    d. Tonic

11. What type of movement/contraction do athletes perform during active assistive lengthening?
    a. Isometric
    b. Eccentric
    c. Concentric
    d. Tonic

12. Proper stroke mechanics for pétrissage would include:
    a. gripping the tissue with curved fingers and thumbs.
    b. squeezing the tissue firmly with extended flat fingers and thumbs.
    c. lifting tissue without allowing the palm of the hand to contact the tissue.
    d. hyperextending the thumbs and fingers to "reach" for a new bundle of tissue each stroke.

13. Which of these tapotement strokes is most appropriate for use in the brachium?
    a. Drumming
    b. Cupping
    c. Pincement
    d. Hacking

14. Which of the basic sports massage strokes is generally contraindicated in post-event massage?
    a. Pétrissage
    b. Friction
    c. Jostling
    d. Tapotement

15. Proper stroke mechanics for pin-and-stretch includes:
    a. pressing the target tissue straight down into the bone before the stretch.
    b. putting the tissue in a lengthened position before pinning it.
    c. scooping the tissue to create light tension before moving the body part to a stretched position.

d. lifting the tissue away from the bone initially, then pressing it down and the stretch is initiated.

16. Inter-event massage is most important in which of these athletic situations?
    a. Between events at a track meet
    b. Halftime at a football game
    c. At the end of a day between a multiday event.
    d. Between innings of a championship baseball game.

17. Which category of sports massage is a full-body massage that is designed to minimize the negative effects of training and reduce the risk of injury?
    a. Event
    b. Maintenance
    c. Treatment
    d. Basic

18. Which of the following athletes would receive an event massage with more focus on the upper body muscles?
    a. Hurdler
    b. Cross-country runner
    c. Soccer player
    d. Tennis player

19. The intention of jostling strokes is to:
    a. stimulate mechanoreceptors to improve muscle tone.
    b. provide kinesthetic feedback to reduce subconscious muscle guarding.
    c. stimulate local circulation.
    d. stretch and loosen the deep fascia in each muscle group.

20. The major contrasts between classic/Swedish massage and basic sports massage include a difference in the intention and pace of the massage, plus the following:
    a. Classic massage is a full-body massage and basic sports massage is not.
    b. Emollients must be used in basic sports massage and is optional in classic.
    c. Basic sports massage uses a completely different set of strokes from that of classic.
    d. Basic sports massage is usually 1 hour long and classic is always under 30 minutes.

REFERENCES

1. Archer PA. Massage for Sports Health Care. Champaign, IL: Human Kinetics, 1999.
2. Kuprian W. Physical Therapy for Sports. Philadelphia: WB Saunders, 1982.
3. Benjamin PJ, Lamp SP. Understanding Sports Massage, 2nd ed. Champaign, IL: Human Kinetics, 2005.
4. King RK. Performance Massage: Muscle Care for Physically Active People. Champaign, IL: Human Kinetics, 1992.
5. Meagher J, Boughton P. Sportsmassage. Garden City: Doubleday & Company, 1980.
6. Tappan FM, Benjamin PJ. Healing Massage Techniques: Classic, Holistic, and Emerging Methods, 3rd ed. Stamford, CT: Appleton & Lange, 1998.
7. Salvo SG. Massage Therapy: Principles and Practice, 2nd ed. St. Louis: Saunders/Elsevier, 2003.
8. Fritz S. Mosby's Fundamentals of Therapeutic Massage, 2nd ed. St. Louis: CV Mosby, 2000.
9. Prentice WE. Therapeutic Modalities for Allied Health Professions. New York & St. Louis: McGraw-Hill, 1998.
10. Field T. Massage therapy. In: Davis CM, ed. Complementary Therapies in Rehabilitation. Thorofare, NJ: SLACK, Inc, 1997.
11. Prentice WE. Therapeutic Modalities for Sports Medicine and Athletic Training. St. Louis: McGraw-Hill, 2002.
12. Field TM et al. Massage reduces anxiety in child and adolescent psychiatric patients. Pediatrics Journal 1996;77(5):135–141.
13. Braverman DL, Schulman RA. Massage techniques in rehabilitation medicine. Physical Medicine and Rehabilitation Clinics of North America 1999;10(3):631–648.
14. Cafarelli E, Flint F. The role of massage in preparation for and recovery from exercise. Sports Medicine 1992;14(1):1–9.
15. Cash M. Sport and Remedial Massage Therapy. London: Ebury Press, 1996.
16. Safran MR, McKeag DB, VanCamp SP. Manual of Sports Medicine. Philadelphia: Lippincott-Raven, 1998.

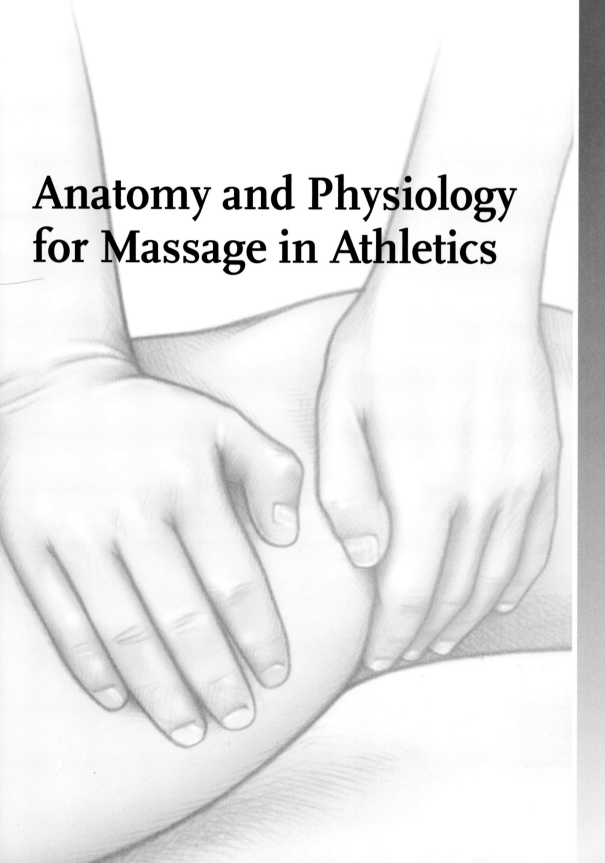

Anatomy and Physiology for Massage in Athletics

Cardiovascular and Lymphatic Systems

After completing this chapter, the reader will be able to:

- Describe the similarities and differences between the cardiovascular and lymphatic systems.
- Name the four types of lymph vessels and describe the structural features of each.
- Compare and contrast mechanisms of fluid flow in arteries, veins, and lymph vessels.
- Define diffusion, osmosis, filtration, and oncotic pressure.
- Identify the Starling forces that create and mediate capillary exchange and edema uptake.
- Define edema, lymphedema, circulatory edema, and traumatic edema.
- Explain edema uptake and distinguish this process from lymph flow.
- Define pre-lymphatic channel, and explain its function in edema uptake and flow.
- Explain and locate the primary catchments and watersheds of the body.
- Describe the physiologic mechanisms that create and influence lymph flow.
- Describe the different routes for lymph flow back into cardiovascular circulation for the torso, upper, and lower extremities.

irculation in the body involves both the cardiovascular and the lymphatic systems. The cardiovascular system is a true circulatory system made up of a closed network of vessels that carry blood to and from the heart. There are three types of blood vessels in the cardiovascular network: arteries, veins, and capillaries. Arteries carry blood away from the heart, and veins carry blood toward the heart (Fig. 3-1). Capillaries are microscopic vessels grouped together to form a complex network called a capillary bed. In a simplistic model, the capillary beds are situated between the arteries and veins and are the theoretical point at which blood flow switches from delivery to return.

Cardiovascular Circulation

If capillary beds are viewed as the transition point for delivery and return of blood, then arterial blood flow is the delivery half of the equation and venous flow the return half.

Blood is moved through arteries and veins via different circulatory mechanisms based on the structural differences between the vessels.

▉ BLOOD VESSEL STRUCTURE

Both arteries and veins have the same three layers of tissue that make up the vessel wall: an outer connective tissue layer, a middle smooth muscle layer, and an inner epithelial layer. In arteries, the muscle layer is thick, making arteries both **elastic** and **contractile.** Veins have neither of these functional characteristics because their muscular wall is thin. However, their connective tissue layer is thick and provides the functional characteristic called **extensibility** to facilitate high volumes of fluid.

The very small arteries that carry blood into the capillary beds are called **arterioles,** and their structure is considerably different from a large artery. In the smallest arterioles

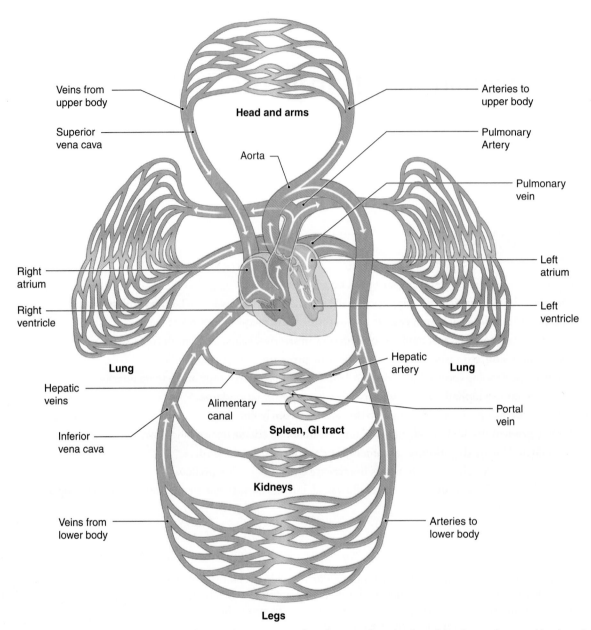

FIGURE 3-1 Cardiovascular system. The cardiovascular system is a closed system that circulates blood away from and back to the heart.

(those closest to the capillary bed), the normal three-layer construction of an artery changes to a single layer of epithelium surrounded by several well-spaced rings of smooth muscle. These smooth muscle wraps ringing the arteriole essentially control the amount of blood flow into the capillary bed by constricting or dilating the arteriole on command from the nervous system or in response to local chemical changes in the tissue. Conversely, the smaller veins that carry blood out of the capillary beds are called **venules.** These transition into the larger veins that carry blood back into the heart. The venules closest to the capillary beds have a two-layer structure similar to that of the arteriole, but the smooth muscle rings are very widely spaced. This means that the venules can adapt to changing

volumes of capillary flow, but do not exert much control over the process. In addition, the venous end of a capillary bed has more vessels than the arteriole end.[1-5]

The capillary beds of the cardiovascular system are the site for the nutrient–waste exchange process with body tissues. This nutrient–waste exchange is possible because of the unique anatomy of capillaries; only a single layer of epithelial cells surrounded by a very thin and porous basement membrane makes up the capillary wall (Fig. 3-2). The diameter of the capillary is just large enough for a red blood cell to squeeze through. There are microscopic openings between the epithelial cells of the capillary inner wall called **intercellular clefts**, which are slightly smaller than the diameter of the average protein molecule. Water mol-

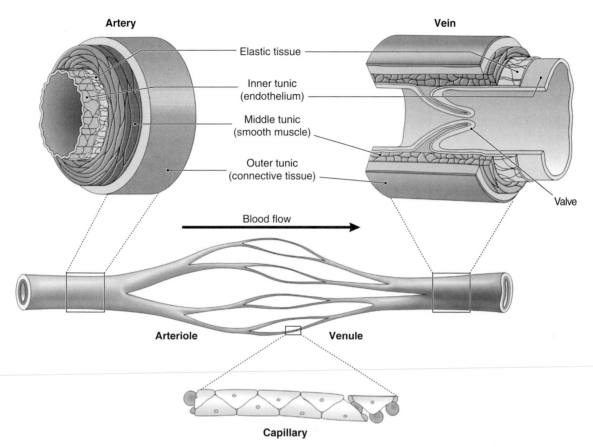

FIGURE 3-2   A comparison of the structural similarities and differences between blood vessels.

ecules, water-soluble ions, and most other small solutes carried in the blood pass easily through the intercellular clefts during nutrient–waste exchange, whereas most plasma proteins remain in the bloodstream. The venous side of a capillary bed is more absorbent because there are more vessels than on the arterial side, and venous capillaries have more numerous intercellular clefts.[2,6–11] However, the intercellular openings in venous capillaries are still too small to allow reabsorption of any protein molecules that do get forced into the interstitium on the arterial side of the bed.

The distribution of capillary beds throughout the body varies greatly and is largely based on the metabolic demands of the tissue. The muscles, lungs, nervous system, and several digestive organs all have high metabolic activity and require a dense capillary network. According to their lower metabolic demands, tendons and ligaments are moderately rich in capillaries, and cartilage and epithelial tissues have no capillaries at all.

◼ ARTERIAL FLOW

Cardiac contraction and the elastic recoil response of arteries provide the force that moves blood through these ves-sels. When the heart contracts and ejects blood into the arteries, the thick muscular wall of the vessels allows them to stretch slightly in response to the extra volume of blood. As the heart is relaxed, the elastic recoil of the stretched arterial wall forces blood onward through the vessel (Fig. 3-3A). This phenomenon of arterial stretch and recoil, measured as blood pressure, is most evident in the larger and more elastic arteries such as the aorta, brachiocephalic, carotid, subclavian, and common iliac.[1–5]

In the peripheral arteries such as the axillary, brachial, femoral, and popliteal, the smooth muscle layer is a little thicker than in the larger aorta and subclavian artery, for example. This layer, innervated by sympathetic nerve fibers, gives the peripheral arteries better contractility and the ability to readily change their diameter. Increased sympathetic stimulus causes **vasoconstriction,** a narrowing of the artery, whereas decreased sympathetic stimulus leads to **vasodilation,** a widening of the vessel. These changes mediate local blood volumes and the overall distribution of blood to the tissues. In addition to sympathetic stimulus, the release of various chemicals, such as histamine, and changes in tissue temperature can cause constriction or dilation of the blood vessels as well. These variables can be intentionally manipulated for therapeutic benefit.

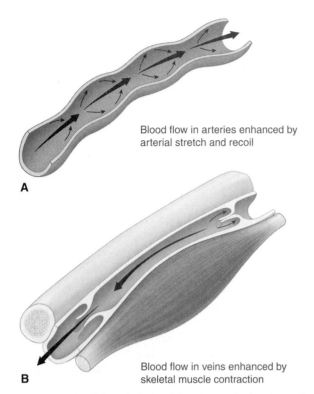

A

Blood flow in arteries enhanced by arterial stretch and recoil

B

Blood flow in veins enhanced by skeletal muscle contraction

FIGURE 3-3 Blood flow. (A) Blood flow in arteries is enhanced by the stretch and recoil of the blood vessel. The force and volume of blood pumped into the artery stretch the vessel wall, and the recoil gives additional force to flow. **(B)** Blood flow in veins is enhanced by skeletal muscle contraction. The contraction applies external compression of the vessel to assist in movement of blood back to the heart.

From the Field

"With the intensity and short duration of the WNBA season, it is vital for our athletes to avoid injury and take care of little aches and pains right away. The regular attention players get from our massage therapist plays an important role in that. I wouldn't even consider trying to get through a season without a qualified massage therapist as a part of my sports medicine team."

AnnMarie Henkel, ATC

Head Athletic Trainer, Seattle Storm

VENOUS FLOW

In contrast to arterial flow, venous blood flow depends on external pressures applied to the vessels. The primary source of external pressure is skeletal muscle contraction. To facilitate movement of blood back to the heart, veins have an internal system of one-way valves that divide a vein into short segments (see Fig. 3-1). These segments hold blood at a certain level within the vein until a contraction of skeletal muscle pushes the blood into the next segment on its way back to the heart (see Fig. 3-3B). Gravity is generally working against venous flow, which makes regular voluntary muscle contraction vital for circulation.

In addition to skeletal muscle contraction, breathing provides another boost to venous blood flow. The contraction and relaxation of the diaphragm change the pressure inside the thoracic and abdominal cavities during ventilation. These changes in pressure facilitate venous flow in the large veins inside the cavities, creating a **respiratory pump**.

CAPILLARY EXCHANGE

Blood flows through the capillaries to link the arterial and venous portions of the cardiovascular loop. However, exploring capillary flow is less important than understanding the process of fluid exchange that occurs between blood and tissue. This fluid movement, or capillary exchange, can be divided into two distinct processes: capillary filtration and reabsorption. **Capillary filtration** is the movement of fluid and dissolved substances from the blood to the interstitium, whereas **capillary reabsorption** is the movement of fluid and dissolved substances back into the blood.

Diffusion, Osmosis, and Filtration

Movement of substances and fluids between tissues can be a *passive* process, which does not require the expenditure of energy, or an *active* process, which requires energy. One of the primary transport mechanisms at work in the capillary beds is diffusion. **Diffusion** is a passive transport mechanism based on *concentration gradients*. When a substance is found in high concentrations on one side of a semipermeable membrane (such as the capillary wall) and low concentration on the other side, movement occurs in a "downhill" manner. The substance moves from the area of high concentration to the area of lower concentration until things are balanced or can no longer move. Most of the nutrients and other important solutes such as oxygen, glucose, and hormones move out of blood and into the interstitium on the arteriole side of the capillary bed via the diffusion process. The outward diffusion of these solutes occurs because their concentrations are higher in the blood than in the interstitial spaces. Diffusion is also the method of transfer for metabolic wastes such as carbon dioxide and ammonia into the bloodstream because the concentration gradient is reversed at the venous end of the capillary bed.[1-4,8,9,12,13]

Osmosis is a specialized form of diffusion, in which only water molecules move. Osmosis occurs when a semipermeable membrane does not allow the solid substances of a solution, the **solutes**, to pass through because the molecules or particles are too large. In this situation, the body seeks balance by bringing more water across the membrane to dilute the high-solute concentration. The high-solute tissue has **osmotic pressure** because it draws water into it in an attempt to balance the solution. When protein molecules, which are veritable water magnets, are the solutes causing the concentration gradient, it is termed **colloidal osmotic**, or **oncotic** pressure. **Plasma,** the fluid portion of blood, is approximately 92% water. The remaining 8% of plasma is composed of high levels of various protein molecules. These plasma proteins are an essential feature of blood and play a vital role in capillary exchange.[1-7]

The passive transport mechanism called **filtration** is based on differences in pressure. Fluids in an area of high pressure are forced through a semipermeable membrane to an area of lower pressure. This hydrostatic pressure gradient is more *mechanical* in nature than osmotic pressure gradients because it is created by weight, fluid volume, or flow force rather than differences in solute concentrations.

Fluid Movement Through the Capillary Membrane

The nutrients and wastes that make up the solutes in blood are exchanged across the capillary wall primarily through diffusion. In contrast, plasma and interstitial fluid movement occurs via filtration and osmosis. Over a century ago, E. H. Starling dissected and carefully described the movement of fluid across the capillary membrane. He divided the differences between hydrostatic and osmotic pressures inside and outside of the capillary bed into four distinct forces.[2] These **Starling forces** are now universally acknowledged as the regulatory mechanisms for capillary exchange of fluid.[2,6,8,10,14-16] The four forces at work in the capillary bed are:

1. **Capillary fluid pressure (CFP)**—hydrostatic pressure created by the water content of the blood in capillaries.

2. **Interstitial fluid pressure (IFP)**—hydrostatic pressure created by the water content in the interstitial spaces of the capillary bed.
3. **Plasma oncotic pressure (POP)**—osmotic pressure created inside the capillary by the protein content of the blood.
4. **Interstitial oncotic pressure (IOP)**—osmotic pressure created in the interstitial spaces by the protein content of the interstitial fluid.[1,2,6,8,10,11,13,15,17]

Both CFP and IOP create movement of fluid out of the blood and into the interstitium (eg, filtration), whereas IFP and POP create fluid movement from the interstitium back into the blood (eg, reabsorption) (Fig. 3-4). In healthy tissue, the dominant Starling force at the arteriole end of the capillary bed is capillary fluid pressure due to arterial blood pressure. This dominant CFP leads to net capillary filtration. In contrast, plasma oncotic pressure is the dominant Starling force on the venule side. This is because most of the plasma proteins are too large to move easily through the capillary membrane and remain in the blood even though most of the fluid has been filtered out of the capillary. The net effect of dominant POP creates a net reabsorption of fluid back into the capillaries.[2,6,7,10,11,13,15]

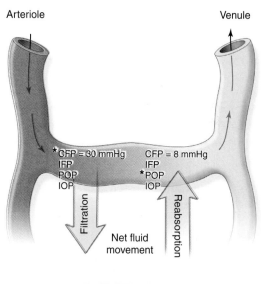

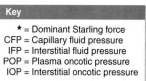

FIGURE 3-4 Capillary pressures and fluid movement. Capillary exchange is influenced and controlled by four Starling forces. High capillary fluid pressure at the arteriole side of the capillary creates a net filtration of fluid outward. Because the proteins in the blood remain high on the venous side of the capillary, the higher plasma oncotic pressure creates a net reabsorption of fluid into the vessel.

Edema

Capillary reabsorption is a vital process for the recovery of the high volume of fluid filtered out at the arteriole end. On a daily basis approximately 30 liters of fluid are filtered out of the capillaries and into the interstitial tissue. Most of the fluid is then reabsorbed; however, even at its best the capillary reabsorption process brings back only 90% of the filtered fluid (approximately 27 liters) into the venous side of the capillary bed. The remaining 10% of the capillary filtrate is the responsibility of the lymphatic system.[4,6,7,10,11,17] If this fluid is not picked up by the lymphatic system, an excess amount of fluid begins to collect in the interstitial spaces, a condition called edema. Left untreated, edema continues to accumulate, and the stagnation of the metabolites and waste products in the fluid eventually compromise the tissue's function and healing.

Simple edema is not itself a disease, but a common sign or side effect of other problems. For example, high blood pressure creates two problems at the capillary bed. It increases the CFP at the arteriole end of the bed, which increases the volume of capillary filtration. The high CFP also tends to remain at the venous side of the bed, decreasing reabsorption because the oncotic pressure of the blood may not be sufficient to overcome the high fluid pressure in the capillary. An example that occurs more commonly in athletics is the traumatic edema associated with sprains and strains. Stretching and tearing of tissue causes proteins to hemorrhage out of the blood and damaged cells, which significantly increases the interstitial oncotic pressure in that area. This increased IOP neutralizes the plasma oncotic pressure so that reabsorption is severely limited and swelling results. These are just two examples of how imbalances in normal capillary filtration and reabsorption lead to edema. There are several other ways in which filtration and reabsorption processes can be disturbed, and several types of edema are discussed later in this chapter with the lymphatic system.[4,6,10]

From the Field

"I feel as though expanding my horizons and becoming a massage therapist has allowed me to not only improve my ability to manage athletic injuries, but also to develop better relationships with the athletes I work with. One of the best ways to indicate to an athlete that you truly are committed to creating an optimal healing environment is by using hands-on manual therapy skills."

Ian McLeod

ATC and Massage Therapist at Arizona State University

Overview of the Lymphatic System

The exact structure and function of the lymphatic system was quite a mystery until the last 30 to 40 years. The first documentation of the existence of the system came from the Greeks. Herophilus and Erasistratus of the Alexandrian Medical School hypothesized about the system in about 300 BC; however, Galen did not believe their theories to be correct, so not much was written. In 1622, Gasparo Aselli, an Italian physician, again described a theoretical second and largely separate part of the circulatory system. In 1653, Bartholin first named the system lymphatics, and Cruikshank and Hewson of the United Kingdom put forward the suggestion that the system was made up of absorbing vessels located over the entire body.[6,10] Several scientists continued to study the structure of the system and formulate theories regarding the formation of lymph over the next 200 years. With the advent of the electron microscope in 1960, scientists were finally able to verify the presence of the lymph capillaries, describe their structure, and confirm the process of lymph formation as absorption of interstitial fluid into the lymphatic capillaries via small openings in the ends of the vessel. The study of why interstitial fluid enters the lymphatic system, how it stays there, and how the system moves the fluid through its vascular network for return to circulation has been ongoing since that time.

The lymphatic system serves two functions: fluid return and immunity. In contrast to the cardiovascular system, the lymphatic system is an *open system* because lymphatic vessels are not connected in a full circuit with each other or with the heart. This makes the lymphatic system capable of fluid *return only* (Fig. 3-5A). The immune functions of the lymphatic system are vital processes, involving the actions of specialized lymphocytes (B cells and T cells) and the specialized lymphoid structures such as the tonsils, appendix, thymus, spleen, lacteals, and Peyer's tissue. However, for sports health care professionals, the system's role in fluid return is of greatest interest and relevance to the application of therapeutic massage in athletics.

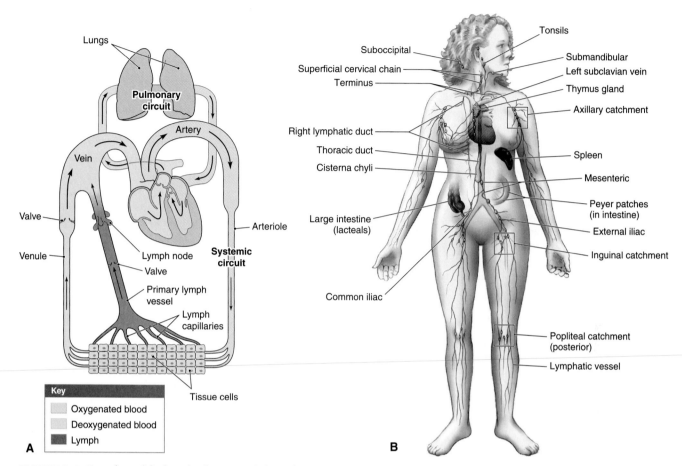

FIGURE 3-5 Overview of the lymphatic system. (A) A schematic representation of the relation between the cardiovascular and lymphatic systems shows the "open" lymphatic system returning fluid from the interstitium to circulation. **(B)** The specialized lymphoid tissues, nodes and vascular network of the lymphatic system.

COMPONENTS OF THE LYMPHATIC SYSTEM

Lymph nodes and the other specialized lymphoid tissues along with a complex network of vessels are the primary components of the lymphatic system (see Fig. 3-5B). Unlike the other specialized lymphatic organs, lymph nodes are a *structural* part of the vascular network because they are interspersed along the length of the primary lymph vessels. This gives the lymph nodes an important role in the fluid return function of the system in addition to their role in the immune response. The nodes have both afferent vessels with one-way valves that carry lymph into the nodes and efferent vessels with valves that prevent back-flow into the lymph node. This structural feature plus the irregular channel network inside the node control both the direction and rate of lymph flow through the nodes.[1–7]

Although each primary lymph vessel has several nodes interspersed along its length, there are a few areas in which several lymph nodes are clustered together forming a bed of lymph nodes, or a **catchment**. Each catchment is respon-

sible for collecting the lymph from a specific region of the body to filter out pathogens and perform the other immune processes specific to the nodes. Generally located at hinge areas of the body such as the axilla, elbow, inguinal and popliteal regions, catchments offer 100 times more resistance to flow than the entire vascular network of the lymphatic system put together.[6] Therefore, the rate of lymph flow through a catchment is significantly slower than through the network of lymph vessels, making them common areas of blockage and essential areas to address for improved lymph flow.

The largest vessels in the network, the **right lymphatic** and **thoracic ducts**, complete the lymphatic network of vessels. The **cisterna chyli**, a small bulge at the base of the thoracic duct, is situated just below the diaphragm approximately at the level of the second lumbar vertebra (Figs. 3-5B and 3-6). It is a passive collecting well for lymph from the lower extremities, which also gives a boost to lymph flow into and through the thoracic duct. Because the cisterna chyli is located in close proximity to the diaphragm, each breath squeezes it and forces lymph into the thoracic duct, similar to the action of a rubber bulb on a turkey baster.

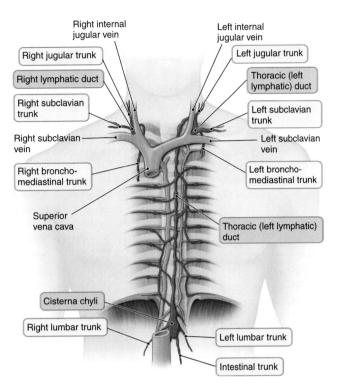

A   Overall anterior view

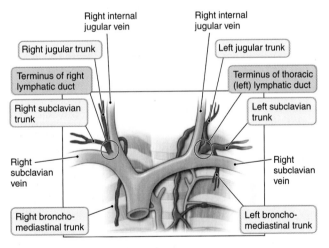

B   Detailed anterior view

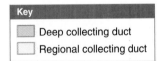

Key	
	Deep collecting duct
	Regional collecting duct

FIGURE 3-6 Right lymphatic and thoracic ducts. (A) The cisterna chyli is located at the base of the thoracic duct just below the diaphragm approximately at L2 vertebral level. **(B)** The inset shows the angulus venosus (terminus) where both lymphatic ducts return fluid to circulation.

■ THE ESSENTIAL ROLE OF FLUID RETURN

Similar to venous return, the lymphatic system works to return fluid from the body back toward the heart (3 to 4 liters per day), but through its own network of vessels.[2,6,7] A good visual that clarifies the individual roles of the cardiovascular and lymphatic systems is to picture a bathtub and shower, as depicted in Figure 3-7.

The shower, tub, drain, and overflow drain represent systemic circulation as a whole. The faucet represents the arterial side of the system pouring water (capillary filtrate) into the tub or interstitium. The drain at the bottom of the tub represents the venous side of the system taking fluid out of the interstitium (capillary reabsorption). The overflow drain in the wall of the tub represents the lymphatic system as a whole. When water rises to the level of the overflow opening, it serves as an additional or emergency drain to remove the excess fluid from the tub. This is analogous to the lymphatic system that serves to return capillary filtrate that cannot be "drained" by capillary reabsorption back into circulation. Even in healthy tissue, capillary filtration always exceeds capillary reabsorption, creating a **lymphatic obligatory load** of approximately 10% of the overall volume of filtered fluid. The lymphatic obligatory load is fluid that also contains many metabolic byproducts and cellular substances that cannot be removed from the inter-

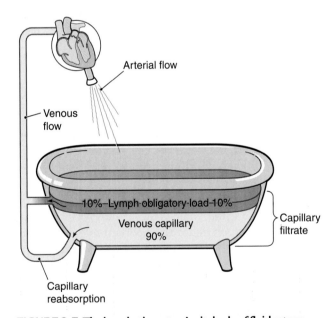

FIGURE 3-7 The lymphatic system's vital role of fluid return. Ninety percent of the gross capillary filtrate is reabsorbed at the venous side of capillary beds. The lymphatic system is required to return the remaining fluid and proteins back into circulation via its own network of vessels. The reabsorption capacity of the capillaries cannot be improved beyond 90%, whereas the lymph systems capacity can be tripled through various therapeutic interventions.

stitium in any other way. Besides water, the obligatory load also includes:

- Plasma proteins and the hormones and enzymes bound to them. Even though some of the plasma proteins that reach the interstitium can be broken down by the macrophages in the connective tissue, most are reliant on lymphatic return because they are too large to be reabsorbed by the capillaries. Lipoproteins are also part of this protein load for the lymphatics.
- Cells such as erythrocytes, macrophages with their contents, dead cells, and cellular debris all are part of the *cell load* for lymphatic pick-up. Cancer cells and other mutated cells are also common components of the obligatory load.
- Foreign substances such as dust, pollen, bacteria, and other environmental particulates.
- Long-chain fatty acids absorbed into lymph by the lacteals of the large intestine. The short-chain fatty acids absorbed into the large intestine go to the liver via the portal vein for metabolism.[2,6,7,10,18]

After interstitial fluid enters the initial vessel, it is called **lymph.** Lymph fluid has approximately the same composition as plasma, containing all the elements from the lymph obligatory load *plus* most of the same electrolytes and organic substances of plasma. Lymph also contains a large number of lymphocytes and white blood cells that are not included in the obligatory load because these immune cells migrate into the system on their own. The protein content of lymph varies from one body region to another, depending on the nutritional and metabolic demands of that tissue. The concentration of lymphocytes in lymph also changes from the vessels of one region to another, with larger lymph vessels containing more lymphocytes. As one might suspect, the concentration of lymphocytes is highest during inflammation and/or infection processes, and after lymph has passed through several lymph nodes where the lymph comes in contact with lymphocytes before the fluid passes out of the node.[6,7,11]

The Lymph Vessel Network

The vascular network of the lymphatic system begins with small vessels enmeshed with the cardiovascular capillaries and continues through a group of larger vessels that eventually join with the jugular veins to return lymph to cardiovascular flow. Structurally, the primary lymph vessels are similar to that of veins, and both vascular networks serve as fluid return pathways. However, a major distinction between the venous and lymphatic networks is that the lymphatic network is organized into *regional flow patterns* rather than the targeted flow pattern of veins. Venous flow

is a targeted pattern because the heart is the target for fluid return from all regions of the body. In contrast, the primary vessels of the lymphatic system are arranged by regions that have specific boundaries. Each region has its individual target, which is the catchment for that specific group of vessels (see Figs. 3-5B and 3-14).

■ LYMPH CAPILLARIES

There are two types of lymph capillaries in the system: initial vessels and collecting capillaries. Although all authors and researchers acknowledge the slight differences in structure and function between these vessels, very few use distinguishing terminology for them, referring to both as lymphatic capillaries.[2–5,7,10,12,16,19] For clarity, this text uses the term **initial vessel** to describe the first capillary in the network (entwined in the cardiovascular capillary bed) and **collecting capillary** to designate the vessel that collects lymph from several of the initial vessels. Initial vessels are described as "blind-ended" because they begin as a snub-nosed tube in the interstitial spaces of the sub-epidermis. Like cardiovascular capillaries, the vessel wall is only a single layer thick (Fig. 3-8). Unlike cardiovascular capillaries, the **lumen** (inside diameter) of an initial lymphatic vessel is four to six times larger, and the basal membrane forming the external covering of the vessel has a much looser weave, making it only a partial membrane. In several areas, the initial vessel has no outer membrane at all.[2,6,7,10,11,15,19] This makes initial vessels much more permeable than cardiovascular capillaries, and therefore functionally more absorbent.

The epithelial cells of the initial vessel overlap each other by approximately one third, (eg, fish scales) and have microscopic fibers called **anchor filaments** that extend into the interstitial tissue. These anchor filaments hold the initial vessel in the interstitial space and pull the ends of the epithelial cells outward when the tissue is stretched (see Fig. 3-8A). The tissue stretch creates an opening between the cells that allows the interstitial fluid to flow into the initial vessel. Once fluid enters the initial vessel, the combination of decreased fluid pressure in the interstitium and the increased fluid volume inside the vessel pushes the epithelial cell flap closed to hold it inside the initial vessel.

The second type of lymph capillary is called a **collecting capillary** because lymph is collected from several of the microscopic initial vessels as they converge into these larger capillaries. Unlike the initial vessel, the walls of the collector capillaries are several layers of epithelial cells thick, and the basement membrane around the outside is much less porous, making the collecting capillaries much less absorbent than the initial vessels. Like the initial vessels, the collecting capillaries are also without valves for most of their length to allow easy lymph flow through them to the primary vessels. However, there is generally

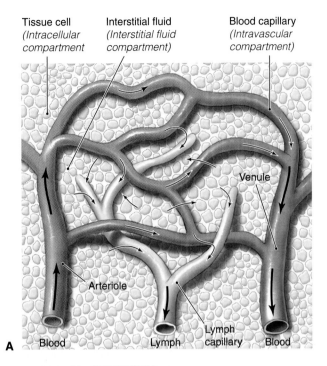

Tissue cell
(Intracellular compartment

Interstitial fluid
(Interstitial fluid compartment)

Blood capillary
(Intravascular compartment)

Venule

Arteriole

A

Blood   Lymph   Lymph   Blood
                            capillary

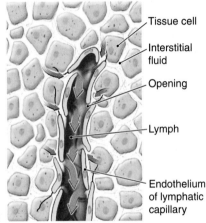

Tissue cell

Interstitial fluid

Opening

Lymph

Endothelium of lymphatic capillary

B

FIGURE 3-8 Initial vessels. (A) The initial vessels of the lymphatic system are entwined in the cardiovascular capillaries. This is the site of "edema uptake." **(B)** Close-up of an initial vessel.

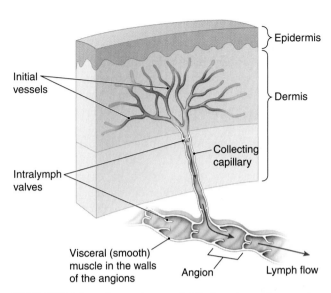

Epidermis

Dermis

Initial vessels

Intralymph valves

Collecting capillary

Visceral (smooth) muscle in the walls of the angions

Angion   Lymph flow

FIGURE 3-9 Lymph vessel network. The lymph vessel network of initial vessels connects to the collecting capillary, then to a primary vessel called a lymphangia. Each segment of the lymphangia is an individual functional unit called an angion.

one valve at the junction between the initial vessel and collecting capillary. In addition, as these capillaries get closer to the large lymph vessels, the number of epithelial layers increase, the connective tissue sheath around the outside becomes complete, and a few more one-way valves are interspersed along the vessel. A one-way valve is always located at the junction between collecting capillaries and the primary lymph vessels (Fig. 3-9). These one-way valves, called **intralymph valves**, prevent lymph backflow and create a slight propulsion pressure within the vessel when they close. Collecting capillaries are located deeper in the dermal–epidermal junction than are the initial vessels. However, collecting capillaries are still superficial, and

fluid flow through them is easily influenced by light manipulation of the tissue.[6,7,10,11,15,17,20]

In several regions of the body, multiple collecting capillaries are arranged in an end-to-end manner similar to that of a capillary bed in the cardiovascular system. This end-to-end arrangement forms a vital structural feature of the lymphatic system called an **anastomosis**. The collecting capillaries in anastomoses are essentially without valves, allowing lymph flow in either direction. The anastomoses connect primary lymph vessels from one tissue region to those in an adjacent region, providing a pathway for lymph to cross from a region of injury and high edema to an area with healthy tissue and less edema as seen in Figures 3-10 and 3-14.[6,7,10,11,15–17,19]

■ LYMPHANGIA: THE PRIMARY LYMPH VESSELS

Several collector capillaries converge into even larger vessels called primary lymphatic vessels. Other authors have referred to these vessels as collectors[6,7,10–12], but this terminology causes unnecessary confusion between the primary vessels and the collecting capillaries. Primary lymph vessels contain a series of one-way *intralymphatic valves* along their length making them structurally similar to veins. The valves are located every 0.6 to 2 cm, dividing each primary vessel into a series of smaller segments so that lymph has to be moved from only one short segment to the next rather than traveling the full length of the primary vessel.[6,7,11,12] Each specific segment within the primary

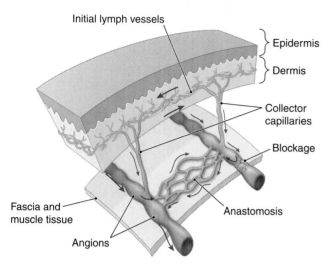

Initial lymph vessels

Epidermis

Dermis

Collector capillaries

Blockage

Anastomosis

Fascia and muscle tissue

Angions

FIGURE 3-10 **Anastomosis between two lymphangia provides an alternate or emergency pathway for lymph when one is blocked or damaged.** Lymph can be directed across the anastomosis to the functioning lymphangia.

lymph vessel is its own functional unit called an **angion** (see Figs. 3-9 and 3-10). Because a primary lymph vessel is actually a series of these smaller angions, another term for the vessel is lymphangia.[6,7,10,11,15,17,19]

Lymphangia have a smooth muscle layer in the vessel wall that spirals around each individual angion, similar to a stripe on a barber pole. Like all smooth muscle, the spiral muscle in the angion is under autonomic control, which stimulates regular rhythmic contractions (similar to peristalsis) to pump lymph through the primary vessels at its own autonomic rhythm (see Fig. 3-12). Because of this autonomic pumping action, angions are sometimes referred to as *hearts* of the lymphatic system. Superficial lymphangia are located between the dermis and the epidermis, and deep lymphangia are in the subdermal layer of skin (see Figs. 3-9 and 3-10) as well as in the deeper fascia. The primary lymph vessels are the lymph pathways from a specific region of the body to the catchments (see Figs. 3-5B and 3-14).

■ CATCHMENTS

As stated earlier, catchment refers to a lymph node bed. Multiple lymphangia carry lymph from a specific body region to a specific catchment for filtering and other immune processes. In the upper body, the *axillary* nodes are the catchment for the entire upper extremity and the thoracic quadrant of the trunk, whereas *cervical* lymph nodes serve as the catchment for the head and face. The *popliteal* catchment receives lymph from the foot and leg, the *inguinal* from the thigh, perineum, lower abdominal regions, and the same-side hip (see Fig. 3-5B). Lymph from the popliteal catchment also flows directly into deep nodes of the inguinal

catchment via deep femoral lymphangia. This deep route from the popliteal to inguinal catchment is a sort of express lane for lymph in the lower extremity. Because the fluid in the popliteal catchment has already traveled through the superficial vessels and multiple lymph nodes, the deep femoral vessels coming out of the catchment have fewer nodes along their length, meaning that lymph travels faster from knee to groin in these deep lymphangia than it does through the superficial vessels. This express lane scenario is further enhanced because the deep femoral lymphangia empty directly into a small group of deep inguinal nodes. Because the lymph does not have to be filtered through *all* of the inguinal nodes, lymph from these deep nodes passes through the inguinal catchment at a faster rate.[6,7,11] Knowing that the popliteal catchment provides a fast lane method of moving lymph from the leg into the cisterna chyli is very important in cases of lower extremity edema.

Each catchment has superficial and deep lymph nodes. The superficial nodes are situated in the subcutaneous adipose layer of the integument, making fluid flow through the superficial nodes fairly easy to influence by light external pressure in the tissue. The deep nodes lie beneath the fascial layers and are generally grouped alongside major arteries such as the aorta, carotid, subclavian, axillary, brachial, mesenteric, iliac, and popliteal.[2,6,7] Because of this positioning, the primary influence on lymph flow through these nodes is the arterial pulse. Therefore, moderately deep manual pressure into the catchments is necessary to influence lymph flow out of the catchments.

■ DEEP COLLECTING TRUNKS AND DUCTS

The primary lymph vessels that exit the catchment areas converge into several larger collecting trunks specific to that body area and catchment. All the deep collecting trunks eventually connect into one of the two **deep collecting ducts:** the right lymphatic duct or the thoracic duct. Similar to lymphangia, deep collector trunks have intralymphatic valves, but they are spaced at wider intervals, approximately every 6 to 10 cm.[14] The **right lymphatic duct** collects fluid from the upper right quadrant of the body, specifically from the *right jugular trunk* (collector trunk for the right side of the head and neck), the *right subclavian trunk* (collector trunk for the right arm via the axillary catchment), and the *bronchomediastinal* trunk (collector for the thoracic organs, muscles and skin). The right lymphatic duct is a very short vessel, ranging from a few millimeters to 1.5 cm. in length, which connects back to the cardiovascular system at the junction of the right jugular and subclavian veins (see Figs. 3-5B and 3-6). This deep collecting duct is actually only present in 5% to 10% of the population. In most cases, the three collecting trunks from the upper right quadrant connect individually to their venous junction.[6,7,10,11]

The **thoracic duct**, situated in the central thoracic and abdominopelvic cavities, is the deep collecting duct responsible for the collection of lymph from the other 75% of the body. The collecting trunks that empty into the thoracic duct are the *left jugular, subclavian, and bronchomediastinum trunks,* which serve as the collectors for the upper left quadrant; the *right and left lumbar trunks* that collect lymph from both lower extremities, and the *intestinal and intercostal trunks* that collect from the remaining 75% of the torso (see Figs. 3-5B and 3-6). Lymph from the abdominal viscera and the lumbar trunks from the legs must first enter the cisterna chyli before passing into the thoracic duct. Deep diaphragmatic breathing gives a boost to lymph flow from the cisterna into the thoracic duct and is vital for edema removal from the lower extremities. Both the right lymphatic and thoracic ducts return fluid to circulation at the lymphovenous junction of the jugular and subclavian veins just posterior to the clavicular head of the sternocleidomastoid muscle (see Figs. 3-6 and 3-11). This junction between the lymphatic and cardiovascular divisions of circulation is called the **angulus venosus or lymphatic terminus.**[2,6,7,10–12,19]

Mechanisms of Lymph Formation and Movement

Over the last 60 years, the mechanisms of edema uptake by the initial vessels and movement of lymph throughout the lymphatic network has been well explained and outlined by several researchers, most notably Casley-Smith,

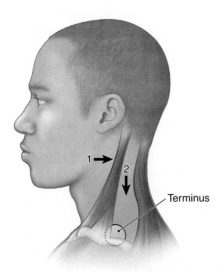

FIGURE 3-11 The lymphatic terminus is supraclavicular and just lateral to the clavicular head of the sternocleidomastoid muscle.

Vodder, and Foldi.[6,7,11,15–17] There is still much to learn, but understanding these basic mechanisms provides the physiologic foundation for proper use of lymphatic techniques in the management of traumatic edema associated with athletic injury.

■ PRE-LYMPHATIC CHANNELS

The beginning of the lymphatic *vascular* network is in the interstitial spaces of the cardiovascular capillary beds where the initial lymph vessels begin as blind-ended tubes. However, in a few areas of the body such as the epidermis and brain, these entwined capillaries do not exist. Instead, the interstitial fluid flows through tissue in unorganized and unstructured pathways called **prelymphatic channels** (Box 3-1). Interstitial fluid moves through prelymphatic channels in the same way in which water drains through sand when a wave washes up on shore. The water first sits on the surface, then quickly seeps down in between the grains of sand. The microscopic spaces between the grains of sand represent the prelymphatic channels, and interstitial fluid movement through these channels is the first step toward fluid absorption into the lymph vessel network.[6,7,10,11,15]

■ FORMATION OF LYMPH: EDEMA UPTAKE

The movement of interstitial fluid into the initial lymphatic vessels, or edema uptake, is based on two factors: (1) the pressure differential between the outside and inside of the initial vessel and (2) the opening and closing of the epithelial flap-valves by the anchoring filaments. In normal healthy tissue, the balance between interstitial fluid pressure (IFP) and pressure inside the initial lymph vessel, the lymph fluid pressure (LFP), shifts slightly during the filtration process. The volume of fluid filtrate from the cardiovascular capillaries creates a brief increase of IFP that pushes against the endothelial cells of the initial capillary to open them slightly. The increased fluid volume in the interstitium also creates a slight stretch in the tissue that pulls on the anchor filaments and opens the valves more fully, making it easier for the interstitial fluid and large proteins to enter the initial vessel (see Figs. 3-4 and 3-8B). After fluid is inside, the increased LFP pushes on and closes the flaps of the initial vessel. When the flaps close, an additional increase in pressure helps push lymph from the initial vessel into the collecting capillary. This repeated pressure change between the interstitium and the initial vessel is necessary for adequate lymph formation and flow throughout the system. Interstitial fluid pressure just above atmospheric pressure (0 mmHg) can increase

BOX 3-1 LYMPHATIC NETWORK SCHEMATIC

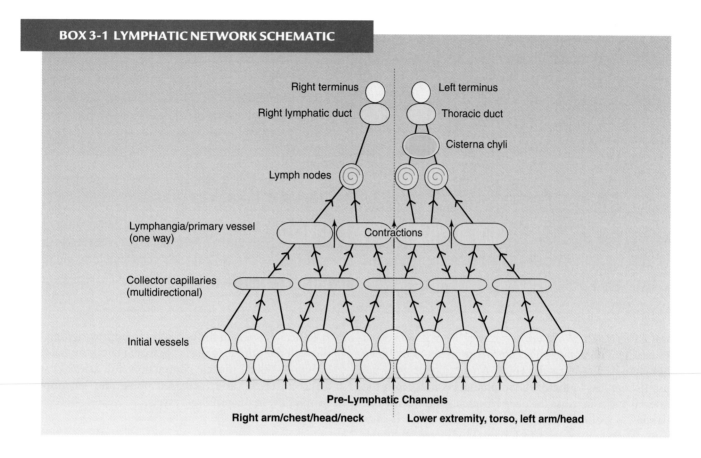

edema uptake more than 20 times higher than normal. However, when IFP increases to 1 or 2 mmHg, edema uptake and flow are actually *diminished* because this level of pressure compresses the fragile initial and collecting capillaries and limits the volume of fluid that can enter these vessels.[5,18] This provides key physiologic rationale for manual lymph facilitation techniques and explains why the strokes are so light and superficial. Lymph facilitation strokes apply light stretch of the superficial tissue to pull the anchoring filaments to open the initial vessel more completely (improve edema uptake) and prevent the deep pressure that actually closes the vessel and diminishes uptake and capillary flow.[2,6–8,10,13,20,21]

Edema uptake is also influenced by activity at the opposite end of the vascular network, the emptying of lymph back into circulation that occurs at the terminus. The rate and volume of fluid return at the terminus create a negative pressure or siphon effect throughout the lymphatic network, which pulls fluid into and through the entire system. This siphon effect created by fluid return at the terminus not only supports edema uptake but provides the driving force for lymph flow through the initial and collecting capillaries into the lymphangia.[4,6,7,10,11,13–17] Once edema uptake has occurred and lymph is formed, fluid movement through the lymphatic network proceeds through the superficial and deep lymphangia.

LYMPH FLOW THROUGH THE LYMPHANGIA

The primary lymph vessels have smooth muscle in the wall of each angion that spirals around each of these individual segments (see Figs. 3-9 and 3-12). The rhythmic autonomic contraction of this smooth muscle creates an internal pump for the primary vessels that is a primary mechanism for the movement of lymph.[11,16–18,22–25] The normal rate of contraction is approximately five to seven times per minute.[11,17,25] An additional intrinsic factor that influences lymph flow through the lymphangia is a type of stretch reflex similar to the reflex contraction that occurs in arteries. When an angion is completely filled and stretched, a reflex contraction is stimulated that pushes the lymph through that segment of the lymphangia into the next. The next angion also reacts with a reflex contraction, and so on throughout the entire length of the primary vessel. The closing of the distal valve before contraction increases the internal pressure of that angion and adds more force to the propulsion of lymph (Fig. 3-12).

In the deep lymphangia, several of the same external mechanisms that move blood through veins are added to the autonomic pump and stretch reflex contractions of the angion to assist in the movement of lymph. Because the primary lymph vessels are segmented by the same one-

A 20-year-old male football player suffered a ruptured anterior cruciate ligament and was scheduled for surgery during the spring break of his university. The certified athletic trainer at his school was recently trained in the lymphatic facilitation techniques and performed three 20-minute sessions on the athlete before surgery, and she taught the athlete how to perform the basic opening protocol for himself. The athlete did not receive any other type of postoperative care—just self-massage with the lymphatic facilitation techniques. When school reconvened at 16 days post-injury and the athletic trainer evaluated the athlete's knee, she was mildly surprised to find that the swelling was almost gone and that the athlete's active range of motion was only moderately limited. The athlete described the first 2 postoperative days as uncomfortable and depressing, until he remembered to do the self-massage. By doing the lymphatic facilitation a minimum of three times a day, he decreased his pain enough to stop medication on the third postoperative day and is now completely without pain for most of the day. The trainer treated the athlete with lymphatic facilitation and general massage twice during the first week he was back at school, and he continued doing his self-massage at least once a day. By the middle of the following week, the swelling was almost completely gone, and his pain-free range of motion was approximately 80% of normal.

way valve system as are veins, it is easy to see how skeletal muscle contraction applies external pressure to the deep lymphangia as well as the veins. An additional "external pump" applied to the deep lymphangia comes from the arterial pulse. Because the deep lymphangia generally run parallel to major arteries, the arterial pulse of the cardiovascular system exerts an additional influence on lymph flow. As arteries expand to accommodate the volume of blood pushed in by the heart, they press against the adjacent primary lymph vessels, pushing lymph through the particular angion in contact with the artery. In this way, the arterial pulse exerts a kind of reverse pump to the deep primary vessels: that is, when the artery fills and extends outward the lymphangia is compressed and emptied and when the artery contracts the lymphangia is allowed to fill again. In this way, lymph movement and rate of flow are directly influenced by the cardiovascular pulse; an increase or decrease in arterial pulse rate creates a concomitant change in lymphangia contractions.[6,7,10,11,15,17,18,20,22,23,25–27] Therefore, active movement in general, and light exercise specifically, is one of the best ways to improve lymph flow through the primary vessels because it combines all these effects—skeletal muscle contraction, full arterial expansion and recoil, and increased pulse rate—to improve lymph flow in the primary vessels.

■ MOVEMENT THROUGH THE DEEP TRUNKS AND DUCTS

The primary mechanism of lymph movement through the deep collecting trunks and lymphatic ducts is through the external pumping action supplied by the arterial pulse and the *respiratory pump* associated with breathing (Fig. 3-13). With each breath, the contraction of the diaphragm expands the thoracic cavity and creates a pressure change that facilitates lymph flow in general. Diaphragmatic breathing, specifically deep inhalation, causes enough of a decrease to intrathoracic pressure to enhance the siphon effect of fluid return at the terminus and to improve lymph flow. In addition, deep breathing applies direct external compression to the cisterna chili, thus adding a boost to the propulsion of lymph into and through the deep thoracic duct. This stimulus of the cisterna chyli is particularly important for drainage of edema from the lower extremity because all lymph from the legs must go through the cisterna chyli before moving into the thoracic duct.[6,7,10,11,15,17,18,20,22]

The formation and movement of lymph through the entire system depend on several anatomic and physiologic factors. Most of these factors can be manipulated to improve edema uptake and the movement of lymph throughout the system. Some key points to remember are the following:

1.   Fluid containing water, plasma, nutrients, and so on, is diffused into the interstitial space of capillary beds.

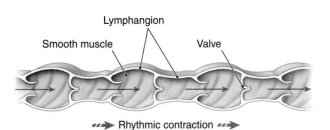

Lymphangion

Smooth muscle   Valve

⟫⟫➤ Rhythmic contraction ⟫⟫➤

FIGURE 3-12   The primary vessels, or lymphangia, of the lymph system have multiple intralymphatic valves that divide the vessel into several segments called angions. Vessel walls have a thin smooth muscle band that spirals around the angions and is controlled by the autonomic nervous system.

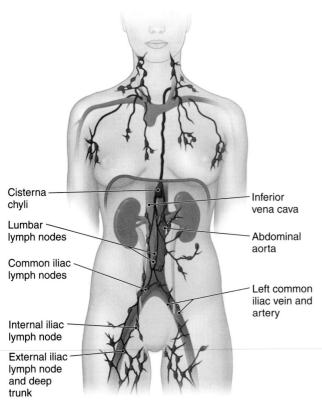

Cisterna
chyli

Lumbar
lymph nodes

Common iliac
lymph nodes

Internal iliac
lymph node

External iliac
lymph node
and deep
trunk

Inferior
vena cava

Abdominal
aorta

Left common
iliac vein and
artery

FIGURE 3-13 The deep nodes, collecting trunks, and ducts of the lymphatic system are closely associated with major arteries. An increased pulse rate in arteries enhances lymph flow through these vessels and nodes.

Approximately 10% of the net capillary filtrate becomes the responsibility of the lymph system (obligatory load).

2. The proteins in interstitial fluid cannot be reabsorbed into the capillary bed, making the initial lymph capillary the only route for protein removal.

3. Edema uptake is dependent on mild stretch of the superficial tissues, and the pressure differential between interstitial fluid pressure (+), and pressure inside the initial lymph capillary (–). The rate of lymph flow back into circulation at the terminus plays a critical role in creating this negative pressure and siphon effect on the system.

4. Each angion of the primary vessel has its own internal pump, an autonomic smooth muscle contraction.

5. The rate of angion contraction increases in response to increases in lymph volume, arterial pulse, skeletal muscle contractions, heat, and diaphragmatic breathing.

6. The arterial pulses and deep breathing have the most influence over lymph flow through the deep collecting trunks, cisterna chyli/thoracic duct, and the right lymphatic duct.

The combination of these factors creates a normal lymph flow rate of approximately 120 milliliters per hour.[7]

Moderate exercise that increases the frequency of muscle contraction and the pulse rate increases edema uptake and flow 20% to 30%. Other factors can increase the rate by as much as 50%.[7,28]

Direction of Lymph Flow

The movement of lymph through the vascular network of the system generally follows a specific and predictable pattern based on how the structural elements are connected and organized. The direction of lymph flow is based on the anatomic connections between vessels called lymphotomes and the regional organization of these pathways into lymphatic watersheds.

■ LYMPHOTOMES

Once edema uptake has occurred and lymph is passed into the lymphangia, the route of the lymph to the catchment is a predetermined pathway. The anatomic connection between a specific group of initial vessels, collecting capillaries and lymphangia, forms a single pathway for lymph flow called a lymphotome. Just as a dermatome carries sensory information from a specific segment of skin via a specific spinal segment, a lymphotome carries lymph from one specific region of tissue via a predetermined network of vessels into a specific catchment. Lymphotomes were discovered and outlined by injecting ink into the system and tracking its progression through the vessels via specialized photography; a process now called lymphoscintigraphy.[6,7,11] As depicted in Figure 3-14, multiple lymphotomes in adjacent body regions carry lymph into the same catchment, and each catchment then directs lymph into specific collecting trunks and ducts.

■ WATERSHEDS

Watersheds are a type of boundary line that give regional organization to the multiple lymphotomes in the body (Figs. 3-14 and 3-15). Structurally, a watershed is a thin area of tissue or stripe between body regions, which contains a high concentration of anastomoses. Because of the anastomoses, a watershed line is more of a directional marker than an actual physical boundary. Imagine the peak of the roof on a house with the north side of the roof representing one lymphotome and the south side a completely different one. Water that falls on the north side of the roof flows to the gutters on that side, which represents the inguinal catchment, for example, and water falling on the south flows to the opposite gutter representing the axillary catchment. The water that falls directly on the peak of the roof can go in either direction. In the case of rain, it is sim-

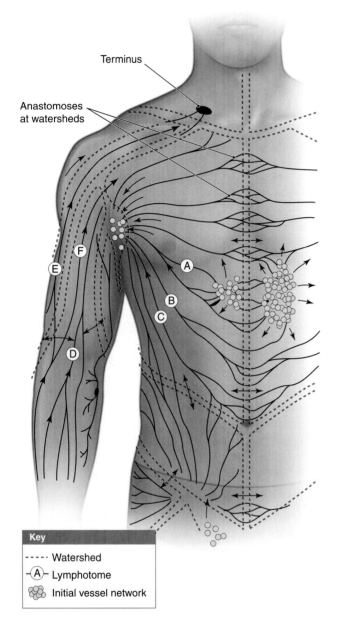

Terminus

Anastomoses
at watersheds

F

E

A

B

C

D

Key
- - - - - Watershed
-(A)- Lymphotome
🍇 Initial vessel network

FIGURE 3-14 Major watersheds and lymphotomes of the upper body. Modified from Foldi M, Kubrik S. Lehrbuch der Lymphologie. Stuttgart: Gustav Fischer Verlag, 1993; and from Casley-Smith JR. Modern Treatment of Lymphoedema. Adelaide, Australia: Henry Thomas Laboratory, Lymphoedema Association of Australia, 1994.

ply a matter of chance whether it rolls into the north or south gutters. A watershed is a boundary line just as a roof peak is a boundary line. Lymph that would normally flow into the right axillary catchment can be taken across a watershed because of the anastomoses, and it will then flow into the left axillary catchment. Therapists can use watersheds to move lymph from an edematous area to another body region with less congested lymphotomes or into an entirely different catchment altogether.[6,10,11,15,17,29,30]

Watersheds of the Torso

In the torso, there are two horizontal watershed lines: one at the level of the clavicles and scapular spines and one at the umbilicus. The torso also has a vertical watershed at the midsagittal line (see Fig. 3-15). These watersheds form six regions: two supraclavicular regions (clavicular watershed), two thoracic regions between the clavicular and umbilical lines (thoracic watershed), and two lower abdominopelvic regions between the umbilical line and inguinal catchments (abdominal watershed). The **supraclavicular watersheds** carry lymph from the head and neck to the terminus catchments, the **thoracic watersheds** drain to the axillary catchments, and the **abdominal watersheds** direct all lymph into the inguinal catchments.

The Extremities

Although multiple lymphotomes and watersheds are in the extremities, this text focuses on only three watersheds in the legs and two in the arms. Because therapists in sports health care are working with athletes that generally have very healthy lymphatic systems, this condensed version of watersheds in the extremities gives sufficient information to safely apply the lymphatic facilitation techniques described in Chapter 7.

In the arms, a single watershed line runs vertically from the base of the thumb to the acromion process, creating a **medial watershed** that is about two thirds the width of the arm, and a **lateral watershed** of the remaining third. Both of

From the Field

"I don't know what you did, but I'm happy. I had been going to the athletic training room for 2 weeks for my sprained ankle (grade 2 inversion) and still was not able to practice or play. After just two sessions (20 minutes each) with the massage therapist at the end of the second week, I was able to practice at 75% and play in the tournament over the weekend with no noticeable problems."

Tommy Mitchell

Starting guard for the Sienna University basketball team 2003

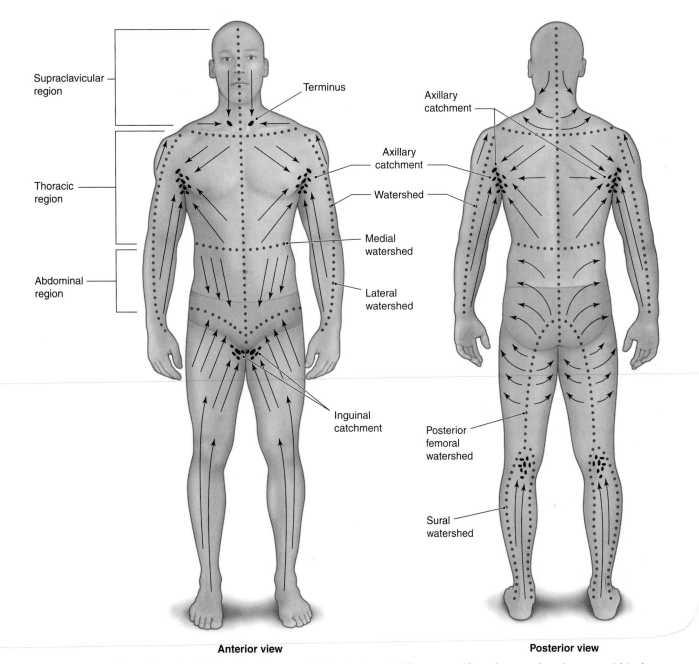

Supraclavicular region

Thoracic region

Abdominal region

Terminus

Axillary catchment

Axillary catchment

Watershed

Medial watershed

Lateral watershed

Inguinal catchment

Posterior femoral watershed

Sural watershed

Anterior view

Posterior view

FIGURE 3-15 The major watersheds and catchments of the body. Lymph follows a specific pathway, or lymphotome, within the watersheds to a specific catchment.

these watersheds have an anterior and posterior surface, and the medial watershed drains into the axillary catchment while the lateral drains more directly to the terminus. In the legs are two watersheds on the posterior surface—the sural and posterior femoral—and one on the anterior surface. The **sural watershed** is defined by a horseshoe-shaped line with the rounded part of the horseshoe beginning in the popliteal space and the two shafts of the horseshoe running down through the medial and lateral malleoli to the first and fifth toes (see Fig. 3-15). The sural watershed directs lymph into the popliteal catchments.

Likewise in the posterior thigh, the **posterior femoral watershed** is defined by a horseshoe shaped line with its apex at the tip of the sacrum and the two shafts running distally through the middle of the posterior thigh to the popliteal space (see Fig. 3-15). The **anterior watershed** actually includes both the lateral and the anterior aspects of the lower extremities, with the sural and posterior femoral watershed lines marking its borders. The posterior femoral and anterior watersheds carry lymph into the inguinal catchments. Watersheds and lymphotomes are the same for both deep and superficial lymphangia, so the direction of lymph movement is the same. Moreover both the superficial and deep nodes in the catchments direct lymph into the same deep collecting structures.[6,7,11,15,17]

Types of Edema

As stated earlier, the simple definition of edema is an excess amount of fluid in the interstitium. Several circulatory mechanisms and/or pathologies lead to edema formation. Some causes of edema are related to cardiovascular dysfunction and others to disruption of normal lymphatic functions.[6,7,14,17,18,26,27,30] It is important to determine whether the problem is more cardiovascular or lymphatic because the root of the problem dictates which treatment modality is most effective and safe. For example, it could be dangerous to address edema related to kidney disease with lymph facilitation techniques designed to enhance fluid flow because the additional flow would add stress to already distressed renal functions. Likewise, most deep tissue strokes can actually inhibit edema uptake because the pressure closes the initial lymphatic vessels. Therefore, it is important to be aware of the most common causes of edema and to use consistent terminology that distinguishes one type from another. There are three basic categories of edema:

1. Circulatory edema
2. Lymphedema
3. Traumatic edema

■ CIRCULATORY EDEMA

Circulatory edema is caused by dysfunction or disease in the cardiovascular system. Some authors refer to this type of edema as dynamic edema, because the excess fluid is the result of an imbalance between the dynamic forces of capillary filtration and reabsorption.[6,11] A few examples of common causes of circulatory edema are hypertension, venous insufficiency (low ratio of veins per cubic centimeter of tissue), kidney dysfunction (leading to proteinuria), and obesity. In the examples of hypertension and obesity, capillary filtrate is excessive and reabsorption is diminished because both conditions tend to increase the capillary fluid pressure (CFP). In venous insufficiency, the volume of fluid reabsorbed is anatomically limited, and in kidney dysfunctions that lead to *proteinuria* (excretion of excess amounts of protein) the plasma oncotic pressure decreases and capillary reabsorption is compromised.[6,7,11,13,15,17,27,30,31]

In circulatory edema, the function of the lymphatic system is presumed to be sufficient, although temporarily overwhelmed by the excess fluid in the interstitium. The cause of the imbalance between capillary filtration and reabsorption must be identified and addressed to fully relieve this type of edema. Examples of appropriate management of circulatory edema might be prescribing medication to reduce blood pressure, correcting proteinuria with changes in nutritional plans, and dieting for weight loss. All these changes in cardiovascular and other systemic functions allow the lymphatic system to "catch up" with its obligatory load and successfully reduce the edema.

Lymphatic facilitation techniques in cases of circulatory edema require considerable caution. If the cause of the edema is not addressed, the increased edema uptake may actually make the swelling increase because the interstitial fluid pressure is decreased, thus allowing more filtration and inhibiting reabsorption. Therefore, the lymphatic techniques described in this text are not appropriate for most cases of circulatory edema.

■ LYMPHEDEMA

Categorizing swelling as lymphedema specifies that there is dysfunction or failure in the lymphatic system, the opposite of circulatory edema. There are two types of lymphedema: primary and secondary. In **primary lymphedema**, a congenital or genetic defect in lymphatic development results in insufficient fluid return function of the system. This type of edema generally becomes evident in early childhood and most often begins as swelling in the legs. This systemic insufficiency is a life-threatening condition that eventually develops into full-body lymphedema, sometimes called elephantiasis.

Secondary lymphedema occurs when the nodes or vessels of the lymphatic system are damaged or destroyed. Scar tissue develops in a lymphotome or catchment that is damaged, and edema uptake and lymph movement are compromised through that pathway. In secondary lymphedema, swelling is pronounced and covers an entire body region like a full arm or leg rather than a small localized area of tissue. Common causes of the damage leading to lymphedema include the following[6,7,10,11,15,17,18,30,31]:

- Surgery
- Radiation/chemotherapy
- Virus/infection
- Repeated compression/restrictions at superficial catchments

Infestation with a parasite called *Filaria* (filariasis) is another cause of secondary lymphedema because the parasite makes its home in the lymphatic system, blocking the lymph vessels and destroying nodes. Filarial infestations are generally limited to poverty-stricken tropical environments and are a rare occurrence in North America and Europe.[6,7,10,11,17]

Treatment of *lymphedema* requires more in-depth knowledge of the anatomy and physiology of the lymphatic system and more precise application of a wider variety of edema removal techniques than is addressed in this text. The complex decongestive therapy required in cases of lymphedema includes the use of carefully measured and regularly altered compression garments and bandages, prescription medications, and strict adherence to detailed edema flow patterns. The information on lymphotomes, catchments, and watersheds described in this chapter is intentionally condensed based on the presumption that sports health care therapists are working with athletes who have a healthy lymphatic system. Therefore, the lymphatic techniques described here are not appropriate for the treatment of lymphedema, and, if used in these cases, the condition is likely to worsen. However, a sports health care therapist must be able to recognize situations in which true lymphedema may develop in athletes and refer the athlete to a lymphedema specialist if it does occur. Situations in which an athlete may develop secondary lymphedema include surgery in a primary catchment area and radiation or chemotherapy treatment for other conditions (cancer). Recognizing the increased risk of secondary lymphedema in these situations can allow the therapist and athlete to take specific preventive measures to avoid the onset and/or advancement of the condition.

■ TRAUMATIC EDEMA

Traumatic edema is the localized and temporary swelling of tissue associated with soft tissue injury and the exertion of exercise, including the acute or chronic sprains, strains, and hematomas common to sports and exercise. There are two types of traumatic edema: primary edema, which is the amount of fluid actually spilled out of stretched and torn soft tissue, and secondary edema, the amount of fluid drawn into the area of damage due to the increased interstitial oncotic pressure of that area.[6,7,10–12,15,17,19,27,28] This is the only type of edema that the lymphatic facilitation technique outlined in Chapter 7 is designed to treat.

The sports health care therapist must recognize that all swelling is not the same and cannot be treated in the same manner. Standard treatments for swelling related to sprains, strains, and contusions such as ice and compression are essential treatment measures for traumatic edemas, but are specifically contraindicated in cases of lymphedema. Cold decreases lymphatic flow and excessive pressure, that is, compression pumps set above 60 mmHg, tight elastic wraps, and deep massage can damage the fragile superficial lymphatic vessels.[11,17,21,30,32] Even when used in traumatic edema, therapists should realize that ice and compression address only the cardiovascular side of edema removal via vasoconstriction and control of the hemorrhage with external pressure. The amount of initial swelling is limited, but edema uptake has not been improved and may have been hampered to some extent by the compression.

The anatomic and physiologic principles set forth in this chapter help therapists to clarify their thinking about "swelling" and supply strong rationale for the use of the manual lymphatic techniques described for the treatment of traumatic edema associated with common athletic injuries.

SUMMARY

The circulatory system has two divisions, cardiovascular and lymphatic, which work together and separately to move fluids throughout the body and carry out complex immune processes. The movement of lymph through its vascular network follows a specific and predictable pattern that can be positively influenced by several factors including heat, muscle contraction, arterial flow, deep breathing, and manual stimulation of the superficial pathways.

- Edema removal is a primary responsibility of the lymphatic system, not the circulatory system.
- There are several types of edema, and therapists must *not* treat all edemas in the same fashion. This text provides lymphatic facilitation techniques that address *only* traumatic edema.
- The *only* route for removal of the protein component of edema is through the lymphatic system. Therefore, reducing/controlling the secondary edema of the acute phase in the healing cycle depends on stimulating the lymphatic system to improve edema uptake and protein removal.
- The initial vessels and collecting capillaries of the lymph vessel network are the most superficial vessels of the network, and fluid flows through them in either direction because they do not have valves. Therefore, manual lymphatic techniques stimulate flow through these superficial pathways by using very light strokes that increase edema uptake and influence the direction of fluid flow.
- Lymph flow is regional and is defined by nonstructural boundaries to each region called a watershed. Because watersheds are made up of a high number of anastomoses, they provide "bridges" between different regions of lymph flow.
- Catchments are lymph node beds that collect all of the lymph from a specific region of the body. Because the lymph nodes must filter the lymph, the catchments increase resistance to flow and slow the movement of lymph in the entire system. Therefore, the catchments must be cleared before the specific area of edema is addressed.
- Lymph vessels from the lower extremities carry lymph into the cisterna chyli. Therefore, stimulating the respiratory pump is a vital part of edema removal for the lower extremities.

Review Questions

SHORT ANSWERS

1. The cardiovascular system functions as a fluid delivery and return, while the lymphatic system is _____ only.

2. What are the two major influences on arterial blood flow?

3. Venous blood flow is dependent on three common factors; gravity, _____, and _____.

4. List the lymphatic vessels from the smallest to largest.
   a.
   b.
   c.
   d.
   e.

5. Define these terms:
   a. Catchment
   b. Watershed
   c. Starling forces
   d. Oncotic pressure
   e. Angion

MULTIPLE CHOICE

6. What is the purpose of the one-way valves in both veins and primary lymph vessels?
   a. Increase the force propulsion of fluid through the vessels.
   b. Prevent backflow of fluid and divide the vessels into shorter segments.
   c. Provide extra surface area in the vessel for nutrient waste exchange.
   d. Create extra resistance to fluid flow to mediate blood pressure.

7. The lymphovenous junction where fluid is returned to the cardiovascular system is called the_____.
   a. lymphatic jugular junction
   b. cardiolymphatic junction
   c. cisterna chili
   d. terminus

8. Which of the following describes the balance of Starling forces that create capillary filtration?
   a. Capillary fluid pressure (CFP) is higher than interstitial fluid pressure (IFP), whereas plasma oncotic pressure (POP) and interstitial oncotic pressure (IOP) are relatively balanced.

   b. POP and IOP are both higher than capillary and interstitial fluid pressures.
   c. Interstitial fluid pressure and oncotic pressure are highest pressures.
   d. CFP is lower than IFP and IOP is higher than POP.

9. What percentage of total capillary filtrate is reabsorbed into the cardiovascular capillaries?
   a. 100%
   b. 50%
   c. 90%
   d. 10%

10. What term describes the volume of capillary filtrate that is the responsibility of the lymphatic system?
    a. Lymph obligatory load
    b. Edema uptake volume
    c. Lymphatic absorption load
    d. Lymphedema capacity

11. Which of the following best describes the function of the cisterna chyli?
    a. Serves as the largest lymph node bed in the body
    b. Serves as a collecting well for lymph that propels fluid through the thoracic duct when squeezed
    c. The heart of the lymphatic system that pumps lymph through the entire system
    d. The lymphovenous junction where lymph is returned to the cardiovascular system

12. One-way valves are important structural features in several lymph vessels but are not found in _____.
    a. lymphangia and deep trunks
    b. collecting trunks and primary vessels
    c. initial and collecting capillaries
    d. thoracic and right lymphatic ducts

13. A group of primary vessels that drain lymph into a specific catchment is called a(n)_____.
    a. lymphangia
    b. angion
    c. deep collecting trunk
    d. lymphotome

14. The major influences on edema uptake include the light stretch of skin to open the initial vessel and _____.
    a. increased cardiovascular blood pressure
    b. decreased volume of capillary filtration
    c. increased capillary reabsorption and venous flow
    d. stimulating the siphon effect of lymphatic system by increasing fluid return at the terminus

15. What is the catchment for lymph from the anterior leg and thigh?
    a. Inguinal
    b. Popliteal
    c. Perineal
    d. Patellar

16. A dysfunction in the lymphatic system that results in swelling of an entire body area is called_____.
    a. edema
    b. traumatic edema
    c. lymphedema
    d. circulatory edema

17. Arterial flow and pulse have a major influence on lymph flow through what portion of the lymph system?
    a. Collecting capillaries and anastomosis
    b. Deep collecting trunks
    c. Initial vessels and collecting capillaries
    d. Lymphangia and catchments

18. Swelling related to hypertension and obesity is called
    a. primary lymphedema.
    b. traumatic edema.
    c. secondary lymphedema.
    d. circulatory edema.

19. What substance/molecule can be returned to circulation only via the lymphatic system?
    a. Lipids
    b. Hydrogen
    c. Protein
    d. Saline

20. Where are the largest number of lymphatic anastomoses located?
    a. Watersheds
    b. Pre-catchment
    c. Post-catchment
    d. In the deep fascia

REFERENCES

1. Premkumar K. The Massage Connection: Anatomy and Physiology, 2nd ed. Baltimore: Lippincott Williams & Wilkins, 2004.
2. Guyton AC, Hall JE. Textbook of Medical Physiology, 9th ed. Philadelphia: WB Saunders, 1996.
3. Tortora GJ. Principles of Human Anatomy, 8th ed. Menlo Park, CA: Benjamin Cummings Science Publishing, 1999.
4. Tortora GJ, Grabowski SR. Principles of Anatomy and Physiology, 8th ed. New York: Biological Sciences Textbooks of HarperCollins Publishers, 1996.
5. Goldberg S. Clinical Anatomy Made Ridiculously Simple. Miami: Medmaster, Inc, 1984.
6. Casley-Smith JR. Modern Treatment of Lymphoedema. Adelaide, Australia: Henry Thomas Laboratory, Lymphoedema Association of Australia, 1994.
7. Foldi E, Foldi M. Textbook of Foldi School. English translation by Heida Brenneke. Self-published, 1999.
8. Brace RA, Guyton AC. Interaction of transcapillary Starling forces in the isolated dog forelimb. Am J Physiol 1977;233(1):H136–H140.
9. Bundgaard M. Transport pathways in capillaries: In search of pores. Ann Rev Physiol 1980;42:325–336.
10. Chikly B. Lymph Drainage Therapy: Study Guide for Level 1. France: UI and self-published, 1996. Revised 1999.
11. Kasseroller R. Compendium of Dr. Vodder's Manual Lymph Drainage. Heidelburg, Germany: Karl F. Haug Publishers, 1998.
12. Chaitow L, DeLaney JW. Clinical Application of Neuromuscular Techniques, vol. 1: The Upper Body. Edinburgh: Churchill Livingstone, 2000.
13. Guyton AC, Granger HJ, Taylor AE. Interstitial fluid pressure. Physiological Reviews 1971;51(3):527–563.
14. Engeset A et al. Studies of human peripheral lymph: Sampling method. Lymphology 1973;6:1–5.
15. Kurz I. Textbook of Dr. Vodder's Manual Lymph Drainage, vol. 2: Therapy, 3rd ed. Heidelburg: Karl F. Haug Publishers, 1986.
16. Wittlinger H, Wittlinger G. Textbook of Dr. Vodder's Manual Lymph Drainage, vol. 1: Basic Course. 6th English translation revised and edited by Robert H. Harris. Heidelburg: Karl F. Haug Publishers, 1998.
17. Kurz I. Textbook of Dr. Vodder's Manual Lymphatic Drainage, vol. 3: Treatment Manual. Heidelburg: Karl F. Haug Publishers, 1986.
18. Badger C. Treating lymphoedema. Nursing Times 1996;92(11): 84–88.
19. Chagnon SE. Carpal Tunnel Massage Program for Yourself and Others. Course workbook. Chagnon Health Institute, Glen Falls, New York, 1999.
20. Shields JW. Central lymph propulsion. Lymphology 1980;13:9–17.
21. Hooker DN. Intermittent compression devices. In: Prentice WE, ed. Therapeutic Modalities for Physical Therapists, 2nd ed. New York, McGraw-Hill, 2002.
22. Olszewski W et al. Flow and composition of leg lymph in normal men during venous stasis, muscular activity and local hyperthermia. Acta Physiol Scand 1977;99:149–155.
23. Olszewski WL, Engeset A. Peripheral lymph dynamics. In: Proceedings of the XIIth International Congress of Lymphology. Tokyo, August 27-September 2. Amsterdam, Excerpta Medica, pp. 213–214, 1989.
24. Grouse LD, Senior ed. Human central lymph propulsion. JAMA 1981;246(18):2066.
25. Wang G-Y, Zhong S-Z. Experimental study of lymphatic contractility and its clinical importance. Annals of Plastic Surgery 1985;15(4): 278–284.
26. Boris M, Weindorf S, Lasinski BB. The risk of genital edema after external pump compression for lower limb lymphedema. Lymphology 1998;31:15–20.
27. Kolb P, Denegar C. Traumatic edema and the lymphatic system. Athletic Training 1983;Winter:339–341.
28. Wallace E et al. Lymphatic system: Lymphatic manipulative techniques. In: Ward RC, ed. Foundations for Osteopathic Medicine. Baltimore: Williams & Wilkins, 1997.
29. Guyton AC, Scheel K, Murphree D. Interstitial fluid pressure III: Its effect on resistance to tissue fluid mobility. Circulation Research 1966;XIX(August):412–419.
30. Mortimer PS. Managing lymphoedema. Clinical and Experimental Dermatology 1995;20:98–106.
31. Browse NL, Stewart G. Lymphoedema: Pathophysiology and classification. J Cardiovasc Surg 1985;26:91–105.
32. Eliska O, Eliskova M. Are peripheral lymphatics damaged by high pressure manual massage? Lymphology 1995;28:21–30.

The Neuromuscular System

After completing this chapter, the reader will be able to:

- Explain the difference between intrafusal and extrafusal muscle fibers.
- Define tonic, isometric, and isotonic muscle contractions.
- Separate skeletal muscles into their appropriate categories of primarily postural or movement oriented.
- Define kinetic chain, and give an example of a lower and an upper extremity chain.
- Describe the function and location of the muscle spindles and Golgi tendon organs.
- Describe the physiologic processes of reciprocal inhibition, stretch reflex, inverse stretch reflex, and gamma gain; explain the therapeutic implications of each.
- Define contractile and tensile stress, and describe the muscle imbalances commonly associated with the upper crossed and lower crossed postural adaptations.
- Define motor tone, muscle tone, length–strength ratio, muscle cramps, muscle spasm, hypertrophy, and atrophy.
- Name and explain the three parts of pain, and describe how massage can moderate each stage.
- Explain the gate control theory of pain reduction.

Although the nervous and muscular systems are individual body systems, the functional link between these systems must be understood when dealing with an active population. This interdependence between the systems is complex; however, only a few key concepts help to clarify the physiologic rationale for the neuromuscular techniques used in therapeutic massage. The goal is to understand the basic functions of both systems and how they interact to initiate, moderate, and adapt the complex movements we call athletics.

The anatomic interface between the nervous and muscular systems is the motor unit. Structurally, the motor unit is a single motor neuron and the multiple muscle fibers it innervates (Fig. 4-1). The actual number of fibers in a motor unit depends on the size and function of the muscle, with fine control muscles having as few as 10 fibers per unit and larger gross movement muscles having several hundred, on average between 100 and 150 muscle fibers per 1 motor neuron.[1,2]

A skeletal muscle is organized from larger to smaller bundles of muscle fibers. Muscle fibers, which are single muscle cells, are composed of multiple bundles of smaller fibers called **myofibrils**, which extend lengthwise through the entire muscle in parallel alignment. A microscopic view of a myofibril shows that it has several alternating light and dark circular bands, which gives the entire muscle cell a striped or striated appearance. These striations are caused by an overlapping arrangement of even smaller fibers inside the myofibril called **myofilaments**. The myofilaments are two different types of protein chains called **actin** and **myosin**. They are arranged in a parallel and overlapping manner that is greater when the muscle contracts and less when the muscle is at rest. The actin and myosin filaments do not extend the full length of a myofibril; rather, they are arranged in short segments called **sarcomeres** and attached end to end along the length of the myofibril (Fig. 4-2). The number of sarcomeres in a myofibril varies according to the length and diameter of the fiber and can be altered by regular use or disuse.[1-6] Muscle contraction occurs when the actin and myosin form a chemical bond and slide over one another to increase the overlap between them. This shortening of the sarcomere causes shortening of the entire muscle fiber and eventually of the full skeletal muscle.

Skeletal Muscle Contraction

The mechanical event that leads to the shortening of the sarcomere is described as the **sliding filament mechanism.** This mechanical sliding of the filaments is initiated as a nervous system command and transmitted via a specific motor neuron to the muscle fibers of any given motor unit. A minimum amount of stimulus, called a **threshold stimulus,** is needed to initiate this physiologic process of contraction. When threshold stimulus is applied by the motor neuron, stored calcium is released from the muscle cell. It is this calcium rich environment that initiates a chemical bonding process between the actin and myosin in the sarcomere. The actin and myosin slide or ratchet closer together and increase the overlap between them. This leads to the shortening of the muscle fiber and creates a pulling action at the attachments. None of the fibers in a motor unit contracts

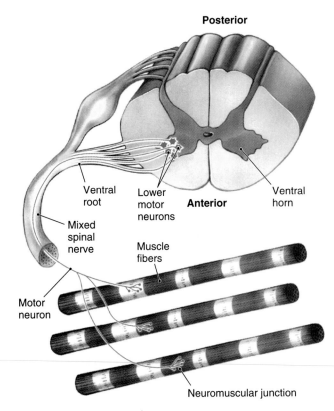

FIGURE 4-1 A motor unit.

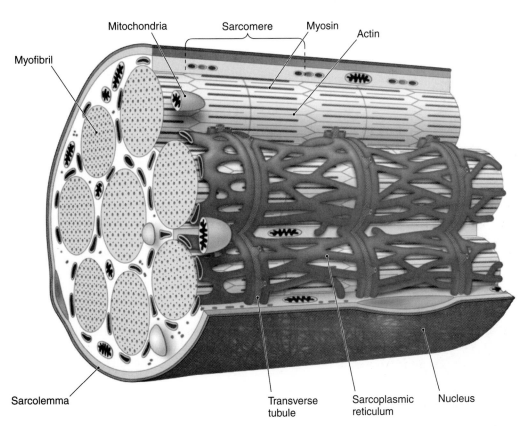

FIGURE 4-2 Microscopic structure of a skeletal muscle fiber. Each muscle fiber contains several myofibrils, which are a series of sarcomeres arranged end to end. Each sarcomere contains the smaller myofilaments, actin and myosin.

until threshold stimulus is delivered, and all fibers must contract in response to this stimulus. This phenomenon is called the **all-or-none response.**

The muscle contraction stops when the stimulus is removed and the calcium dissipates and is actively transported back into storage.[1,2,5,7–9] This physiologic process of muscle contraction is always the same regardless of the resultant mechanical changes in the muscle length as a whole. In other words, muscle fibers always shorten and create tension. However, this increase in tension may or may not result in movement of a body part.[3,9–11]

Each skeletal muscle contains many motor units to allow regulation of the total force of contraction. For example, only one motor unit is stimulated when a minimal contraction is needed as in lifting a pencil, and hundreds of motor units are engaged to lift a 50-pound barbell. The regulation of muscle effort by increasing or decreasing the number of motor units stimulated is called **graded response** or muscle recruitment. These changes are based on central nervous system command and spinal reflexes.[1,2,7,9]

Types of Muscle Contraction

Muscular contraction is classified according to the mechanical changes in a muscle as a whole, not the cellular shortening that is constant in all types of contractions. Two constant mechanical actions occur when a muscle contracts: (1) tension is created by the shortening of the sarcomeres to generate a pulling force at the attachments, and (2) the middle of the muscle tends to broaden or bunch as a result of overlapping myofilaments (Fig. 4-3). There are three basic categories of muscle contraction: tonic, isometric, and isotonic.

■ TONIC CONTRACTIONS

A tonic contraction is a constant low-grade tension in the muscle that registers neuromuscular activity on electromyography (EMG), but is not strong enough to create movement. This low-grade tension caused by the contraction of only a few motor units is called muscle tone by many authors.[1,2] Chaitow and DeLaney[12,13] suggest using the term *motor tone*. This term, first used by Ledderman,[14] in 1998, accurately describes muscle tension related to neuromuscular activity. In contrast, the term muscle tone describes the natural state of firmness in a muscle, even at rest, which does not register neuromuscular activity on EMG. Muscle tone is a natural firmness due to the structural components of the muscle such as the intramuscular fluids, fascia, and other connective tissue that is unrelated to tension in the contractile cells.

The distinction between motor tone and muscle tone is an important one for the soft tissue therapist because it clarifies that a muscle does not need to be contracted or short to feel tight and stiff. For example, anterior compartment syndrome and adhesive capsulitis are conditions that display tight and stiff muscles, not because the muscles are contracted but because of problems in the fluid and connective tissue elements of the muscle. These are examples of muscle tone dysfunctions, not motor tone issues. Therefore, the more appropriate treatment modalities are lymphatic and/or myofascial techniques (described in Chapters 7 and 9) rather than the neuromuscular techniques in Chapter 8, which address motor tone dysfunctions.

■ ISOMETRIC CONTRACTIONS

An isometric contraction occurs when the resistance to movement is greater than or equal to the amount of force that can be generated by contraction of all muscle fibers in a muscle. Because the physiology of contraction remains the same (eg, shortening of the sarcomeres), both tension on the attachments and bunching of the muscle occur. However, there is no overall change in muscle length, and no movement occurs. When range of motion is limited because of injury, isometric exercise is an effective way to maintain muscle strength within the safe pain-free range. However, isometric exercise has limited value as a strength-training method for athletes because strength cannot be developed through the full range of motion.

■ ISOTONIC CONTRACTIONS

During isotonic contraction, the distance between the attachments of a muscle changes, creating movement of body parts. A muscle can either shorten or lengthen as a

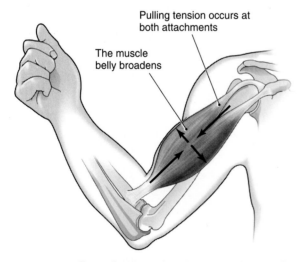

Pulling tension occurs at both attachments

The muscle belly broadens

FIGURE 4-3 All muscle contractions generate two natural forces. A pulling tension is increased in line with the muscle fibers, and the middle of the muscle bunches and broadens. The extent of both of these changes depends on the type of contraction, that is, tonic, isometric, or isotonic.

whole, whereas the tension and force of the contraction remain constant. When the length of a muscle is shortened, the attachments move closer together, creating a concentric isotonic contraction. This is the type of contraction used to pick up a book or cup of tea and is typically what comes to mind when the term "muscle contraction" is used. An eccentric isotonic contraction occurs when the attachments move farther apart and a muscle lengthens. The biceps brachii must eccentrically contract to allow an athlete to lower weight plates back to the stack after arm curls. Similarly, the quadriceps eccentrically contract when a football player squats down to assume a three-point stance. Eccentric muscle work is a good method of generating rapid strength gains in muscle. However, there is also a much higher incidence of muscle soreness and strain injuries with eccentric contraction because of the high tension demands created during the contraction.[1–3,5,7,9,15,16]

Functions of Skeletal Muscles

The muscular system has hundreds of individual muscles. Normal movement is created when muscles work in well-coordinated groups, with some muscles stabilizing and opposing the movement and others creating it. All motions and postural adjustments require synchronized activation and continuous monitoring by the nervous system and muscle proprioceptors of each muscle involved. **Proprioceptors** are specialized sensory receptors in the musculoskeletal systems that constantly monitor changes in muscle tension, length, and joint movement.

■ MOVEMENT: A COORDINATED EFFORT

Skeletal muscles attach to the bones on either side of a joint. The attachment, called the **origin** remains relatively fixed during movement and the **insertion** of the muscle is the attachment to the bone(s) that move during contraction. The type of joint that a muscle crosses determines what kind of movement will be created when the muscle contracts. **Hinge joints** allow flexion and extension motions; **condyloid joints** allow flexion, extension, abduction, and adduction; **pivot joints** allow rotation; and **ball-and-socket joints** allow all five of these movements. The muscle's shape, line of pull, angle at which it crosses the joint, and the site where it attaches on the bone dictates which direction the muscle can pull the bone and the amount of force it can contribute to the movement.

Movement Assignments

The muscle that has the primary responsibility in creating a specific movement is called the **agonist** or prime mover. The agonist is usually the largest muscle that crosses a joint, or the muscle with the best architecture to create the most powerful angle of pull across the joint. When a muscle is playing the role of agonist, it contracts concentrically. It is not uncommon for more than one muscle to be considered a prime mover in any one motion. For example, in the movement of hip extension the gluteus maximus and all three of the hamstrings could be considered agonists because all are large, powerful muscles with efficient angles of pull.

Very few body movements occur as the result of a single muscle contracting. Assisting muscles called **synergists** are signaled to contract with the agonist, creating a well-coordinated and smooth motion. The synergists may be smaller and less powerful than the agonist or may cross the joint in a manner that gives it a poor pulling angle on the bone. Sometimes the assisting role played by a synergist is to stabilize an intermediate joint for the agonist. An example of this can be found in hand muscles. The finger flexor muscles also cross the wrist joint, which must be stabilized by the synergist muscles for the movement of finger flexion to occur without the wrist also flexing.

From the Field

"When teaching clinical approaches and applications, I find it is especially important to help students develop their critical thinking skills. A clear understanding of anatomy and physiology provides a sound foundation from which to make therapeutic choices. Otherwise, it is too easy for students to give in to the temptation to simply memorize treatment protocols or techniques, rather than truly understand what they are doing and why."

Lisa Nelson, LMP

Faculty Supervisor and Learning Strategist
Brenneke School of Massage
Seattle, WA

An **antagonist** is a muscle that contracts to oppose a particular motion. When a muscle is assigned the role of antagonist, its job is to create tension in the opposite direction of the agonist, acting as a brake to control that movement. Because the antagonist is functioning in opposition to the prime mover, it is contracting eccentrically, which increases its risk of strain.[5,15,16] In fact, Lieber states that ". . . muscle injury and soreness are selectively associated with eccentric contraction."[5] Examples of antagonist injury abound in athletics, ranging from hamstring strains when a soccer player kicks a ball or a sprinter jumps out of the starting blocks to abdominal strain on the non-throwing side of a javelin thrower.

The Kinetic Chain

The organization of muscle function into the categories of prime mover, antagonist, flexor, or extensor is necessary for learning, but oversimplifies the complexity of normal motion. It is not possible to assign one specific role to any given muscle because of the myriad body movements we go through on a daily basis. Each time we raise an arm, almost every other muscle in the upper extremity contracts at some level, and many in the torso and legs also contract to stabilize intermediate joints, assist and oppose the arm movement, and keep us from falling over when our center of gravity shifts with the outstretched arm. Every contraction is mediated and movement is coordinated by the cerebellum. The series of muscles involved in a movement has a pattern of muscle recruitment that represents a kinetic chain associated with that movement.[3,6,7]

The kinetic chain concept was first used by mechanical engineers in the 1970s and called a link system to describe a series of rigid beams joined together and fixed at both the top and bottom.[3] In this link system, when either the top or the bottom moved, there was equal movement in all the joints. In the human body, completely closed chains do not exist, but when the distal joint of an extremity is engaged and weight bearing, it sufficiently simulates a closed kinetic chain. By closing the kinetic chain, the cerebellum receives more sensory information to guide muscle recruitment resulting in a smooth and well-coordinated movement.

The concept of the kinetic chain has implications for injury prevention and rehabilitation. When an athlete complains of a tight or injured muscle, tension and limitation in that muscle can spread through the kinetic chain and lead to subtle or overt changes in the athlete's biomechanics. This may affect the athlete's performance (think about a professional golfer with a tight neck muscle) and increase the risk of injury or increase the severity of injury from overload strain to synergists and other muscles in the chain. Therefore, the full kinetic chain should be evaluated, and soft tissue treatment is often necessary in areas far removed from the tight or injured muscle.[6,7,17–19]

■ POSTURE

To maintain the body's upright position against gravity, several muscles must maintain variable levels of tonic contrac-

tions at all times, making them **postural muscles** (Fig. 4-4). Postural muscles are still voluntary and thus capable of creating movement when commanded to do so. However, their primary role is based on well-established neuromuscular pathways that are subconsciously controlled by the cerebellum.[6,12,13]

Basic Muscle Reflexes

The nervous system signals and regulates muscle contraction in response to specific sensory input. All three portions of the brain—cerebrum, cerebellum, and brain stem—play some role in creating movement. The **cerebrum** contains the primary motor center that commands voluntary muscle activity. The **cerebellum** works with and through the primary motor center, but on an unconscious level, to stimulate and coordinate muscle contractions necessary to maintain our balance and posture, and it rotates the work load required in this ever-changing effort between the motor units within each muscle. The cerebellum also orchestrates the sequence of agonist, synergist, antagonist stimulation to create smooth efficient movement and dictates the muscle recruitment pattern through the kinetic chain. The **brain stem**, which also operates below conscious levels, is where most afferent neurons from the proprioceptors terminate. As a whole, the musculoskeletal system receives more of the efferent outflow from the central nervous system than any other body system. The musculoskeletal system is also the source for most of the sensory input to the brain and spinal cord, with reports coming from thousands of muscle, joint, and fascial receptors.[2,7,20] Inside the spinal cord, specific neuronal pathways link sensory and motor neurons to create instantaneous motor responses to specific sensory input without integration of that input by the brain. These are called **reflex arcs.** Without these reflex loops, there could be no purposeful movement. As stated by Guyton and Hall, ". . . there is no neuronal circuit anywhere in the brain that causes the specific to-and-fro movement of the legs that is required in walking. Instead, the circuits for these movements are in the cord, and the brain simply sends command signals to set into motion the walking process."[2] The reflex pathways between skeletal muscle and the spinal cord are unique because muscles serve as both the sense receptor that reads muscle length and tension and the effector that responds to the motor command, thereby moderating its own activity on a subconscious level.

■ RECIPROCAL INHIBITION

For coordinated movement to occur anywhere in the body, contraction of an antagonist muscle must be sufficiently inhibited to allow the agonist to create the desired move-

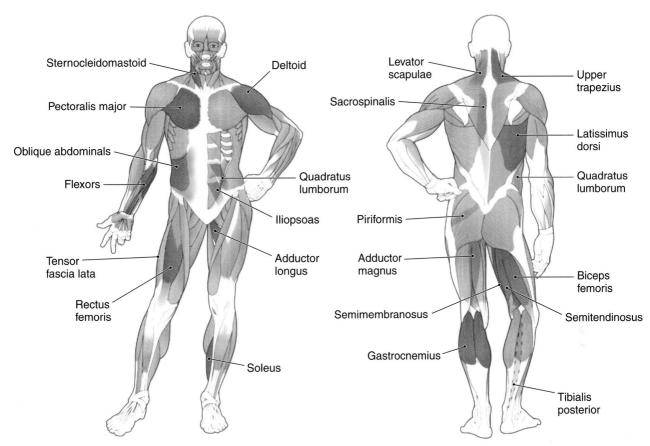

FIGURE 4-4 The postural muscles of the anterior and posterior body.

ment. This is accomplished by a reciprocal innervation between the agonist and the antagonist that coactivates both muscles when a motor command is given. Simply stated, smooth movement requires a coordinated contraction in the agonist and a slight relaxation in the antagonist (Fig. 4-5), but not complete inhibition of the antagonist that results in an uncontrolled motion. The reflex mechanism that coordinates this effort between agonist and antagonist is called *reciprocal inhibition*. This muscle reflex can be used for therapeutic benefit to decrease muscle cramps and spasms.

■ THE STRETCH REFLEX

The stretch reflex, also called the myotatic reflex, is a protective mechanism in skeletal muscle that signals a concentric contraction in response to rapid lengthening of a muscle. This contraction is meant to protect the muscle from tearing by restoring normal fiber length. This reflex is signaled and mediated by a group of proprioceptors located within the muscle called **muscle spindles.** Muscle spindles, also called intrafusal fibers, are named for their

shape, which is similar to a textile thread spindle; bulging in the middle with two tapered ends. They are located within the muscle belly between the standard or extrafusal fibers of the muscle. The intrafusal fibers have connective tissue attachments to the extrafusal cells, which allows them to sense and respond to changes in length occurring in the muscle.

Voluntary motor commands for skeletal muscles are signaled through a neuronal pathway made up of a group of motor neurons that innervate all muscle fibers. This pathway is designated as an **alpha pathway.** The alpha pathway is the means by which the primary motor center of the cerebrum and cerebellum control and coordinate voluntary movement. Muscle spindles have a second neuronal pathway that is a reflex arc in which the muscle spindle plays a dual role as receptor and motor effector. This reflex arc is called the **gamma loop** (Fig. 4-6). A full 30% of all motor nerve fibers innervating skeletal muscle are the **gamma efferents** in this reflex arc.[2] Both alpha and gamma pathways must be used to produce smooth well-coordinated movements.[2,12,20]

The gamma afferent pathway in the muscle spindle is far more sensitive to the rate of lengthening than the

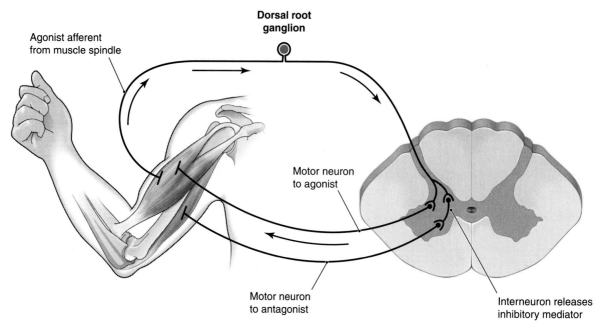

FIGURE 4-5 Reciprocal inhibition. When the agonist is contracted, the tension of the antagonist is inhibited.

actual length change. Rapid lengthening of a muscle stimulates the gamma afferents in the spindle and creates an immediate and bold protective contraction of the muscle. A stretch reflex contraction is also stimulated by slow, sustained lengthening, although this sensory information is carried on the alpha afferent neurons from the muscle spindle. The protective contraction stimulated by slow,

sustained lengthening is not as bold as the one stimulated by sudden stretch.[1,2,5,12,20–23] In other words, the intensity of the report from the muscle spindle to the spinal cord is directly proportional to the rate at which stretch occurs. Moreover, if the muscle has been static for an extended period of time, the sensitivity of the muscle spindle to sudden lengthening is significantly increased. This increased sensitivity of the muscle spindle is referred to as **gamma gain** or gamma loading.[12,20,24]

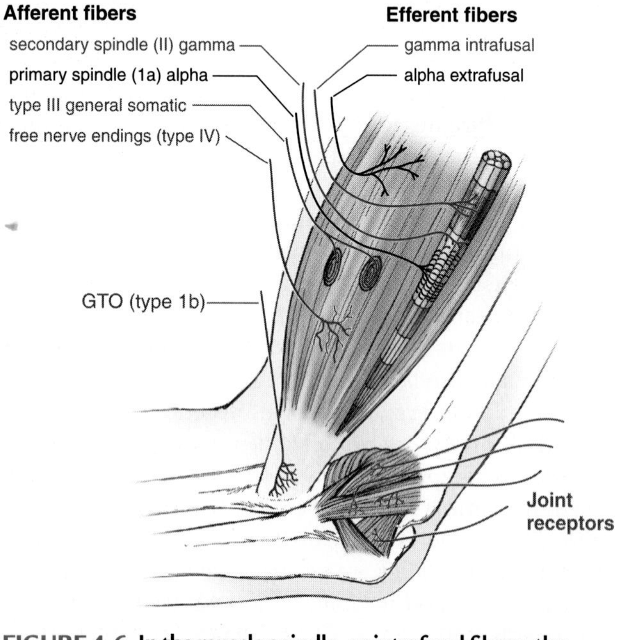

THE INVERSE STRETCH REFLEX

In addition to muscle spindles, muscles also contain another type of proprioceptor called the **Golgi tendon organ** (GTO). These proprioceptors are sensitive to tension in the muscle and respond to increased tension by inhibiting contraction. This reflex is called the inverse stretch reflex, because the response of the muscle is opposite that of the stretch reflex. Although a few GTOs are scattered throughout the muscle, the highest concentration of these proprioceptors is in tendons and musculotendinous junctions (Fig. 4-7). Because tension is created by all muscle contraction, the GTOs serve as monitors of the force of contraction and protect muscles and their tendons from tearing due to excessive tension.

The activities of the muscle spindles and GTO are responsible for providing the sensory information and motor adjustments to muscle tone for posture. More important to athletes, these proprioceptors are necessary for the continuous modulation of the muscle length, tension, and power needed for well-coordinated movement. Understanding these muscle reflexes provides the physiologic

Afferent fibers

secondary spindle (II) gamma
primary spindle (1a) alpha
type III general somatic
free nerve endings (type IV)

Efferent fibers

gamma intrafusal
alpha extrafusal

GTO (type 1b)

Joint receptors

FIGURE 4-6 In the muscle spindle, or intrafusal fibers, the *alpha afferents* **are sensitive to lengthening of the muscle, and the** *gamma afferents* **are most sensitive to the rate of lengthening.**

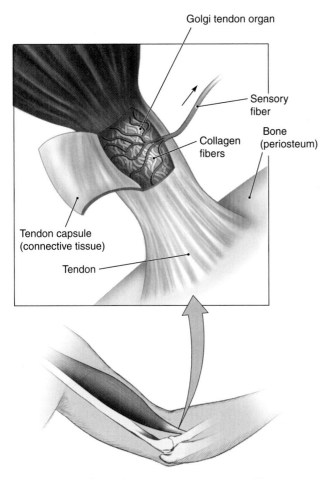

FIGURE 4-7 Golgi tendon organs (GTOs) are sensitive to increased tension and inhibit the muscle tension when stimulated.

rationale for many everyday athletic practices such as the use of static stretching over ballistic methods. Sports health care therapists can use these same rationales to direct their therapeutic applications of the neuromuscular techniques for maximum benefit.

Skeletal Muscle Response to Abnormal Stress

Skeletal muscles adapt very quickly to the use, dis-use, and abuse of everyday activities. Constant remodeling of length, diameter, vascular supply, metabolic processes, and connective tissue elements can completely transform fiber characteristics of a muscle, even shifting it from movement to postural duties. Under normal circumstances, the contractile proteins of a muscle can be totally replaced in as little as 2 weeks.[2] Athletes' exercise and training routines are designed to create predictable muscle adaptations relevant to their sports. However, in the course of training, some

undesirable adaptations may occur. For example, a tennis player will develop greater strength and muscle size in the racket arm. This is a desirable outcome. However, the quadratus lumborum, psoas, and obliques on the opposite side may shorten, which most would consider a negative adaptation that may lead to injury.

■ POSTURAL ADAPTATIONS

Muscles that are held in shorter or longer than normal positions for extended periods of time undergo adaptive changes that can diminish muscle performance. Muscles maintained in a contracted and short position lose sarcomeres at the end of the myofibril. Conversely, muscles held in a stretched or lengthened position add sarcomeres to the end of the chain.[2,6] Both of these adaptations affect the muscle's ability to generate power and withstand tension and compression stresses, and can generate tension and strain throughout the myofascial chain.[1,2,5–7,10,12,18,19,25,26]

Vladimir Janda[12,18,19,27] has presented several articles over the years on postural adaptations that have identified common patterns that can cause movement dysfunction and chronic pain. His work has been validated and supported by the more recent works of several authors and researchers.[6,12,13] Called **cross-patterns**, these adaptations can be identified and correlated to several chronic and persistent pain syndromes.[6,11–13,18,23,27] For example, the common postural position of forward head, depressed chest, rounded shoulders and increased kyphosis creates the **upper crossed syndrome** (Fig. 4-8). Common pathologies related to this upper crossed pattern include headaches, thoracic outlet syndrome, scapular dyskinesis, and shoulder impingement syndromes.[28–31] The **lower crossed syndrome** is typified by excessive lordosis and a protruding belly and can be related to conditions such as sciatica, sacroiliac dysfunction, and chronic low back pain.[6,12,18,19,28]

Contractile and Tensile Stress

Cross patterns show the lines of stress created by short-tight muscles on one side of a body hinge creating long-tight muscles on the other side. For example, in a lower crossed syndrome, tight iliopsoas and lumbar erector spinae muscles are countered by lengthened upper abdominals and gluteals. The shortened muscles are concentrically contracted and feel tight when palpated. The lengthened muscles are also tight when palpated, but for a different reason—they are contracting eccentrically to hold the body upright. The short-tight muscles are appropriately described as being under contractile stress, whereas the long-tight muscles are under tensile stress. Although palpation reveals tight muscles on both sides of the crossed patterns, the athlete is often only aware of pain and tension in the tensile

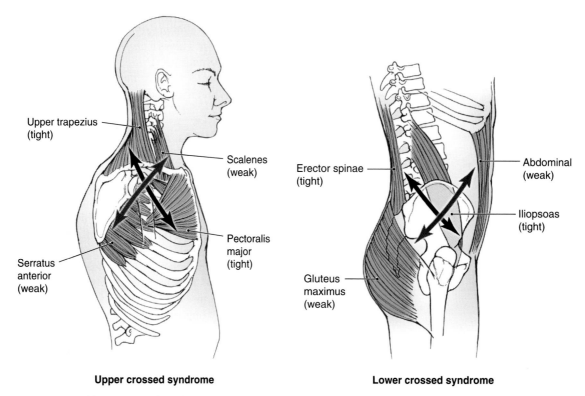

Upper crossed syndrome

Lower crossed syndrome

FIGURE 4-8 Upper and lower crossed syndromes.

stressed muscles, because eccentric contractions require more effort to sustain and these muscles are easily fatigued, most likely as the result of a combination of increased energy demands and ischemia (local restriction to blood flow) created by the hypertonicity.[1,2,5,7,10,12,25,26] In addition, the tensile stressed muscles often have a fibrous or gritty feel to them owing to the connective tissue adaptations.

Because a tight muscle may already be too long and under strain, it is clear that stretching is not always an appropriate choice for treatment. In addition, even the shortened muscles under contractile stress tend to resist normal static stretching. This is related to the gamma gain theory, which makes it clear that stretching before reducing the aberrant muscle tension will be ineffective.[12,20,24,32–34] Instead, neuromuscular techniques must be applied to reduce muscle tension in the contractile stressed muscles before the strain on the tensile stressed muscles can be relieved.

Length–Strength Ratio

When postural adaptations hold a muscle in sustained contractile or tensile stress, the strength of that muscle's contraction is affected. Because a muscle contraction requires actin and myosin to slide over one another, the strength of contraction is directly affected by the number of bonding sites available to the myofilaments. For example, a shortened muscle cannot contract with as much strength as a muscle at normal resting length because the actin–myosin

bonding sites have been used.[1,2,5–8,10] Try a heel raise in a standing position with knees extended, then squat down and repeat the heel raise from this position. It is clear that the first contraction is much stronger than the second. This is because the gastrocnemius is shortened in the repetition and therefore limited in its ability to create a strong plantar flexion contraction.

On the opposite end of the spectrum, a muscle that has been stretched too far beyond normal resting length also has a weak contraction because the actin–myosin overlap has been decreased so that there is no access to the bonding sites. Normal resting length of muscle is the optimal position for a maximum strength contraction. The strength of contraction is weakened both when muscle is held too short and when it is too long.[1,2,6,10] These length–strength ratios have significant performance implications for athletes. Athletes should focus equal amounts of time on building strength and improving flexibility if they hope to achieve powerful muscle contractions through a full range of motion. Therapeutic massage can help return muscles to their normal resting length after the exertion of a practice or game.

■ HYPERTROPHY AND ATROPHY

Muscles adapt to increased or decreased demand by adding or removing sarcomeres from the chain of units that make up the fibrils and by increasing or decreasing the number

A 42-year-old woman with a diagnosis of carpal tunnel syndrome was scheduled for surgery in 3 weeks. She experienced a constant aching pain and intermittent tingling sensations in several different areas of her affected arm. Her grip strength was good, but her pain increased significantly when she was asked to squeeze a ball 10 times consecutively. She went to a massage therapist on her own to seek some stress relief and general muscle relaxation after the surgery was scheduled. During the health intake, she told the therapist about her diagnosis and upcoming surgery, and the therapist carried out a thorough evaluation of her complaint. Findings were as follows:

- Wrist flexors and extensors were tight and fibrous, and trigger points (TrPs) were located in both muscle groups.

CASE STUDY 4-1

- Scalenes, sternocleidomastoid, and the pectoral muscles were also tight and tender.
- Compression of a central TrP in the scalenes reproduced the tingling pain the client often experienced.
- Negative Tinel's test, and positive Roos test.

The therapist released the TrP in the scalenes and sternocleidomastoid first and continued with general full-body massage. At the end of the first session, the client reported good general relaxation and a significant reduction in the arm pain/tingle. After the second session, her symptoms were gone, and she was able to cancel her surgery.

and size (diameter) of myofilaments. Muscle hypertrophy is an increase in size and strength of the muscle fibers in response to exercise. It is generally developed through isotonic muscle work. Both concentric and eccentric training create hypertrophy, but eccentric exercise stimulates hypertrophy at a faster rate.[2,5] However, the benefit of developing strength and hypertrophy rapidly by using eccentric work also increases the risk of muscle strain during training. This is because the eccentric contraction requires maximal contraction during mechanical lengthening of the muscle because it is acting as a brake. Therefore, a balance between the amount of eccentric and concentric exercise is always desirable. In addition, extreme muscle hypertrophy can actually diminish an athlete's performance if adequate attention is not given to maintaining appropriate flexibility along with the size and strength gains.

In contrast, atrophy is a decrease in size and strength of the muscle fibers from lack of use or denervation. In muscle atrophy, the actin and myosin myofilaments get thinner and decrease in number within the sarcomere. In some cases, the actual number of sarcomeres at the end of the chain also decreases. When an athlete's injury requires surgery or immobilization, sports health care professionals understand that some atrophy is expected and utilize various exercise and treatment modalities to limit or prevent the process. However, muscle atrophy can also occur in completely healthy athletes. When athletes are not using proper skill mechanics, some intrinsic muscles that are not being properly recruited can start to atrophy. Whether it is a case of poor skill development or short muscles on one side of the joint inhibiting muscles on the opposite side, the risk of injury is increased when the problem is not identified and corrected.[1–3,5,7,9]

From the Field

"I've treated hundreds of athletes with a multitude of injuries and complaints, and I find that my soft tissue skills are of great value in the athletic setting. For example, I've never treated an athlete with iliotibial band syndrome who doesn't have an associated trigger point or tender point in the tensor fascia latae, gluteus maximus, or both. My greatest treatment success comes from first relieving this point, then addressing the fascial restrictions in the iliotibial band itself. By addressing the neuromuscular tension first, the direct work on the iliotibial band is less intense for the athlete and less work for me."

Benny Vaughn, LMT, ATC, NCTMB, CSCS

Founder and Director of Neuro-kinetics®

■ CRAMPS AND SPASMS

Muscle cramps are acute involuntary muscle contractions that generally last for several minutes (Table 4-1). A knot in the belly of the muscle can be seen or felt as the entire muscle or a large section of the muscle contracts. The most common causes of cramping are muscle fatigue and metabolite imbalances. Although cramps can be stimulated by psychological stress, they are more often of metabolic origin. As an acute condition, cramps do not present any long-term problems to the athlete. However, if cramps are not managed properly before the athlete returns to activity, the risk of muscle strain may be increased.[9,35] Methods of cramp management are discussed later in Chapter 8.

Spasms are also involuntary muscle contractions, but these contractions are sustained over hours, days, weeks, or months and often affect specific motor units within a muscle. When a muscle is in spasm, it registers increased motor tone (EMG activity) and may or may not feel tight to the athlete. Both contractile and tensile stressed muscles can be described as being in spasm. However, contractile stressed muscles are often not spontaneously painful, but are tender or painful to touch, whereas tensile stressed muscles are painful with or without palpation.[12,13,18,19,24,27,28,32–34] Muscle spasms can be part of the etiology for many chronic pain syndromes, the result of musculoskeletal trauma, and/or an indicator of a local neuromuscular dysfunction.

Muscle spasms restrict the blood vessels and compress the free nerve endings within the muscle, interfering with normal nutrient delivery and waste exchange as well as causing pain that then helps sustain the spasm. The self-perpetuating nature of muscle spasm and pain is especially true for tensile stressed muscles, making early identification of postural changes and other functional adaptations important (Box 4-1). Muscle spasms can also lead to faulty biomechanics and movement patterns for an athlete, which decreases performance potential and may lead to pain or injury.

■ TRIGGER POINTS

When a muscle spasm is localized to a very small area or nodule of a muscle, it is often characterized as either a trigger point or tender point. A trigger point (TrP) is a hyperirritable nodule within a skeletal muscle that gives rise to extreme pain with only moderate compression. When compressed, a TrP stimulates a characteristic referred pattern of pain into surrounding and sometimes far reaching tissues.[12,13,28,36–38] There are several different mechanisms that lead to the development of a TrP, but the clinical characteristics of the point (always in a taut band, always radiates pain) suggest that although development may be initiated via different mechanisms, the actual pathophysiology of the point is the same. The most common precipitating events for development or activation of TrPs include[7,11–13,19–21,27,28,36,39]:

1. *Increased mechanical strain.* The very nature of sports is to repeat a particular motion, and this repetitive stressful motion adds mechanical strain that often causes TrPs. For example, an athlete who over-pronates creates excess strain on the medial head of the gastrocnemius. This mechanical strain can cause a TrP to develop in the gastrocnemius.

TABLE 4-1	Key Characteristics of Cramps, Spasms, TrPs, and TePs	
	Etiology	**Characteristics**
Cramps	Muscle fatigue Metabolic imbalance	Visible and palpable contraction in full muscle or large segment Short term
Spasms	Injury Emotional stress Mechanical strain Postural adaptation	Contractile or tensile stress Palpable tension and fibrous adhesions Sustained contraction leading to ischemia and pain
TrPs	Motor end plate stimulates "calcium spill" into sarcomere leading to actin-myosin bonding	Palpable nodule in a taut band of muscle Hypersensitive to mechanical pressure Pressure reproduces pain complaint in a predictable pattern Cause muscle to be hypersensitive to stretch
TePs	High gamma gain in muscle spindle signals contraction in response to sudden lengthening	May or may not be palpable Hypersensitive to mechanical pressure No referred pattern of pain; Often silent until compressed Cause muscle to be resistant to stretch

TePs, tender points; TrPs, trigger points.

BOX 4-1 SELF-PERPETUATING CYCLE OF MUSCLE SPASMS

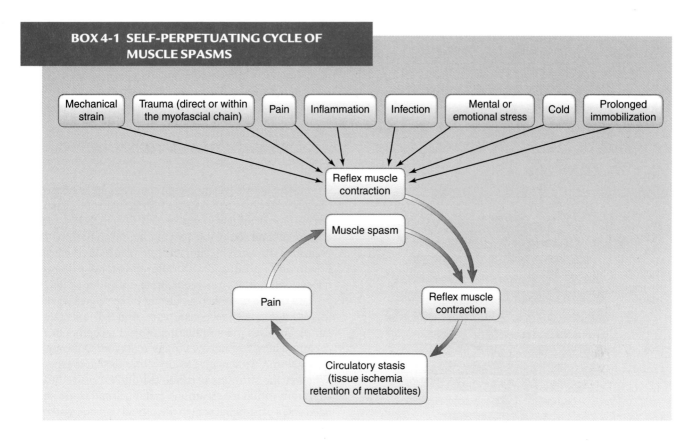

2. *Impaired circulation (ischemia).* When circulation is impaired, an area can become hypoxic and painful, stimulating a localized spasm and TrP. The cause of ischemia can be either pathologic, as when muscle tension constricts arterial flow or chemical releases (serotonin, histamine) cause vasoconstriction, or anatomic, as in hypovascular areas such as the supraspinatus and infraspinatus tendons and the midsection of the levator scapula where it twists before ascending to the cervical attachments.

3. *Trauma/local inflammatory response.* The hemorrhage and chemicals released with tissue damage stimulate nociceptors to cause pain, which triggers localized muscle spasm.

4. *Dis-use or prolonged immobility.* This is related to impaired circulation and fibrous tissue changes that occur with dis-use.

5. *Mental/emotional distress.* Simply put, when the mind is stressed the muscles are tight, and when the mind is relaxed so are the muscles.

Chaitow and DeLany[12] summarized this group of precipitating factors as over-use, mis-use, dis-use, or abuse. When one or more of these factors is at work, the common result is the development of TrPs. Regardless of what precipitating event is at work, the initial event in TrP development is believed to be a dysfunction at the synapse between a motor neuron and the muscle fiber. Irritation

or overload stress causes increased acetylcholine (neurotransmitter) to be released to the motor end plate, the muscle fiber side of the synapse, stimulating the sarcoplasmic reticulum (SR) to release calcium within the muscle fiber. It is also possible that the SR itself may sustain a microscopic tear that leads to a "calcium spill" over several sarcomeres. In either case, the localized presence of calcium ions causes actin–myosin bonding, and several sarcomeres in the area shorten, creating a **contraction knot** in several muscle fibers, but not in the entire motor unit.[36] The contraction knot is palpated as a nodule in a taut band of muscle, a key characteristic of all trigger points (Fig. 4-9).

The sustained contraction of a trigger point creates a maximum energy demand that uses up the stored energy source of the sarcomere (adenosine triphosphate [ATP]) at the same time it constricts blood flow thus decreasing any new energy supply (Fig. 4-10). This creates a metabolic crisis leading to early muscle fatigue.[12,21,35,36,39] The combined influences of motor end-plate dysfunction, metabolic crisis, and a low-grade inflammatory response to microtearing explains how and why TrPs develop their characteristic taut band, palpable nodule, and hypersensitivity.[36,40]

◼ TENDER POINT

Like a TrP, a tender point (TeP) is also a hypersensitive spot in the muscle. However, a TeP does not occur in a taut

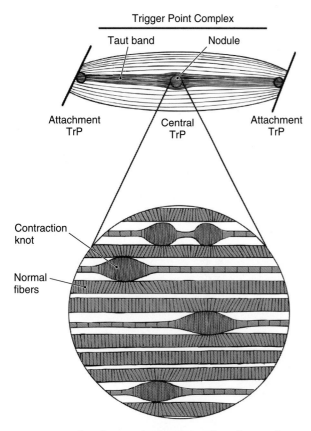

Trigger Point Complex

Taut band   Nodule

Attachment   Central   Attachment
TrP   TrP   TrP

Contraction
knot

Normal
fibers

FIGURE 4-9 The trigger point (TrP) complex. The attachments and middle of a muscle are common sites for trigger points. Several muscle fibers have developed contraction knots, giving the trigger point its nodular feel, taut band, and hypersensitivity.

band of muscle, feel like a fibrous nodule in the muscle, or create referred pain when compressed. Instead, a TeP is a small zone (about 1 cm) of tense and exquisitely tender myofascial tissue caused by a small neurologically generated local muscle spasm.[12,20,32,34,40] TePs commonly occur at muscle attachments and are often located in contractile stressed muscles. Athletes may be unaware of the presence of TePs because they are more conscious of the pain and tension in tensile stressed muscles.

TeP development is most likely due to a false stretch reflex signal. If a muscle is held in a shortened position for an extended period of time and then suddenly lengthened, a stretch reflex contraction will occur even though the muscle is not being stretched. Theoretically, this occurs because the gamma gain process "facilitates" the muscle spindle making it hypersensitive to sudden lengthening (Box 4-2).[11,12,20,34,40] In contrast, if a muscle is slowly stretched or gradually returned to normal length, the muscle spindle shifts easily from dynamic to static reporting and does not signal a protective contraction (Fig. 4-11). The protective spasm caused by the false stretch reflex signal puts strain on the opposing muscle and causes the facilitated muscle housing the TeP to be resistant to lengthening until the

reflexive contraction can be relieved. Efforts to either actively or passively force the muscle in spasm into a longer position are strongly resisted by the motor tone of the muscle, thus explaining why stretching often fails to relieve the pain and restriction experienced by an athlete.[12,32,34,40]

Theories of Pain Reduction

Pain is the body's warning sign that damage is occurring. However, because persistent muscular pain and spasm are so common in athletics, athletes often begin to view pain as a "normal" and acceptable part of training and competition, instead of the warning sign it is intended to be. A review of how pain is produced and relieved can help therapists choose appropriate treatment strategies and modalities.

Pain can be described as having three stages: (1) signal, (2) message, and (3) response/perception.[26] The signal stage simply involves the stimulation of pain receptors or nociceptors. These free nerve endings are scattered throughout all tissue and are sensitive to any stimulus that is excessive. Whether the stimulus is tissue tearing, excessive heat, or cold from eating ice cream too fast, nociceptors are stimulated and a pain signal sent to the central nervous system for as long as the stimulus is present.[1,9,26,37]

The message stage of the pain experience occurs at the spinal gate in the dorsal horn of the spinal cord.[1,9,12,26,41,42] The afferent neurons stimulated by nociceptors, along with other somatic afferent neurons, enter the spinal cord at this location. The response of the cord to afferent stimuli at the spinal gate gives rise to the gate control theory of pain reduction. This theory states that when sufficient levels of somatic stimulus (touch, temperature, pressure, movement) are provided to the body, it will block the spinal gate to pain. This is due both to differences in the speed of impulse transmission along the afferent neurons and to the cord's limited ability to attend to multiple sources of sensory stimuli at any given time. Because somatic afferent neurons have a larger diameter than general pain neurons, they can transmit impulses faster to the cord. The cord only attends to the somatic information it receives first, and so the pain message to the brain is effectively blocked by somatic stimuli and there is no sensation of pain. This is why animals lick their wounds and why athletes often hold or rub an injured area as an initial response to pain. Although gate control is effective at blocking dull aching pain, it cannot suppress an acute sharp pain message. These sharp pain messages are carried on specific sensory neurons with very large diameters. When tissue damage is of sufficient severity, the pain message wins the race through the spinal gate.[9,36,41,42]

The final stage of the pain experience—perception and response—takes place in the cerebral cortex. If a pain message passes through the spinal gate in the second stage, it

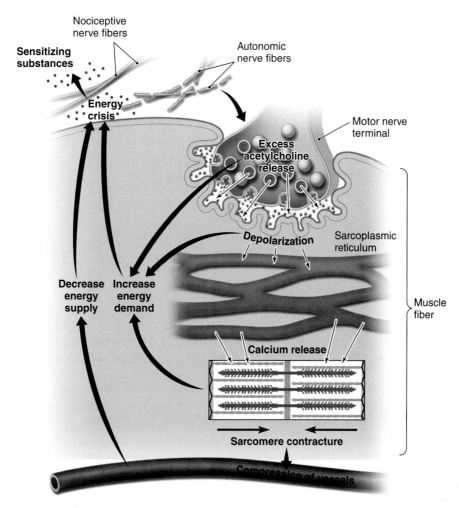

FIGURE 4-10 Myofascial trigger points (TrPs). TrPs are believed to be caused by dysfunction of the motor end plate. The dysfunction results in an abnormal increase in production and release of acetylcholine at rest. This results in depolarization of the sarcolemma with release of calcium from the sarcoplasmic reticulum and sustained shortening of sarcomeres (taut band). The shortening of muscle fiber compresses the local blood vessels, reducing the nutrient and oxygen availability. This, in turn, results in release of substances that sensitize pain receptors (pain).

can be recognized by the brain and a response can be sent back through efferent neuronal pathways. Pain does not truly exist unless this final stage is completed. In other words, if the sensory input is not translated by the brain and perceived as pain, pain does not exist. In addition, pain-inhibiting neuropeptides called **enkephalins** are produced and released in the brain and modulate the pain experience. The presence of these substances seems to inhibit the transmission of pain along nerve fibers. Production of enkephalins and differences in perception help to explain the huge variations in a human's tolerance to painful stimulus. For example, when an athlete is intensely focused both physically and mentally on an activity, he or she can effectively abolish the perception of pain. This explains how athletes in competition are less likely to feel the pain of a moderate strain than when they are in practice and why elite athletes often have a higher pain threshold than every-

day athletes. It is not differences in the type or level of painful stimuli, but differences in individual perception and response to painful stimuli that vary.[26]

Although the exact mechanism has not been unequivocally determined, massage has long been acknowledged as an effective modality for reducing pain. Because massage creates a significant amount of somatic stimulus including pressure, movement, and warming of the tissue, it seems logical to presume that massage closes the spinal gait to pain. Another significant mechanism of pain reduction probably comes from the reduction of myofascial trigger points and neuromuscular tender points. Both of these methods of pain reduction interrupt the initial pain message. Massage may also change an athlete's perception of pain by creating a sense of well-being or by bringing good feelings and memories to consciousness. Clearly, what goes on in an athlete's mind has an important effect on how pain is perceived and

BOX 4-2 UNDERSTANDING THE GAMMA GAIN PHENOMENON

A simple analogy for understanding the gamma gain phenomenon in the muscle spindle is to think of the gamma afferent pathway from the spindle as the volume control knob on a radio. When a muscle is held in a shortened position for a period of time, the volume (tension reporting) is very low; therefore, the brain is not receiving any tension reports from the muscle. During this period of not reporting, the brain does some fine tuning to the gamma afferents and turns up the volume from the muscle spindle to prepare for any sudden lengthening of the muscle. This increase in the volume setting is similar to the gamma gain experienced by the muscle spindle. The muscle spindle has been sensitized to sudden stretch and now has a "hair trigger" that will fire if the muscle is suddenly lengthened. This sudden dynamic lengthening of the muscle is the same thing as plugging in a radio with the volume knob already turned to full blast. In the case of the radio, a listener would be startled and would respond dramatically. In the case of the muscle, the spindle signals a stretch reflex contraction even though the muscle is not being stretched.

how it affects the individual. The take-home lesson is that even if massage only helps an athlete "feel good," this may actually be a profound therapeutic intervention to pain.

SUMMARY

Control, coordination, and development of the neuromuscular system are at the very heart of all athletic endeavors. Most athletes experience problems with this system in the form of muscle tension, soreness, and low-grade strain. When athletes express that a muscle feels tight and sore, therapists must recognize the particular causes of these symptoms to make appropriate therapeutic choices.

- Muscle contraction is a *physiologic* process of actin and myosin bonding. The *mechanical* changes that always occur in the muscle as a whole are (1) increased tension (pull) at the attachments and (2) a bunching or widening of the muscle belly. Muscles must be able to do both for optimal function.
- A tight muscle is generally not a singular problem because tension is transmitted across body planes and regions and can inhibit and weaken other muscles. All

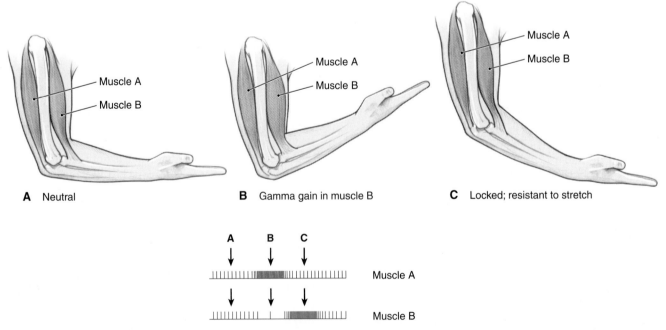

A Neutral   **B** Gamma gain in muscle B   **C** Locked; resistant to stretch

FIGURE 4-11 Gamma gain. When muscle B is held in a short position for a sustained period of time, the neurologic report of tension is very low. The brain facilitates this pathway, a process called gamma gain. When B is suddenly lengthened, as depicted in the third panel, the muscle spindle signals a stretch reflex contraction that locks the muscle into a shorter than normal position.

of this tends to compound the athlete's sense of tension and strain.

- A muscle that feels tight and sore to an athlete can be under either contractile stress or tensile stress. Therefore, stretching is rarely the best therapeutic intervention for addressing tight muscles.
- Engaging normal muscle reflexes such as reciprocal inhibition, the stretch reflex, and reversing high gamma gain allows therapists to intervene into the self-perpetuating cycle of muscle tension.
- Trigger points (TrPs) and tender points (TePs) have been identified as common causes of muscle tension and pain, and they also occur in response to muscle strain and repetitive use. In either case, full relief of the problem might only be achieved when TrP and/or TeP techniques are included in the treatment plan.
- The transitional tissue areas such as musculotendinous junctions and tenoperiosteal junctions are common sites for strain, TrPs, and TePs to occur. Excess and/or unbalanced muscle tension can be a causal factor in these conditions and *always* occurs as a response to them.
- In addition to muscle and tendon pathologies, excessive muscle tension also leads to compression of joints and may be a significant part of pathologies like bursitis, chondromalacia, and capsulitis.
- TrPs and TePs seem to have different physiology origins and may require different therapeutic approaches for complete relief.

Review Questions

SHORT ANSWERS

1. Define the following terms:
   Muscle tone
   Motor tone
   Tensile stress
   Contractile stress
   Atrophy
   Hypertrophy

2. Name three key characteristics of a trigger point.

3. What are the two mechanical changes that occur in a skeletal muscle during any type of contraction?

4. List four initiating or sustaining factors for muscle spasms and trigger points.

MULTIPLE CHOICE

5. A motor unit is made up of a single motor neuron and
   _____.
   a. all the fibers in a muscle
   b. a single muscle fiber
   c. several muscle fibers
   d. two muscle fascicles

6. What is the smallest contractile unit of a muscle?
   a. Fascicle
   b. Motor unit
   c. Muscle fiber
   d. Sarcomere

7. Another term for a muscle spindle is _____.
   a. fascial fiber
   b. intrafusal fiber
   c. extrafusal fiber
   d. Golgi tendon fiber

8. A muscle spindle is sensitive to what type of stimulus?
   a. Rapid lengthening
   b. Rapid shortening
   c. Increased tension
   d. Decreased tension

9. A Golgi tendon organ is sensitive to what type of stimulus?
   a. Rapid lengthening
   b. Rapid shortening
   c. Increased tension
   d. Decreased tension

10. According to reciprocal inhibition, what muscle is inhibited when the biceps brachii is contracted?
    a. Brachioradialis
    b. Coracobrachialis
    c. Deltoid
    d. Triceps brachii

11. What mineral is needed for the actin and myosin bonds to form and create a muscle contraction?
    a. Potassium
    b. Sodium
    c. Calcium
    d. Magnesium

12. The force of a muscle contraction is effected by the length and tension of that muscle before contraction. This theory is called _____.
    a. length–strength ratio
    b. positional force variance
    c. tension contraction modulation
    d. contraction differentiation

13. A muscle generates a more forceful contraction when it is in a(n) _____ position.
    a. fully shortened
    b. partially shortened
    c. overstretched
    d. slightly stretched

14. When the muscle spindle is stimulated, what change occurs in the muscle?
    a. Tension is inhibited.
    b. The muscle contracts.
    c. Circulation is increased.
    d. The muscle lengthens.

15. When the Golgi tendon organ is stimulated, what change occurs in the muscle?
    a. Tension is inhibited.
    b. The muscle contracts.
    c. Circulation is increased.
    d. The muscle lengthens.

16. Gamma gain occurs in a muscle spindle when it is held in _____ for an extended time?
    a. a lengthened position
    b. eccentric contraction
    c. a shortened position
    d. tetanic contraction

17. Which statement is true about muscles with myofascial trigger points?
    a. They have a higher force production.
    b. They are more sensitive to stretch.
    c. They are hyperemic.
    d. They exhibit increased range of motion.

18. Which phrase best describes a tender point?
    a. Contraction knot
    b. Metabolic crisis
    c. Always occurs in a taut band of myofascial tissue
    d. Local muscle spasm indicating a sensitized muscle spindle

19. Voluntary motor commands for skeletal muscles are signaled through what kind of neuronal pathway?
    a. Alpha
    b. Beta
    c. Gamma
    d. Delta

20. The three phases of pain are the stimulus, the message, and _____.
    a. reception
    b. perception and response
    c. signal
    d. activation

REFERENCES

1. Tortora GJ. Principles of Human Anatomy, 8th ed. Menlo Park: Benjamin Cummings Science Publishing, 1999.
2. Guyton AC, Hall JE. Textbook of Medical Physiology, 9th ed. Philadelphia: WB Saunders, 1996.
3. Prentice WE. Rehabilitation Techniques in Sports Medicine, 2nd ed. St. Louis: Mosby, 1994.
4. Hubbard DR, Berkoff GM. Myofascial trigger points show spontaneous needle EMG activity. Spine 1993;18(13):1803–1807.
5. Lieber RL. Skeletal Muscle Structure and Function: Implications for Rehabilitation and Sports Medicine. Baltimore: Williams & Wilkins, 1992.
6. Sahrmann SA. Diagnosis and Treatment of Movement Impairment Syndromes. St. Louis: Mosby, 2002.
7. Juhan D. Job's Body: A Handbook for Bodywork, expanded edition. Barrytown, NY: Station Hill, 1998.
8. Huxly AF. Prefatory Chapter: Muscular Contraction. Ann Rev Physiol 1998;50:1–16.
9. Premkumar K. The Massage Connection Anatomy and Physiology, 2nd ed. Baltimore: Lippincott Williams & Wilkins, 2004.
10. Gordon AM, Huxley AF, Huxley FJ. The length tension diagram of single vertebrate striated muscle fibers. Proceedings of the Physiological Society. 1964;February:28–31.
11. Korr IM. Somatic dysfunction. JAOA 1986(2):109–114.
12. Chaitow L, DeLany JW. Clinical Application of Neuromuscular Techniques, vol. 1: The Upper Body. Edinburgh, New York: Churchill Livingstone, 2000.
13. Chaitow L, DeLany JW. Clinical Application of Neuromuscular Techniques, vol. 2: The Lower Body. Edinburgh, New York: Churchill Livingstone, 2000.
14. Ledderman E. Fundamentals of Manual Therapy. Edinburgh: Churchill Livingstone, 1998.
15. Armstrong RB, Warren GL, Warren LA. Mechanisms of exercise-induced muscle fiber injury. Sports Medicine 1991;12:184–207.
16. Friden J, Leiber RL. Structural and mechanical basis of exercise-induced muscle injury. Med Sci Sports Exercise 1992;24:251–530.
17. Denegar CR. Persistent pain and kinetic chain dysfunction: Making the link. Proceedings of NATA Annual Meeting and Clinical Symposium, June 2002.
18. Hendrickson T. Massage for Orthopedic Conditions. Baltimore: Lippincott Williams & Wilkins, 2003.
19. Greenman PE. Principles of Manual Medicine, 3rd ed. Philadelphia; Lippincott Williams & Wilkins, 2003.
20. Korr IM. Proprioceptors and somatic dysfunction. JAOA 1975; 74(March):638–650.
21. Walsh GE. Clinics in Developmental Medicine #25: Muscles, Masses, and Motion; The Physiology of Normality, Hypertonicity, Spasticity, and Rigidity. Oxford: MacKieth Press, 1992.
22. Johansson H, Djupsjobacka M, Sjolander P. Influence of gamma-muscle afferents stimulated by KCL and lactic acid. Neuroscience Research 1993;16:49–57.
23. Liebenson C. Muscular imbalance: An update. Dynamic Chiropractor Website http://www.chiroweb.com/dynamic.
24. Johansson H, Sojka P. Pathophysiological mechanisms involved in genesis and spread of muscular tension in occupational muscle pain and in chronic musculoskeletal pain syndromes: A hypothesis. Medical Hypotheses 1991;35:196–203.
25. Woo SL-Y, Buckwalter JA, eds. Injury and repair of the musculoskeletal soft tissues. American Academy of Orthopedic Surgeons Symposium Workshop. Savannah, GA, 1987.
26. Brand P, Yancy P. The Gift of Pain: Why We Hurt and What We Can Do About It. Grand Rapids, MI: Zondervan Publishing House, 1993.
27. Janda V. Muscle spasm: A proposed procedure for differential diagnosis. Journal of Manual Medicine 1991;6:136–139.

28. McLeod I, Mistry D, Archer P et al. Massage therapy utilization and application in the treatment of myofascial trigger points. Advanced track seminar, June 2005; NATA Annual Meeting.

29. Su KP, Johnson MP, et al. Scapular rotation in swimmers with and without impingement syndrome: Practice effects. Medicine and Science in Sports and Exercise 2004;1117–1123.

30. Cools AM, Witvrouw EE et al. Scapular muscle recruitment patterns: Trapezius muscle latency with and without impingement syndromes. Am J Sports Med 2003;31(4):542 549.

31. Lucas KR, Polus BI, Rich PA. Latent myofascial trigger points: Their effects on muscle activation and movement efficiency. Journal of Bodywork and Movement Therapies 2004;8:160–166.

32. Chaitow L. Positional Release Techniques. New York: Churchill Livingstone, 1996.

33. Chaitow L. Muscle Energy Techniques. New York: Churchill Livingstone, 1996.

34. D'Ambrogio KJ, Roth GB. Positional Release Therapy: Assessment and Treatment of Musculoskeletal Dysfunctions. St. Louis: Mosby, 1997.

35. Anderson MK, Hall SJ, Martin M. Sports Injury Management, 2nd ed. Philadelphia: Lippincott Williams & Wilkins, 2000.

36. Simons DG, Travell JG, Simons LS. Myofascial Pain and Dysfunction: The Trigger Point Manual, 2nd ed. vol. 1; Upper Half of Body. Philadelphia: Lippincott Williams & Wilkins, 1999.

37. Mense S. Peripheral mechanisms of muscle nociception and local muscular pain. Journal of Musculoskeletal Pain 1993;1.

38. Travell JG, Rinzler S. The myofascial genesis of pain. Postgraduate Medicine 1952, May 11:425–434.

39. Smolders JJ. Myofascial Pain and Dysfunction: Myofascial Trigger Points. Hammer WI, ed. Functional Soft Tissue Examination and Treatment by Manual Methods: The Extremities. Gaithersburg, MD: Aspen Publishers, 1991.

40. Kusunose RS. Strain and Counterstrain for the Upper Quarter. Course syllabus, 1990.

41. U-Mass Medical School. Complexities in the nervous pathways carrying pain: from "silent" C-fibers to cingulate gyrus. Serial on line doc. 7. http://courses.umassmed.edu/mbb1/Limbic/CentralPain.cfm.

42. Spine-health.com. Modern ideas: The gate control theory of pain. 1999–2005.

5 The Myofascial Network

After completing this chapter, the reader will be able to:

- Define and explain the implications of muscle architecture.
- Define fascia, describe the three layers of the body-wide fascial system, and name and locate the three layers of fascia found in all skeletal muscles.
- Describe the complexity and comprehensive nature of the fascial system.
- List the three common components of all forms of connective tissue.
- Define tensegrity and thixotropic.
- Name and locate the 11 superficial body bands of fascia in the body.
- Name and locate the four deep horizontal planes of fascia.
- Define myofascial chain, and name all of the myofascial chains in the body.
- Identify the primary myofascial connections and boney attachments of the superficial front and back lines of the body.
- List five common causes of fascial dysfunction.

Connective tissue is the most abundant and widely distributed tissue in the body. The general purpose and function of connective tissue are to bind and hold structures together, to offer general insulation and protection to the body as a whole, and to provide a framework for the passage of blood vessels, lymph vessels, and nerves. To the sports health care professional, it is the organized dense connective tissues such as tendons and ligaments and the less organized or dense irregular connective tissue-like fascia, joint capsules, and periosteum that are of greatest interest. Together, these fibrous connective tissues serve to compartmentalize and connect all musculoskeletal structures into a unified locomotor system and to connect all other organs and body systems.

Connective Tissue

Different types of connective tissue vary in thickness, rigidity, tensile strength, elasticity, and viscosity, giving each type unique functional abilities. This versatility in form and function comes from combining different ratios, concentrations, and patterns of cells and matrix. The specific quality and content of the matrix provide the major distinctions between the form and function of different types of connective tissue.

The **matrix** is the background substance for the cells, composed of ground substance and fibers (Box 5-1). Ground substance is a clear fluid of 70% water, some carbon mol-

BOX 5-1 DESCRIPTION OF THE MATRIX

"Where we find mostly fluid and few fibers, we have a watery intercellular medium that is ideal for metabolic activities; with less fluid and more fibers, we have a soft, flexible lattice that can hold skin cells or liver cells or nerve cells into place; with little fluid and many fibers, we have the tough, stringy material of muscle sacs, tendons, and ligaments" (3:66)

ecules, and other chemicals common to general intercellular fluids.[1-4] Functionally, the ground substance serves as a spacer and lubricant between the fibers of the matrix. There are four types of cells common to all types of connective tissue: macrophages, plasma cells, mast cells, and fibroblasts.

CONNECTIVE TISSUE CELLS

Macrophages and **plasma cells** play vital roles in our body's specific immune response; the first acts as a phagocyte and the latter produces antibodies. Because high numbers of macrophages are present in connective tissue, specifically fascia, we begin to understand that the network of connective tissue in our body serves not only as a vital *structural* component giving us support and form, but also as a key *functional* element for a multitude of physiologic processes ranging from immune responses and healing to translating muscle contraction into movement.

Mast cells are distributed throughout all types of connective tissue and are most abundant around blood vessels. They produce two chemicals, histamine and heparin, which play important roles in the healing cycle. When tissue is damaged or stressed the mast cells release **histamine**, which causes two changes in the surrounding tissue: blood vessel vasodilation, and increased capillary permeability. These two changes allow easy passage of clean-up and repair cells into an injured area, which are vital steps of the inflammatory process and healing. The normal function of **heparin** is to serve as an anticoagulant. However, the heparin from mast cells is in the form of a proteoglycan, which weakens its effectiveness as an anticoagulant. Because proteoglycans hold water in the ground substance of connective tissues, it is theorized that the heparin in mast cells may serve more as a binding substance for other intracellular constituents.[1-4]

The most abundant connective tissue cells are **fibroblasts.** These cells secrete the protein substances that make up the ground substance, and the fibers that crisscross through it to form the matrix for most varieties of connective tissue. For this reason, fibrous connective tissues, that is, ligaments, tendons, joint capsules, periosteum, and fascia all have very high numbers of fibroblasts. Fibroblasts are the only cells in our body that exhibit a lifelong ability to migrate to any point in the body, then to secrete the specific form of connective tissue needed for repair in that area. Owing to this remarkable versatility, fibroblasts are the key cells for tissue regeneration and repair for the entire body, and they are most active during growth and the healing process.[1-5] Simply stated, it is the fibroblasts that synthesize connective tissue. The type of protein fibers secreted by the fibroblasts and the rate of their production varies according to the type of tissue they are in and the mechanical stresses placed on the cells in that tissue. It is the fibroblasts' response to mechanical stresses that provides the rationale for establishing pain-free movement as early as possible in the healing process.

CONNECTIVE TISSUE FIBERS

There are three varieties of connective tissue fibers: (1) collagen, (2) reticular, and (3) elastic. These fibers, made up of protein chains secreted by fibroblasts, are embedded in the ground substance of connective tissues and provide variable amounts of strength, support, and elasticity, depending on the ratio and pattern of fiber arrangement. Of the three types of fibers, collagen is the thickest, strongest, and most abundant.

Collagen fibers are very tough and resistant to stretch because of the structure of the fibers, a bundle of thinner protein fibrils in parallel arrangement similar to the structure of a muscle fiber. To fully understand the functional strengths and limitations of collagen, its microscopic structures must be examined more closely. The smaller fibrils within a collagen fiber are composed of a specific protein molecule called **tropocollagen**, which is produced by the fibrocytes (Fig. 5-1). Each of these molecules is a long chain of amino acids that has a natural corkscrew appearance. When three of these tropocollagen molecules are bound together, they form a triple-helix collagen molecule very similar in appearance to DNA. Several collagen molecules linked together form a **collagen fibril**, which retains the spiral shape of the collagen molecules inside.[1-4,6]

This spiral arrangement is carried through to the collagen fiber itself. It gives collagen fibers a natural ability to lengthen when tension is applied by unwinding these multiple spirals. When complete unwinding occurs and the full length of the fiber is reached, it cannot lengthen further

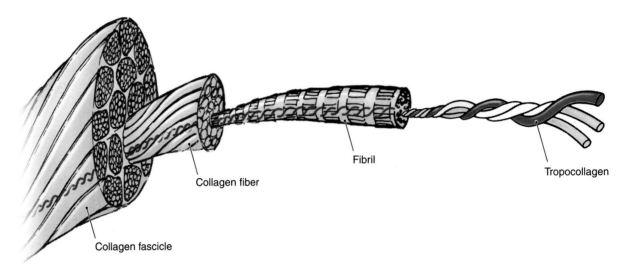

FIGURE 5-1 Tendon or ligament structure. These fibrous connective tissue structures parallel the structures of a muscle. They are made of bundles of collagen fibers called fascicles. Each collagen fiber is made of smaller bundles of fibrils, which are made up of bundles of microscopic filaments called tropocollagen. The spiral structure of tropocollagen is reflected throughout the full collagen fiber.

without structural damage. A helpful analogy is to visualize a hemp rope because it has a "natural give" and appears to stretch when gradual tension is applied. However, like collagen fibers, the rope is not actually stretching, but unwinding. Once the rope is pulled taut, having unwound as much as possible, no further lengthening occurs without the rope beginning to fray or tear. If sudden, forceful tension is applied, the rope firmly resists extension because the fibers cannot unwind. The same is true for collagen fibers: they unwind and extend when gradual tension is applied, but resist sudden application of force. The ground substance between collagen fibers allows fascia and other connective tissues to slowly return to their original length when tension is removed. For this reason, myofascial massage techniques affect change by applying slow and gradual stretch to the fascia. When connective tissue is subjected to sustained and repeated tension, such as in stretching exercises, collagen fibers do not become more elastic, but increase their resting length by stimulating fibrocytes to produce more chains of the tropocollagen. This provides a rationale for frequent stretching exercises and explains why improvements in range of motion immediately after a massage cannot be sustained beyond a few hours.

The **reticular fibers** of connective tissue are very similar to collagen in structure and function, but thinner and more delicate. Reticular fibers form the network of connective tissue that surrounds and gives support to smooth and skeletal muscle cells and to nerve fibers, and they form the connective tissue framework for organs. Like collagen, reticular fibers are slightly extensible and tolerate moderate to high levels of tensile stress without tearing.

Elastic fibers are made up of a protein called elastin rather than the collagen protein, making them much smaller but more "stretchy" than either collagen or reticu-

lar fibers. When tensile stress is applied, these fibers have the unique ability to stretch up to 150% of their normal length without tearing; then they quickly recoil to normal resting length when the tension is released.[1] Therefore, connective tissues high in reticular and elastic fibers such as skin, lungs, and blood vessels are much more flexible and resilient than connective tissues such as tendons and ligaments that are very high in collagen.

From the Field

"In athletics, the optimum health of soft tissues that governs movement can make the difference between a long and healthy career or one plagued by nagging minor injuries. The skilled hands of a therapist deliver site-specific results that impact the full body. It is no wonder that athletes the world over routinely tout the benefits of massage for maintaining their health and performance."

Whitney Lowe, LMT

Director, Orthopedic Massage Education & Research Institute Sisters, OR

■ GROUND SUBSTANCE

Ground substance is the intercellular fluid in all connective tissues. It is mostly water, but it also contains a unique protein and polysaccharide chain called GAGs (glycoaminoglycans) that serve as water magnets for the ground substance. The presence of these GAGs keeps the ground substance fluid and allows it to fulfill its function as the spacer and lubricant in connective tissue. When connective tissue is dehydrated or injured, the diminished capacity of ground substance causes fibers to stick to one another and form **adhesions.**[3,7,8]

■ FIBROUS CONNECTIVE TISSUE

Fibrous or dense connective tissues contain thicker and more densely packed collagen fibers, less ground substance, and few cells, thus making them strong and resistant to tensile stresses. The collagen fibers in ligaments and tendons are parallel with one another and arranged to stabilize the joints or withstand the contractile stress produced by muscle contraction. Ligaments contain slightly higher numbers of elastic fibers than tendons because light stretch is required for the joints to achieve full range of motion. In contrast, the fiber arrangement in fascia and joint capsules is less organized and not always parallel. The multidirectional stresses placed on these tissues result in fibers running in several directions and a more sheet-like arrangement rather than the ropes of collagen found in the ligaments and tendons.[1–4]

Skeletal Muscle Architecture

Muscle architecture is the arrangement of muscle fibers along the line of pull for that muscle as well as how the connective tissue layers weave, group, and divide these fibers. Any full-body diagram of the muscular system illustrates the many shapes, sizes, and fiber arrangements of muscles and shows the multiple layers and groupings of muscles common to each body area. It is the different shapes and arrangements of muscle fibers that make some muscles more powerful than others and dictates the role that each muscle plays in creating specific movements. For therapists, the muscle architecture defines fiber direction.

■ THE CONNECTIVE TISSUE ELEMENTS

All skeletal muscles have the same three connective tissue layers regardless of their shape or size. The most superficial layer of connective tissue wraps around the outside of the whole muscle and is called the **epimysium.** The epimysium

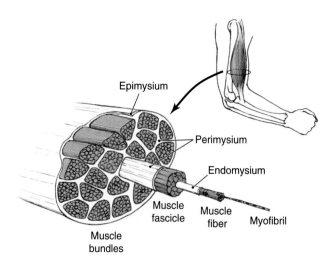

FIGURE 5-2 Fascial layers within skeletal muscles.

plays a major role in separating one major muscle from another to give some independent action to muscles within the same group or in surrounding areas. The next layer, the **perimysium,** divides the muscle into several different internal compartments by wrapping around a bundle of several muscle fibers to make a *fascicle*. This structural arrangement gives each muscle a distinct shape and appearance and allows the fascicles to act independently. The third layer of connective tissue in a skeletal muscle is the **endomysium.** This is the connective tissue covering the outside of each individual muscle fiber or cell. All three of these layers extend beyond the ends of the muscle fibers and feed into a common cord forming a **tendon** (Fig. 5-2). These connective tissue layers not only give shape and structure to a muscle, but also contribute to its functional capacity. It has been demonstrated that the strength of muscle contraction is diminished by almost 15% when a small slit is made in the epimysium.[9]

■ MUSCLE SHAPES AND FIBER ARRANGEMENT

Skeletal muscles have several shapes and fiber arrangements, defined by the connective tissue elements that divide, surround, and weave into each muscle. Some muscles are broad and flat with attachments that cover large areas of the bone, and others are more spindle-shaped with cordlike attachments at either end. In addition, the fiber arrangement within each muscle is variable; some with vertical alignment and others with shorter fibers in an oblique alignment to the bone (Fig. 5-3). Shape and fiber arrangement are used to classify muscles into one of five categories: parallel, fusiform, pennate (with three subclasses of unipennate, bipennate, and multipennate [Fig. 5-4]), circular, or triangular.[1,2,4] A muscle's architecture determines what role

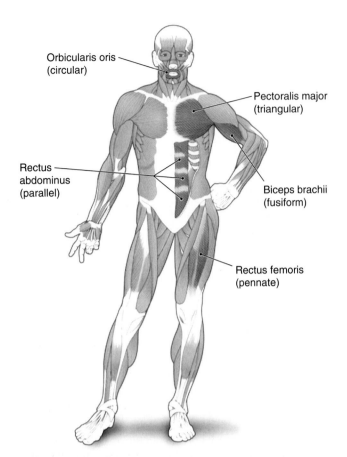

FIGURE 5-3 Examples of muscle architecture in different areas of the body.

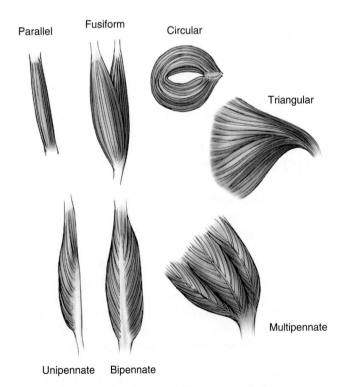

FIGURE 5-4 Individual views of different muscle shapes.

each muscle plays in creating specific body movements, the amount of power a contraction can generate, and the range of motion a full muscle contraction can produce. For example, muscles with long fibers in parallel arrangement tend to produce a greater range of motion, whereas muscles with short fibers in a pennate arrangement produce greater power over a small range of motion.[2,3,6]

Understanding the shape, fiber direction, and fascial divisions within a muscle has several therapeutic implications. The shape of a muscle helps therapists identify likely stress points, fiber direction is used to guide therapists in the choice between cross fiber and linear friction strokes, and fascial divisions and junctions in the muscle are probable sites for restrictions, adhesions, and lesions to develop. These areas of stress, restriction, and adhesions can limit a muscle's functional capacity, and thus an athlete's ability to perform at their best.

MUSCLE ATTACHMENTS

Skeletal muscles attach to bone via a tendon, or a broad, flat sheet of fibrous connective tissue called an **aponeurosis**, which weaves into the tougher and less extensible outer covering of bone called the **periosteum**. Two important transition zones are associated with muscle attachments. The **musculotendinous junction** is the area where muscle transitions to the fibrous connective tissue of the tendon, and the **tenoperiosteal junction** is where the fibrous connective tissue of the tendon weaves into the periosteum (Fig. 5-5). These two junctions are areas of high stress and common sites of muscle injury. The tension created by muscle contraction, together with torsion or compression forces created by movement, challenge these zones to quickly and efficiently absorb and adapt the force to prevent injury to the muscle.[1,2,6–8,10]

The Fascial Network

The fascial system is a multidimensional network extending from just below our skin to deep within our bones and internal organs. Barnes and Juhan[3,7,11] suggest that the fascial system is the *only* body system and that all other organs are merely specialized components within this multipocketed and continuous connective tissue web. The fascial web weaves together the less organized fascial layers in muscles (epimysium, perimysium, endomysium) and the more organized fibrous connective tissues (ligaments, tendons, and periosteum) as simply the thicker and more fibrous extensions of the muscle's investing fascial layers. If fascia is viewed as the unifying medium for all components of the body's locomotor system, we can see how *localized trauma* is often reflected in distant tissues and organs.[6–8,10,12] Fascia

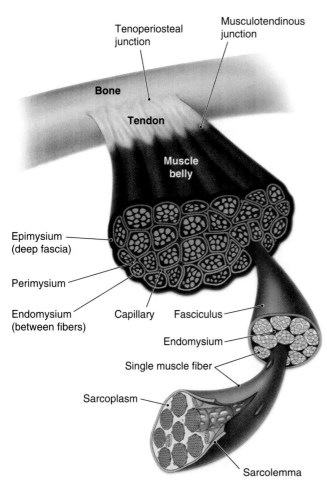

Tenoperiosteal junction

Musculotendinous junction

Bone

Tendon

Muscle belly

Epimysium (deep fascia)

Perimysium

Endomysium (between fibers)

Capillary   Fasciculus

Endomysium

Single muscle fiber

Sarcoplasm

Sarcolemma

FIGURE 5-5 **The musculotendinous and tenoperiosteal junctions are areas of high stress and are common sights of injury and stress points (trigger points and tender points).**

is also rich in sensory neurons and plays a vital role in reflecting and generating both proprioceptive and pain responses.[1,3,6-8,10,12,13] In fact, the amount of proprioception that occurs in fascial sheaths is third in line, coming only after joint and muscle spindle input.[4] Shifts in posture and biomechanical patterns are common responses to injury that may be related to this proprioceptive nature of fascia. Individuals with fibromyalgia or myofascial pain syndromes often describe body-wide aching and shifting pain. Because this pain is rarely associated with mechanical dysfunctions, fascial considerations may provide the missing link to understanding these syndromes (Box 5-2).

■ TENSEGRITY AND THIXOTROPY

Tensegrity is an architectural term coined by Buckminster Fuller, which describes a structure that maintains structural integrity by continuously adjusting tension and compression. The opposite structural form is one of continuous compression, such as a brick wall. In a brick wall, each brick is stacked one on top of the other to create a rigid structure held together by the weight, or compressive force, of each part. If one end of the wall is overloaded, that area may collapse but the rest of the wall may still stand. The stability of a tensegrity model, such as a suspension bridge, is not as firm as the brick wall, but it is much more resilient. When a big heavy truck is on the bridge, the entire structure may compress and/or pull, and some sections may actually be damaged but not necessarily the sections that were loaded. The human body is a complicated system of guidewires, rigid beams, and pulleys. The bones are held together by connective tissue that is, in turn, pulled taut by the muscles and fascia. The bones serve as rigid beams, or spacers, but it is the tension produced by the muscles and fascia that maintains our upright position and holds the body together.[3,6-8,10-18]

In tensegrity models, stress is reflected throughout the system rather than being confined to the precise point of stress. Imagine wearing a full-body stretch suit with one sleeve that is one size smaller than the rest of the suit. When the arm in the smaller sleeve is raised, the movement creates compression and pulling across the upper body and down into the hips. Moving the opposite arm or hip also creates some compression and pull across the body (Fig. 5-6). In other words, because of tensegrity muscle tension is easily transmitted from one area to another, and fascial restrictions can create strain in distant structures.

Another unique quality of fascia is its **viscoelastic** properties of extension and rebound. The fibers of the matrix provide the tensile strength of fascia, whereas the ground substance protects against compression forces. Because ground substance is *colloidal* (particles suspended in a fluid medium) when it is cold and/or stagnates, the ground substance becomes more viscous and solid—gel. When it is warm and/or moving, it becomes less viscous and more liquid—sol. This ability of ground substance to change between the gel and the sol state gives fascia its **thixotropic** nature. An everyday example of how these thixotropic changes affect movement is when we exercise in cold temperatures. At first, our bodies feel stiff and tight, but after a short period of movement, we feel looser and suppler. Long-term spasms that lock muscles into long or short positions also create these changes, leading to muscle stiffening (Box 5-3).

■ FASCIAL LAYERS AND PATTERNS

Fascia consists of two layers, the *superficial fascia,* which anchors the dermis of the skin to the underlying structures, and the *deep fascia,* which surrounds individual muscles, bones, and organs. Because both the superficial and deep fascia carry nerves, blood, and lymph vessels throughout the body, it is easy to see how fascial tension can negatively affect a multitude of organs and system functions. Blood and lymph flow can be restricted or diverted, and pain

BOX 5-2 UNDERSTANDING FASCIA'S LAYERING AND WRAPPING PATTERN: A SLICED ORANGE

The continuous and complex layering and wrapping pattern of the fascia in our body is analogous to an orange that has been sliced open. The white "connective tissue" of the orange holds the peel to the fruit and continues into the thick central core, dividing the fruit into several segments along the way. The connective tissue that surrounds each segment extends into the fruit dividing each segment into individual "cells" surrounded by a thin film.[5] This same multiple layering and weaving of connective tissue can be seen here in a transverse section of a human leg.

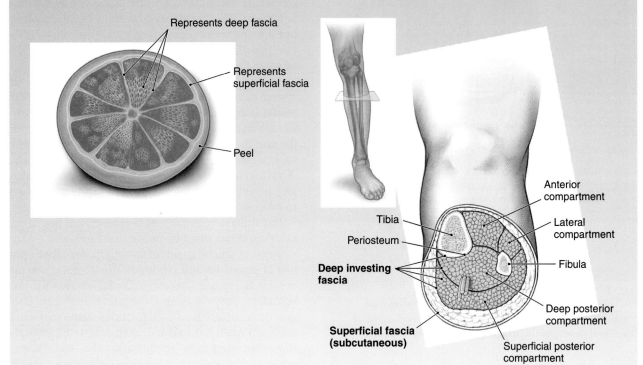

receptors can be stimulated directly by compression and tension or indirectly by ischemia.[1-4,6-8,10]

Some fascial components are difficult to characterize as strictly superficial or deep structures. For example, the thick and broad connective tissue sheets such as the *lumbosacral aponeurosis* and *iliotibial band* are firmly anchored to the skin, as well as to the muscles and bones. Therefore, these structures are part of both the superficial and deep fascial layers. It is not as important to label structures as superficial or deep as it is to recognize that all tissues are three dimensional and connected.

Fascia is not only layered, it is also organized into well-defined fascial chains and horizontal planes. These fascial patterns provide the necessary tension, counterbalances, and directed force to keep us upright as well as to create smooth, coordinated movement. Recognition of these chains and planes and understanding of how their connection affects a wide range of structures can help therapists establish more comprehensive plans for injury prevention and treatment.

Superficial Body Bands

Louis Schultz and Rosemary Feitis outline seven horizontal lines of superficial fascia, referred to as body straps in their text *The Endless Web*.[10,12,19] These seven lines, also identified in the *Journal of the Rolfing Institute* as Rolf lines, are considered large retinaculi for the torso that function in the same manner as the retinaculi of the wrists and ankles (Fig. 5-7). As part of the superficial layer of fascia, these horizontal straps tend to restrict fat deposition so they are fairly easy to identify in a postural assessment. They appear as flattened bands of tissues within the normal adipose contours of the torso, and their precise location varies from one individual to another. In addition to their superficial appearance, each band can be correlated to a specific spinal junction.[3] Figure 5-7 shows the general location and appearance of the bands and Table 5-1 numbers and describes the approximate path through the tissue for each band. Both table and diagram should be considered as

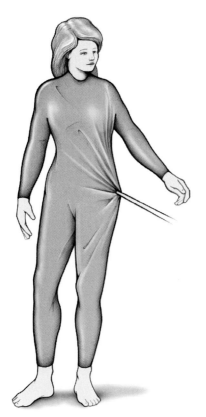

FIGURE 5-6 **The superficial fascial can be likened to a full body suit of connective tissue.** When stress or tension is applied in one area of the body's fascial suit, it is reflected throughout the network.

guidelines because it is not uncommon for the bands to curve slightly after individual body contours rather than progressing along a straight horizontal line.

The horizontal fascial bands can be viewed as tie-straps that hold the softer, rounder anterior torso closer and more firmly to the vertical and semirigid spine, just as a gardener might tie a bushy vertical plant to a supporting pole. Even though the bands are structurally necessary, the plant may be damaged if the ties are too tight, which is also the case with these body bands. Injury or immobilizations can cause them to thicken and adhere, leading to restrictions in

breathing, movement, and the body's general sense of ease. The fascial bands also create pressurized segments in the body to help maintain the upright position. Juhan[3] uses the imagery of a water balloon to explain this phenomenon. While resting on the ground, a water balloon is a simple oval sphere. When the balloon is wrapped with several rubber bands, the sphere is transformed into a more cylindrical structure that can be made to stand vertically (Fig. 5-8). The shape and rigidity of the cylinder can be modified by adding more bands and/or tightening the existing bands. This model is completely congruent with tensegrity because tension and pressure, not rigid beams, play the dominant role in creating form and function.

Deep Horizontal Planes

The deep fascia that weaves into and through the skeletal muscles and wraps around our organs and bones also forms multiple horizontal fascial planes all over the body. Each joint line represents a deep horizontal plane by connecting the periosteum, joint capsule, and articular cartilage in a continuous fascial sheet. On an even deeper level, the anterior and posterior body cavities each have two horizontal fascial planes that divide and support the internal structures (Fig. 5-9). The four horizontal planes are[6–8,20]:

1. *Cranial base*—separates the spinal and cranial cavities; covers the foramen magnum, and weaves into the meninges.
2. *Thoracic inlet*—crosses the opening at the top of the rib cage running from sternum to the cervical thoracic junction of the spine over the superior aspect of the first ribs.
3. *Diaphragm*—separating the thoracic and abdominopelvic cavities, this domed skeletal muscle is wrapped in several fascial layers that are attached to the vertebrae and inside of the rib cage.
4. *Pelvic diaphragm*—forms a floor for the pelvic girdle.

The purpose of these horizontal planes is similar to that of the superficial bands, that is, to increase the pressure

BOX 5-3 UNDERSTANDING FASCIAL RESPONSES TO MANUAL MANIPULATION: CORNSTARCH MIXTURE

A simple mixture of 2 parts cornstarch and 1 part water provides therapists with a helpful analogy for understanding fascial responses to manual manipulation. When you place your fingertips on the surface and press down quickly into the mixture, you feel resistance to pressure and your fingers only create a slight indentation in the surface. In contrast, the application of slow and shifting pressure is not resisted, and your fingers gradually sink to the bottom of the container.

TABLE 5-1	Fascial Bands	
Name and Number	**Soft Tissue Zone**	**Connecting Spinal Junction**
#7 Eye	Originates on the nose, goes around the eyes, above the ears, and along the occipital ridge, ending just above the occipital ridge	Sphenobasilar
#6 Chin	Broad line that includes the tissue between the mandible and hyoid, passing just below the ear and ending at the junction	Occipital-atlas
#5 Collar	From the manubrium out the subclavius to acromion through supraspinatous fossa to cervical-thoracic junction of the spine	Cervicothoracic
#4 Chest	Around rib cage approximately at the lower margins of pectoralis major on the front, under the armpit, and along the upper horizontal edge of the latissimus dorsi to a firm attachment at T6	Midthoracic or dorsal hinge of the ribcage/spine
#3 Umbilical	Either exactly at umbilicus or midway between umbilicus and costal arch; in both cases lateral—posterior portions of the band cross at the level of the floating ribs and attach at the spine	Thoracolumbar
#2 Inguinal	Follows crest of ilium from posterior superior iliac spine to anterior superior iliac spine, then dips down to follow the inguinal ligament and join just above the pubic bone	Lumbosacral
#1 Groin	Begins at pubic bone, curves around the lateral sides of the torso at greater trochanters before meeting again at sacrum and coccyx	Sacrococcygeal

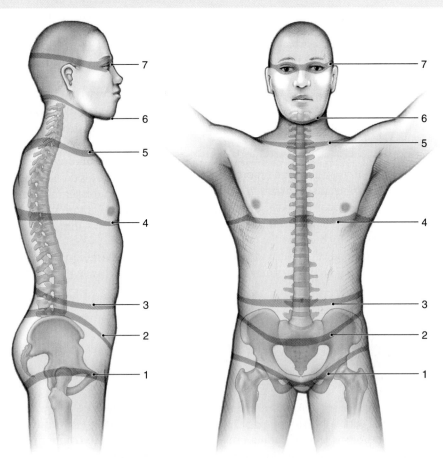

FIGURE 5-7 Seven horizontal bands around the body.

CASE STUDY 5-1

A 45-year-old female triathlete was referred to a sports massage therapist by another athlete she competed with. Her complaint was of constant, aching pain over the anterior aspect of both ankles, which occasionally progressed to aching throughout her anterior compartment. The athlete also said that she sometimes gets aching in her knees and hips and that she has cut her training back because of the pain. The therapist confirmed that there was no numbing or tingling in the foot and that pedal pulses were normal before evaluating the soft tissue. There were multiple trigger/tender points throughout the lower extremity with the most active points being in the anterior tibialis, peroneus longus, hamstrings, and gastrocnemius. The retinaculi of the ankle, fascia of the leg, iliotibial band, and lumbosacral aponeurosis were fibrous and adhered. The massage plan combined myofascial techniques (skin rolling and linear shift) with neuromuscular techniques (trigger point deactivation and contract–relax) from the low back through the plantar fascia. The massage sessions lasted approximately 1.25 hours and were scheduled weekly. The athlete reported an immediate improvement in the intensity of the pain after the first session, although the pain returned about halfway through her next workout. Within 4 weeks, the athlete was completing her full training schedule without pain. The therapist and athlete discussed additional stretches and self-treatment techniques to reduce the muscle tension and established an every other week massage schedule that successfully maintained the treatment results for her full year's schedule of triathlons.

within the body cavities and provide structural strength to the rather "hollow" torso. Each horizontal plane of fascia surrounds and supports major blood vessels, nerves, and organs and connects them to the surrounding muscles and bones. For example, the trachea, esophagus, aorta, vena cava, and thoracic duct of the lymph system all pierce through the thoracic inlet and diaphragm. Clearly, tension or restrictions in the horizontal planes have profound effects on the structures they surround. For example, any excess tension or strain from the scalenes can be translated through the thoracic inlet plane into tension and/or compression of the subclavian artery and brachial plexus. Similarly, tension from the hip adductors and external rotators can translate through the pelvic floor and contribute to sciatic nerve irritation.

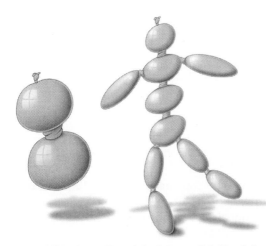

FIGURE 5-8 Horizontal bands in the superficial fascia increase hydrostatic pressure within body regions to help hold us upright.

From the Field

"Myofascial release is an invaluable assessment and treatment tool for my specialty area. When golfers begin taking lessons and making changes in swing mechanics, they may get sore or injured if the new biomechanics exceed their physical capacity at the time. I always evaluate the golfer for specific restrictions in their shoulders and torso and apply the appropriate releases to my students as a part of my instruction. Regular myofascial <u>massage</u> gives most golfers more efficient and effective motion to improve their game and reduces their risk of injury."

Patty Curtiss, MS, ATC

LPGA Teaching Pro

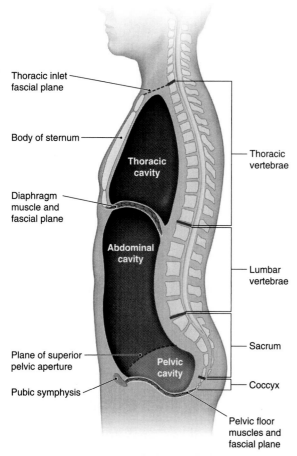

Thoracic inlet
fascial plane

Body of sternum

Thoracic
cavity

Thoracic
vertebrae

Diaphragm
muscle and
fascial plane

Abdominal
cavity

Lumbar
vertebrae

Sacrum

Plane of superior
pelvic aperture

Pelvic
cavity

Pubic symphysis

Coccyx

Pelvic floor
muscles and
fascial plane

FIGURE 5-9 Deep fascia forms four horizontal planes across the dorsal and ventral cavities.

Myofascial Chains

Look at any full-body muscle chart, and you can visually follow a continuous line of fascia/connective tissue from the foot to the head and sometimes over it (Box 5-4). This visible line represents a superficial fascial chain that explains how tension and restriction in one muscle can lead to problems in distant areas—they are connected. The concept of myofascial chains differs slightly from the familiar kinetic chain model, because a kinetic chain is referring only to the transference of contraction force from one muscle to

another. In contrast, a myofascial chain describes the anatomic connective tissue links among muscles, bones, and fascial membranes. These myofascial chains, both superficial and deep, are vertically aligned either as a straight line in the coronal or sagittal planes or as a spiral vertical line traversing all three planes. They provide a pathway for the mechanical communication of tension and compression throughout the body that is tensegrity.[10] For example, the points of attachment for a muscle, the origin and insertion, are not the end points of movement for that muscle because the fascia continues beyond that to the next muscle and bone. The muscle attachments direct a certain percentage of the contractile force directly to the point of attachment, and a portion of that contractile energy is carried beyond that point to the bones and organs connected to that muscle via the fascial network. The key concept is that tension and compression strain in one area of the body is passed through the body along specific myofascial lines that connect far-ranging structures. Knowledge of these myofascial chains provides therapists with a "map" guiding them to a more global view for assessment and treatment of muscle tension and fascial restrictions.

Through numerous dissections and other studies, Thomas Myers[10] has given therapists a clear and concise picture of the anatomic cohesion in the locomotor system and the absolute impossibility of separating function from structure. He also cautions us that these myofascial chains are not *the* one correct analysis of structure and should not be considered as comprehensive explanations of our body's posture, movement, or muscle action. Therapists are encouraged to simply add this information to their present knowledge of musculoskeletal anatomy and kinesiology as a way of increasing their understanding of movement dysfunctions and developing more comprehensive and three-dimensional treatment plans.

For example, 1 of the 11 myofascial chains, the superficial back line (SBL), has two myofascial sections—from toes to knee and knees to forehead. These two sections function as one unit when we are weight-bearing and the knee is extended (Fig.5-10). The SBL plays a vital role in maintaining posture and has the overall function of creating and maintaining *body extension*.[10] Conditions such as plantar fasciitis, Achilles and hamstring tendonitis, chronic low back strain, and even headaches can be related to one another through this SBL.

BOX 5-4 MYOFASCIAL MERIDIANS

Meyers' 11 myofascial meridians (chains) are:
- Superficial back line
- Superficial front line
- Lateral line
- Spiral line

- Arm lines (4: superficial and deep front, superficial and deep back)
- Functional lines (2: anterior and posterior)
- Deep front line

Myofascial chain   Bone attachments

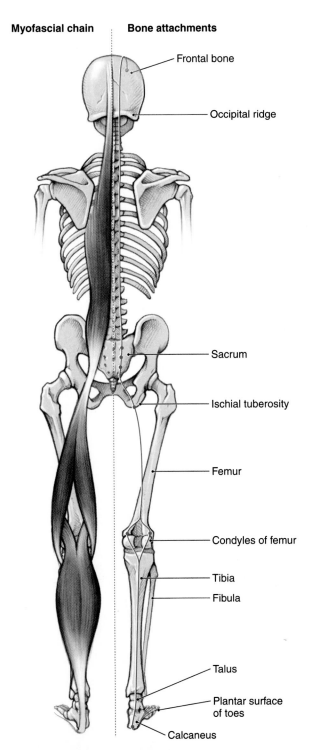

- Frontal bone
- Occipital ridge
- Sacrum
- Ischial tuberosity
- Femur
- Condyles of femur
- Tibia
- Fibula
- Talus
- Plantar surface of toes
- Calcaneus

FIGURE 5-10 Superficial back line (SBL). Myofascial connections of the SBL include the tendons of the toe flexors, the plantar fascia, Achilles tendon, and investing fascia of the gastrocnemius, hamstrings, sacrolumbar aponeurosis, erector spinae, and scalp fascia.

Myofascial chain   Bone attachments

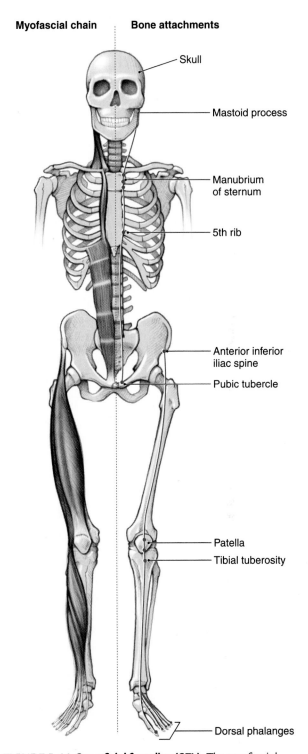

- Skull
- Mastoid process
- Manubrium of sternum
- 5th rib
- Anterior inferior iliac spine
- Pubic tubercle
- Patella
- Tibial tuberosity
- Dorsal phalanges

FIGURE 5-11 Superficial front line (SFL). The myofascial connections of the SFL include the toe extensors, full anterior compartment of the leg, patellar ligament and tendon, rectus femoris (to the anterior inferior iliac spine) and full quadriceps group, rectus abdominis, sternalis/sternochondral fascia, sternocleidomastoid, and the scalp fascia.

Working in opposition to the SBL to maintain posture, the superficial front line (SFL) connects the entire anterior surface of the body. Like the SBL, the SFL really is two segments; from toes to pelvis and pelvis to head (Fig. 5-11). Again, when a person is standing with hips extended, the SFL functions as one integrated line of muscles and fascia. The overall movement function of the SFL can be described as maintaining the general *flexion tension* of our body.[10] Conditions such as tibial stress syndrome, patellar tendonitis, pubic symphysitis, and again headaches all can be related to each other through the superficial front line.

The Functional Myofascial Chains

The functional myofascial chains are made up of muscles and fascial elements that are already included in the superficial chains. However, functional lines are more about powerful movement and not simple standing posture. During dynamic movements, the muscles in the functional line are quite active, both in generating force for the movement and in providing stability and counterbalance to the opposite side. We see athletes combine muscle groups from different regions of the body all the time. For example, dancers connect and balance movements of their feet to the position of head and shoulders, javelin throwers connect the powerful leg muscles to their arms with a twisting movement through the torso, and golfers change the trajectory of their swing (for better or worse) by altering the flex in their knees and weight transference in the feet. These complex movements are accomplished through the functional lines of muscles and fascia. These lines can be described either as carrying the arm line across the torso to the opposite hip and leg, as in pitching, or from the other direction as coming up from the leg and hip across to the opposite shoulder, as in golfing. Figure 5-12 depicts the myofascial connections for the back and front functional lines.[10] By recognizing and considering these functional myofascial lines, therapists can connect the relevance of an old ankle sprain to the throwing mechanics of a baseball pitcher.

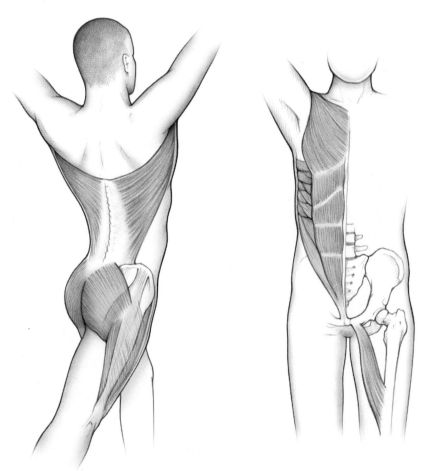

FIGURE 5-12 Anterior and posterior functional lines.

SUMMARY

No sprain, strain, or fracture is simply a local trauma. Myofascial anatomy and the tensegrity concept tell us that ligaments, tendons, periosteum, fascia, and muscles are woven together to form one body-wide system that acts and reacts together.

- Once a specific structural element of a myofascial chain is injured, the other structures in that chain reflect that injury, and need to be investigated and treated to return the athlete to full function.[3,6-8,10-12,15,16,21-24]
- The reality of myofascial chains is that lower extremity structures are connected to the back and beyond. This suggests that athletes may experience a more complete recovery, and reduce their risk of re-injury if myofascial treatment of the full back and hip is included in their treatment.
- Because of the thixotropic nature of all connective tissue, subtle and slow movements of the tissue can lead to profound changes in tissue flexibility, regardless of whether range of motion in a joint is affected. In some cases, the therapeutic goal may simply be to provide a greater sense of ease during movement, and in cases of specific injury, the goal may be to eliminate one or two specific adhesions that are restricting full range of motion.[21-24]
- The fluid properties of connective tissue, and fascia specifically, require that it be fully hydrated to maintain optimal function. When dehydrated, ground substance loses its ability to space and lubricate the fibers within the connective tissue, and thick and adherent tissue is a common result. This is a more probable rationale for recommending increased water intake after a massage than the idea of "flushing out toxins."
- Connective tissue is the very substance for repair and healing. Improperly aligned scar tissue combined with other myofascial chain restrictions leads to changes in biomechanics, range of motion, and muscle power and can create compression and pain in joints.
- Because fascia is rich with proprioceptors and pain receptors, all athletic endeavors rely on the health and vitality of this system. This provides compelling rationale for the regular inclusion of myofascial techniques in the conditioning and treatment regimes for all athletes.

Review Questions

SHORT ANSWERS

1. List the four types of cells common to all connective tissue.

2. Describe the functional relationship between the superficial front and back myofascial chains.

3. Name four muscles in the posterior functional line.

4. Name five of the bony stations/attachment points in the superficial back chain.

5. Name the four horizontal planes of fascia in the body.

MULTIPLE CHOICE

6. Which statement best summarizes the functional importance of muscle architecture?
   a. It determines the line of stress/pull for the muscle and direction of cross-fiber friction for the therapist.
   b. It dictates which muscles are agonist and antagonist for each joint.
   c. It gives the muscle unique shape that distinguishes it from synergists
   d. It dictates the length–strength ratio for each muscle and what type of connective tissue surrounds it.

7. Which of these is an example of organized dense connective tissue?
   a. Fascia
   b. Blood
   c. Tendon
   d. Areolar

8. Fascia is an example of what type of connective tissue?
   a. Organized dense
   b. Disorganized dense
   c. Semipermeable
   d. Organized loose

9. The connective tissue matrix is made up of _____.
   a. cells and molecules
   b. fibrinogen and collagen
   c. elastin and reticulin
   d. fibers and ground substance

10. What is the primary component of ground substance?
    a. Water
    b. Collagen
    c. Fibers
    d. Carbon molecules

11. The ability of fascia to change from a firm and stiff gel state to a soft and pliable sol state is summarized by the term _____.

a. tensegrity
b. semisolid
c. thixotropy
d. extensibility

12. What specialized cell in connective tissue has the ability to migrate to any point in the body and synthesize the specific type of connective tissue used in that area?
    a. Mast cell
    b. Macrophage
    c. Tropocollagen cell
    d. Fibrocyte

13. Which specialized cell is found in all types of connective tissue and releases histamine when stressed or damaged?
    a. Mast cell
    b. Macrophage
    c. Tropocollagen cell
    d. Fibrocyte

14. Tensegrity is best defined as _____.
    a. maintaining structural integrity by shifting/balancing tension and compression
    b. a structure that relies on density and compression to maintain integrity
    c. the hydrostatic tension that holds connective tissue matrix together
    d. the tension component of a muscle's length–strength ratio

15. Which myofascial chain connects the plantar surface of the foot to the frontal bone in the skull?
    a. Deep back line
    b. Superficial back line
    c. Lower functional line
    d. Spiral line

16. What are the most common points of stress/strain in skeletal muscles?
    a. Endomysium and perimysium
    b. Muscle belly and the middle of tendons
    c. Musculotendinous and tenoperiosteal junctions
    d. Epimysium and perimysium

17. What is the functional relevance of the 11 horizontal fascial bands of the body?
    a. They stabilize the spine and attach the appendages to the torso.
    b. They provide hydrostatic tension around the torso to add rigidity and firmness.
    c. They support and separate the abdominopelvic organs.
    d. They provide a medium for force transmission between body regions.

18. What is the purpose of the four horizontal planes of fascia in the body?

a. They transmit force and compression from skeletal muscle contraction to all body regions.
b. They serve as the primary spacers and tension strut between organs in the cavities.
c. They provide broad and deeply invested attachments for thoracic and abdominal muscles.
d. They structurally divide both anterior and posterior cavities and support blood vessels and nerves.

19. Which of these statements best describes a collagen fiber?
    a. Extensible with slow return to original length
    b. Elastic with rapid recoil
    c. Rigid and inflexible
    d. Tough and contractile

20. When histamine is released, what two physiologic responses occur in the surrounding tissues and capillaries?
    a. Increased viscosity and decreased flexibility
    b. Decreased nociception and increased flexibility
    c. Vasodilation and increased membrane permeability
    d. Vasoconstriction and hypoxia

REFERENCES

1. Tortora GJ. Principles of Human Anatomy, 8th ed. Menlo Park, CA: Benjamin Cummings Science Publishing, 1999.
2. Guyton AC, Hall JE. Textbook of Medical Physiology, 9th ed. Philadelphia: WB Saunders, 1996.
3. Juhan D. Job's Body: A Handbook for Bodywork, expanded ed. Barrytown, NY: Station Hill, 1998.
4. Premkumar K. The Massage Connection Anatomy & Physiology, 2nd ed. Baltimore: Lippincott Williams & Wilkins, 2004.
5. Kottke FJ. Therapeutic exercise to maintain mobility. In: Kottke FJ, Lehmann, JF. eds. Krusen's Handbook of Physical Medicine and Rehabilitation, 4th ed. Philadelphia: WB Saunders, 1990.
6. Manheim C. The Myofascial Release Manual, 3rd ed. Thorofare, NJ: Slack, 2001.
7. Barnes JF. Myofascial Release I: Seminar Workbook. Self-published by MFR Seminars, Paoli, PA, 1989.
8. Chaitow L, DeLany JW. Clinical Application of Neuromuscular Techniques, vol. 1: The Upper Body. Edinburgh, New York: Churchill Livingstone, 2000.
9. Barnes JF. The elasto-collagenous complex. Physical Therapy Forum, 1988.
10. Myers TW. Anatomy Trains: Myofascial Meridians for Manual and Movement Therapists. Edinburgh, London, New York: Churchill Livingstone, 2001.
11. Barnes JF. Myofascial Release: The Missing Link in Traditional Treatment. In: Davis CM, ed. Complementary Therapies in Rehabilitation. Thorofare, NJ: Slack, 1997.
12. Schultz RL, Feitis R. The Endless Web: Fascial Anatomy and Physical Reality. Berkeley: North Atlantic Books, 1996.
13. Staubesand J. Zum feinbau der fascia cruris mit berucksichtigung epi-und intrafaszialar nerven. Manuella Medezin 1996;34:196–200.
14. Levin SM. The importance of soft tissues for structural support of the body. In: D'Ambrogio K, Roth GB, eds. Positional Release Therapy. St. Louis: Mosby-Elsevier, 1997.
15. Levin SM. Continuous tension, discontinuous compression: A model for biomechanical support of the body. From Biotensegrity.com.

16. Roth GB. Matrix repatterning™: The structural basis of health. The Roth Institute, Toronto, 2001.

17. Hendrickson T. Massage for Orthopedic Conditions. Baltimore: Lippincott Williams & Wilkins, 2003.

18. Ingber DE. The architecture of life. Scientific American 1998:1. p. 4–8

19. Chaitow L. Soft-Tissue Manipulation: A Practitioner's Guide to the Diagnosis and Treatment of Soft Tissue Dysfunction and Reflex Activity. Rochester, VT: Healing Arts Press, 1988.

20. Zink G, Lawson W. An osteopathic structural examination and functional interpretation of the soma. Osteopathic Annals 1979;12(7): 433–440.

21. Greeneman PE. Principles of Manual Medicine, 3rd ed. Philadelphia: Lippincott Williams & Wilkins, 2003.

22. Sahrmann S. Movement and muscle impairments of the lower extremity. Advanced Track Seminar, NATA National Convention and Clinical Symposium, Nashville, 2000.

23. Denegar CR. Persistent pain and kinetic chain dysfunction: Making the link. Proceedings of NATA Annual Meeting and Clinical Symposium, 2002.

24. Sahrmann SA. Diagnosis and Treatment of Movement Impairment Syndromes. St. Louis: Mosby, 2002.

The Physiology of Healing

After completing this chapter, the reader will be able to:

- Name the three phases of tissue healing.
- List the key physiologic events that mark each stage of healing.
- Explain hematoma organization and granulation tissue formation.
- Define and distinguish primary edema from secondary edema.
- Name at least three variables that affect the extent of signs and symptoms in each phase and the overall rate of healing.
- Name the estimated time frames for each stage of healing.
- Name the therapeutic goals for each stage of healing.
- List at least two signs and symptoms for each stage of healing.
- Name the separate goals of the first and latter halves of the maturation stage of healing.

When athletes are injured, sports health care professionals can choose among many therapeutic modalities for management of that injury. Although some modalities are better suited for pain relief, some for increasing circulation, and others for enhancing balance and strength, all modalities share at least one goal—to facilitate the body's natural healing process and return the athlete to full function. Selecting appropriate treatment modalities and designing a rehabilitation sequence that helps an athlete return to full activity relies on a solid understanding of the predictable physiologic events that occur during the repair process and recognizing their signs and symptoms.

Although healing is a single continuous process, dividing it into three stages—acute, subacute, and maturation—is a helpful organizational tool for discussion and learning. Each stage has a set of key physiologic events that mark its beginning and often overlaps with the ending of the previous stage. These physiological events involve three types of processes: (1) chemical,

(2) vascular, and (3) cellular. These three processes allow the body to clean up debris, create repair tissue, and protect the injured area from infection and further trauma.

The time that it takes the body to progress through the stages of healing varies widely. Type of tissue damaged, severity of the injury, and the individual's general health and immune response are just a few variables that can affect healing time. An estimated time frame for each stage of healing can serve as a helpful subjective indicator to the therapist in determining an appropriate course of treatment. However, more objective indicators should always take precedence over the estimated time frame.

Although the process of healing is generally the same for all tissue, this chapter specifically focuses on healing of skeletal muscles, ligaments, tendons, and fascia. These are the tissues most commonly injured in athletics, as well as most directly affected by the therapeutic massage techniques described in this text.

The Acute Stage

The first stage of healing is the acute or inflammatory phase. It begins at the time of tissue damage and lasts from several hours to 3 or 4 days, depending on the severity of the trauma and the type of tissue(s) that are damaged. The key physiologic events of the acute stage are:

1. hemorrhage and inflammation
2. secondary edema formation
3. pain and muscle spasm
4. hematoma or substrate organization

When strain, sprain, and/or compression trauma occur, blood, intracellular, and interstitial fluids are spilled, or **extravasated**, out of damaged cells, vessels, and tissues. This collective spill, called **exudate**, includes the **hemorrhage** and the resultant collection of fluids to form the **primary edema**. The vascularity of the damaged tissue and the severity of the injury dictate the amount of primary edema. The more extensive the damage, the more exudate formed and the more extensive the repair process will need to be. The vascular response at the time of injury is an immediate vasoconstriction designed to protect against excessive bleeding. Depending on the severity of the tissue damage, the vasoconstriction is brief, ranging from several seconds to several minutes. The blood-clotting process is immediately initiated, and in most cases, the hemorrhage of fluids is controlled within 5 to 10 minutes. This helps the body limit the primary edema to the damaged tissue as best as possible (Fig. 6-1).

The key cellular components in the exudate are platelets, leukocytes, phagocytes, and fibroblasts. Platelets are vital for the clotting process, whereas leukocytes and phagocytes provide immune system protection and clean up dead cells and tissue in the area. The fibroblasts gather during the acute stage to begin repairing tissue as soon as the clean-up crew (leukocytes and phagocytes) is finished.

The **inflammation** part of the acute stage can also be described as **chemical activation.** A plethora of chemicals are released by damaged cells or secreted by surrounding tissues in response to the injury. Chemicals such as kinins, prostaglandins, serotonin, and histamine become a part of the exudate, and each plays a role in creating vasodilation and increasing the permeability of the vessels

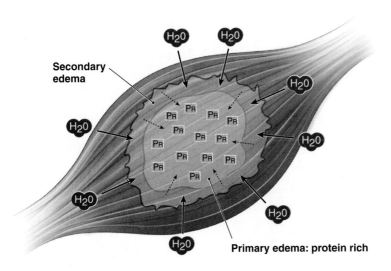

FIGURE 6-1 Primary and secondary edema in the acute stage. Primary edema is the hemorrhaged fluid, cells, and chemicals from the damaged tissue. It includes histamine, plasma proteins, leukocytes and phagocytes, red blood cells, and bradykinins. Secondary edema is the fluid "pulled" from the surrounding healthy tissue due to the increased oncotic pressure of the interstitium. This is why swelling may continue well after the clotting process has stopped the initial hemorrhage.

and tissues in the injured area. The purpose of the vasodilation and increased permeability is to flood the area with the cellular components for healing. The increased permeability also allows large amounts of protein to pass out into the interstitial spaces where they are needed to support the healing process.

The exudate in damaged tissue contains extra cells and fluids from the initial hemorrhage and therefore a high concentration of proteins. This causes an increase in oncotic pressure in the area. Therefore, the primary edema now creates a siphoning effect on the surrounding healthy tissue and pulls fluid out of previously undamaged cells and capillaries in an effort to dilute the large quantity of protein in the initial exudate. This increases the fluid in the interstitium to create **secondary edema** (see Fig. 6-1) and explains why an area of trauma can continue to swell for 24 to 48 hours after initial injury. Secondary edema can dramatically increase the amount of healing/repair that must occur and lead to the unnecessary build-up of repair tissue in surrounding healthy tissue. This can lead to restrictions in range of motion and/or decreases in tissue flexibility.

When tissue is damaged, free nerve endings or pain receptors (nociceptors) that are densely scattered throughout the tissue are exposed and stimulated both by the chemical activation process and by pressure exerted by edema formation. The pain signal to the brain initiates a protective motor response that causes a reflex contraction of the muscles surrounding the injured area. This **muscle splinting** is stimulated in an effort to hold the area still and protect it from further damage. In the acute stage of healing, this protective response should be respected as necessary and normal because it allows the clotting process, cleanup, and hematoma organization to go on undisturbed. Unfortunately, the muscle tension of splinting squeezes the pain receptors and blood vessels, restricting blood flow to the area leading to more pain. This pain leads to further muscle spasm and more pain, establishing the cycle of pain and spasm. If allowed to continue beyond the acute stage, the pain–spasm–pain cycle can hamper the healing process.

After secondary edema formation is controlled and all cellular and chemical components are activated, the exudate begins to get organized. During this process, the leukocytes and phagocytes finish their clean-up and begin to migrate out of the area. The fibroblasts that have been spilled out and called to the area play two important roles in this organization process. First, their presence creates a clotting process in the interstitium within the first several hours of the trauma that isolates the area of inflammation. This is particularly important when the inflammation occurs owing to the presence of pathogens. Second, as the phagocytic actions decrease, fibroblasts begin to move to the perimeter of the exudate and establish a loose-knit net around the exudate. This provides a boundary, or margin, for the repair work that needs to be done (Fig. 6-2). The body has now formed a **hematoma**, which is the last step in the acute stage of the healing cycle.

CASE STUDY 6-1

A good example of the importance of understanding the healing process occurred when one of Karen's regular massage clients limped in for her appointment. The client had sprained her ankle for the third time in a recreational soccer game two nights earlier. She did not want to miss her appointment and was hoping Karen could help her reduce the moderate pain and swelling she was experiencing. Karen asked a few questions and did a quick inspection of the ankle before planning her massage. Yes, she had seen her physician and the diagnosis was a moderate sprain—no fracture. Her doctor put an elastic wrap around the ankle and told her to stay off her feet and ice it for 48 hours. Karen's inspection showed moderate swelling with bright red–purple color around the lateral malleolus, which also felt a little warm to touch. Her client's active range of motion was about half that of the opposite ankle. Karen's massage plan for today:

- A 30-minute session with the client lying supine and the affected leg elevated. Ice was wrapped around the ankle for the first 20 minutes of the massage, and Karen instructed the client to actively move her ankle and foot through whatever pain-free range of motion she had when the ice was removed.
- Ten minutes of classic/Swedish massage for the neck and head, and 10 minutes on the unaffected leg. On the affected leg, Karen performed 20 effleurage strokes from the proximal leg through the thigh and up to the hip, followed by 5 minutes of pétrissage over the same region, and finished with another 20 effleurage strokes.
- Karen gave her client written instructions on how to ice and exercise her ankle over the next few days, and they agreed on another appointment in the following week.

By correctly identifying the acute stage of healing, Karen was able to provide immediate comfort, reduce the pain and swelling, and assist in a rapid and full recovery for her client.

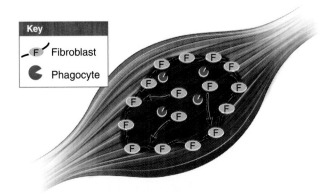

FIGURE 6-2 Margination and hematoma organization.
Numbers of phagocytes and leukocytes decrease as the number of fibroblasts increase and migrate to the perimeter of the exudate. This is the last part of the acute stage and the beginning of the subacute stage of healing.

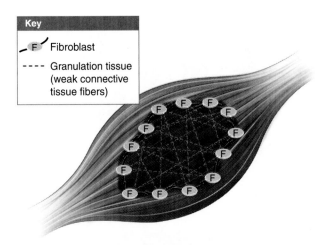

FIGURE 6-3 Formation of granulation fibers. Fibroblasts begin the repair process by forming fragile and disorganized fibers within the hematoma.

The Subacute Stage

The subacute stage, also called the proliferative stage, is considered to be the beginning of true healing. This is when repair connective tissue fibers actually appear in the hematoma. This stage begins around day 4 after the trauma and may continue for up to 6 weeks. It is impossible to determine the exact moment in which hematoma organization is complete and the proliferation of repair tissue begins because the two processes overlap completely. The simultaneous and overlapping physiologic events that mark the subacute stage of healing are:

1. Reabsorption
2. Proliferation of granulation tissue
3. Beginning of collagen remodeling

The term "reabsorption" is used to describe the process of leukocytes and phagocytes returning to circulation via the lymphatic and venous capillary systems after cleaning up the debris from the trauma. This process is very active during hematoma organization, making it the major overlap phase between the acute and subacute stages. As reabsorption is slowing down, the fibroblasts forming the perimeter net around the hematoma begin to synthesize fragile thread-like fibers called **granulation tissue** throughout the hematoma. The granulation tissue is disorganized at first, with fibers cast in every direction across the hematoma (Fig. 6-3). This marks the beginning of the healing process. Once granulation tissue has fully inundated the hematoma, collagen remodeling can begin.

Collagen remodeling is the process of thickening and strengthening the fragile granulation fibers that now crisscross the hematoma into full-strength collagen fibers. The process is called remodeling because some of the granula-

tion threads are dissolved, and those substances are recycled to thicken other fibers. The fibers that thicken are those that are best aligned with the normal lines of stress within the healing tissue. In other words, muscles that have a vertical fiber alignment get the vertical granulation fibers thickened, and those with a horizontal or oblique fiber direction thicken fibers that run along those lines of stress. However, if the healing tissue is not moved within its active pain-free range of motion, normal lines of stress cannot be recognized by the body, and all the granulation tissue threads tend to thicken. Therefore, it is essential to provide pain-free movement during the subacute stage of healing to avoid the development of thick, poorly aligned, and matted repair patches, especially when muscles, ligaments, and tendons are damaged. Disorganized repair patches can disrupt normal tissue function and irritate surrounding healthy tissue (Fig. 6-4).

The Maturation Stage

The key physiologic event in this stage of healing is the continuation and completion of the collagen remodeling process. The granulation tissue has been completely dissolved and recycled by this stage, and fibrocytes are working to produce more collagen to return the area to full tensile strength. The time estimate for the maturation stage can vary widely, ranging from 3 months to a full year before full pain-free function is restored to the area. During the first half of this stage, many collagen fibers are still slightly fragile. Great care must be taken to avoid re-injury to the area, and rehabilitation should focus on creating flexible well-aligned repair tissue and improving pain-free range of motion. In the latter half of this stage,

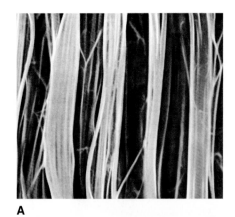

A

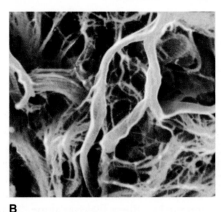

B

FIGURE 6-4 Collagen fiber organization in ligament.
(A) Organized fiber of a ligament in the maturation stage of healing. **(B)** Disorganized arrangement of collagen fibers during the subacute stage.

more vigorous massage and exercise can be used because the collagen fibers have matured and thickened and can withstand more tensile stress.

Signs and Symptoms of Healing

Therapists cannot look inside an area of trauma to identify the physiologic processes actually occurring. Instead, external indicators must be carefully assessed. Because external indicators cannot tell the entire story, therapists must be sure to consider all the objective evidence before moving the treatment forward to modalities appropriate for the next stage of healing.

The external indicators of musculoskeletal trauma and the physiologic processes of healing can be summarized by the mnemonic S.H.A.R.P.

S = swelling
H = heat
A = a loss of function (or asymmetry as an indicator of injury)
R = redness
P = pain

It is important to remember that it is most often the combination of several of these indicators that best points to the stage of healing, no single sign or symptom is a reliable indicator by itself.

■ SIGNS AND SYMPTOMS OF THE ACUTE STAGE

In the acute stage, swelling begins at the initial time of injury (hemorrhage) and continues as long as secondary edema formation is ongoing (generally 24 to 72 hours). Whether this is a first or second injury, the severity of the injury and the type of tissue involved in the trauma are variables that determine how much swelling is associated with the acute stage. For example, mild damage to avascular tissue like the menisci of the knee leads to very little swelling. In contrast, a second-degree ankle sprain results in significant swelling in the joint.

The presence or absence of swelling in the injured area is more meaningful when associated with heat, redness, and sharp pain with movement. Heat and a reddened appearance (*erythema*) over the area of damaged tissue is a clear indicator of the inflammatory process. These two signs are in response to the vasodilation and chemical activation that serves to both irritate the area and increase cellular activity. Although these two indicators generally occur together, the presence of heat alone is enough to indicate acute stage physiology (Box 6-1). There is often a distinct loss of function and sharp pain at the limits of active movement and a dull aching pain at rest in moderate to severe injuries. In contrast, a mild injury generally causes very little loss of function and has limited swelling and pain.

■ SIGNS AND SYMPTOMS OF THE SUBACUTE STAGE

As the subacute stage begins, the amount of swelling starts to decrease. This continues until the end of the subacute stage, when swelling is minimal but may increase slightly after activity. The palpable heat also gradually subsides until there is no difference in temperature between the damaged tissue and the surrounding areas. The reddened appearance of the tissue subsides, and if there was substantial hemorrhage the color changes from red to deep purple and then yellow-green as clean-up and reabsorption continue. Active pain-free range of motion gradually improves to more than 50% of normal before sharp pain is experienced. There is no longer any aching pain at rest, but a mild residual aching may occur after activity.

BOX 6-1 HEMORRHAGE VERSUS INFLAMMATION

Hemorrhage and inflammation should be considered as two different physiologic processes:

Hemorrhage—blood, interstitial/intercellular fluids, and cellular debris poured into the area from damaged tissue; indicated by swelling/edema

Inflammation—the physiologic processes initiated in response to tissue damage, including chemical activation, phagocytosis, and cellular migration; indicated by erythema and increased temperature in the tissue

It is possible to have inflammation without swelling, and either of these signs must be considered as acute-stage indicators even when the other is not present.

From the Field

"In my physical therapy clinical position, I use my manual soft tissue skills on a daily basis. I find myofascial techniques useful when treating patients with chronic pain conditions and believe them to make a significant contribution to the patient's recovery."

Nancy Diehl, MS, PT, ATC

Physical Therapist, Blue Valley SportsCare
Shawnee Mission Medical Center, Overland Park, KS

■ SIGNS AND SYMPTOMS OF THE MATURATION STAGE

The last stage of the healing process continues long after the athlete has returned to activity and may last from 3 months to 1 year. When the athlete demonstrates pain-free active range of motion that is approximately 80% of normal, this indicates maturation-stage physiology. At this point, there is little or no swelling or pain even after activity, and some sport-specific skills can be demonstrated. If the initial injury was to ligaments, testing should confirm that the joint is stable. If there is pain with resistance at the end feel (80% normal range of motion), it indicates that the collagen fibers are not thick and strong enough yet and that healing continues. The collagen remodeling is considered complete when the full range of motion is returned and there is no pain with resistive tests through the full range of motion. Although healing of the injured tissue is now considered complete, the athlete may still require continued functional, kinesthetic, and/or aerobic rehabilitation before full return to activity.

Therapeutic Goals for Each Stage of the Healing Cycle

The overall goal for sports health care therapists is to enhance the body's normal healing process and avoid exacerbation of the injury. Therefore, the goals for each stage of healing are to facilitate the key physiologic processes outlined in the preceding sections.

A general statement of acute-stage treatment goals is to *control and stabilize*. The therapist wants to control the hemorrhage and swelling, decrease pain, and protect the area from further trauma to allow appropriate hematoma organization to occur. In the subacute stage, the therapist attempts to *improve and enhance* the ongoing physiologic processes. The goals are to increase circulation and edema uptake and improve active pain-free movement to encourage well-aligned repair tissue. Continued reduction in pain to interrupt the pain–spasm–pain cycle is also a primary goal in this stage.

In the first half of the maturation stage, the primary goals are to improve pain-free active range of motion and tissue flexibility. During the second half, when approximately 80% of full range of motion has returned and there is no pain with resistance at this point, the goal is to strengthen the repair tissue in the area. Table 6-1 is a summary that compares the physiologic process with the signs and symptoms and outlines the treatment goals for each stage in the healing process.

SUMMARY

- The physiologic process of tissue healing is relatively the same for all tissues and has three phases or stages: acute, subacute, and maturation.
- There is a great deal of overlap between the beginning and ending of each stage in the healing cycle, which is difficult to discern by evaluating the external signs and symptoms.
- The signs and symptoms that help determine the stage of healing are swelling, heat, asymmetry and/or a loss of function, redness, and the quality and intensity of pain.

TABLE 6-1	Summary of Healing Process	
Signs and Symptoms of Each Stage of Healing	**Key Physiological Events in Each Stage**	**Therapeutic Goals/Focus**
Acute (0–4 days)		
Swelling	Hemorrhage	
Erythema and heat in tissue	Inflammation	
Swelling continues	Secondary edema	↓ Secondary edema formation
Sharp pain before tissue resistance	Pain–spasm cycle	↓ Pain (interrupt the pain–spasm cycle)
Swelling has softly defined perimeter	Hematoma organization	Initiate edema uptake
Subacute (day 4–6 weeks)		
Swelling decreases and no heat	Resorption of exudate	Continue ↓ edema and spasm
Discoloration deepens to purple/yellow	Granulation tissue forms	Facilitate formation of flexible and well
↑ Range of motion; pain only at tissue resistance	Decreased pain–spasm	aligned repair fibers
Maturation (3 months–1 year)		
80% Normal pain-free range of motion	Collagen remodeling	Prevent adhesions
Pain with resistance in first half		Facilitate collagen remodeling
No pain with resistance marks second half of this stage		

Modified from Archer PA. Three clinical sports massage approaches for treating injured athletes. Athletic Therapy Today 2001;6(3).

- Although injuries progress through the healing cycle at different rates, an approximate time frame for the acute stage is from several hours to 4 days, whereas the subacute stage is estimated to begin about 4 days after the injury and continue for up to 6 weeks.
- Depending on the severity of an injury and the tissues involved, the maturation stage of healing ranges from 3 months to a full year.

- The treatment goals for the acute stage of healing are to control and stabilize the physiologic processes. The subacute goals are to improve and enhance these processes.
- The first half of the maturation stage of healing is focused on improving flexibility and returning full pain-free movement. Once 80% of the normal pain-free range of motion has returned, the goal shifts to improving strength.

Review Questions

SHORT ANSWERS

1. What does the mnemonic S.H.A.R.P. stand for?

2. Explain the pain–spasm cycle.

3. Define primary and secondary edema, and explain how each is formed.

MULTIPLE CHOICE

4. What stage of the healing cycle has the goals of increasing circulation and preventing the development of adhesions?
   a. Acute
   b. Subacute

   c. Maturation
   d. Chronic

5. In the acute stage of healing, the key physiologic events include hemorrhage, inflammation, and _____.
   a. phagocytosis and a decreasing pain–spasm cycle
   b. reabsorption and collagen remodeling
   c. secondary edema formation and hematoma organization
   d. granulation tissue formation and secondary filtration

6. The approximate duration of the subacute stage of healing is _____.
   a. from day 4 post-trauma to 6 weeks
   b. 24 to 72 hours

c. 3 weeks to 6 months

d. 3 months to 1 year

7. What is the term used to describe the first fragile repair fibers?
   a. Collagen
   b. Fibrocytes
   c. Reticulin
   d. Granulation

8. Which of these signs indicate inflammation in the acute stage of healing?
   a. Sharp pain at tissue limits
   b. Swelling
   c. Purple discoloration in the tissue
   d. Erythema and heat

9. The key physiologic process of the maturation stage of healing is_____.
   a. collagen remodeling
   b. granulation tissue formation
   c. proliferation
   d. margination

10. How much pain-free range of motion should an athlete have before considering the healing process to be in the last stage?
    a. 50%
    b. 75%
    c. 80%
    d. 100%

11. Three variables that affect both the extent of external indicators of healing and the rate of progression through the process include the individual metabolic rate, type of tissue damaged, and _____.
    a. location of the injury
    b. method of evaluation
    c. severity of injury
    d. the medications used on regular basis

12. Which phrase best summarizes the therapeutic goal for the acute stage of healing?
    a. Improve and enhance
    b. Stabilize and control
    c. Strengthen and stretch
    d. Intervene and eradicate

13. Which of these objective measurements would best indicate the readiness of the injured area for a dynamic strengthening program?
    a. No residual swelling after exercise
    b. No pain with resistance at 80% normal range of motion
    c. 80 % normal range of motion
    d. 50% normal range of motion and strength

14. What physiologic event is the end of the acute stage and the overlap to the beginning of the subacute stage?

a. Secondary edema formation

b. Reabsorption of exudate

c. Collagen remodeling

d. Hematoma organization

15. What is the primary influence on secondary edema formation?
    a. Increased oncotic pressure of the interstitium
    b. Histamine release from the mast cells
    c. Volume of primary edema
    d. The immediate vasodilation in the injured tissue

16. To avoid formation of adhesions and encourage strong and flexible repair of the tissue, therapists should_____.
    a. use only heat modalities after the first 48 hours of an injury
    b. encourage pain-free active range of motion throughout the healing process
    c. begin cross-fiber friction massage in the acute stage of healing
    d. start isometric resistive exercises in the acute phase

17. Leukocyte and phagocyte activity is highest in what stage of healing?
    a. Acute
    b. Late maturation
    c. Subacute
    d. Early maturation

18. What is the primary treatment goal for the first half of the maturation stage?
    a. Improve strength
    b. Reduce swelling
    c. Interrupt the pain-spasm cycle
    d. Increase the pain-free active range of motion

19. The swelling related to the amount of exudate from the damaged tissue is called _____.
    a. primary edema
    b. lymphedema
    c. secondary edema
    d. extracellular fluid

20. What type of pain descriptors are commonly used in the subacute stage of healing?
    a. Sharp pain with passive movement
    b. Throbbing pain with active movement
    c. Sharp pain at the end of tissue limits
    d. Constant dull aching pain

REFERENCES

1. Anderson MK, Hall SJ, Martin M. Sports Injury Management, 2nd ed. Philadelphia: Lippincott Williams & Wilkins, 2000.

2. Arnheim DD, Prentice WE. Principles of Athletic Training, 8th ed. St. Louis: Mosby, 1993.

3. Booher JM, Thibodeau GA. Athletic Injury Assessment, 3rd ed. St. Louis: Mosby, 1994.

4. Chaitow L, DeLaney JW. Clinical Application of Neuromuscular Techniques, vol. 1: Upper Body. London: Harcourt Publishers/ Churchill Livingstone, 2000.

5. Guyton AC, Hall JE. Textbook of Medical Physiology, 9th ed. Philadelphia: WB Saunders, 1996.

6. Green E. Tissue healing and massage therapy. Massage Therapy Journal Summer 1987.

7. Hendrickson T. Massage for Orthopedic Conditions. Baltimore: Lippincott Williams & Wilkins, 2003.

8. Kisner C, Colby LA. Therapeutic Exercises: Foundations and Techniques, 2nd ed. Philadelphia: FA Davis, 1990.

9. Knight K. Cryotherapy in sportsmedicine. In: Scribner K, Burke EJ. eds. Relevant Topics in Athletic Training. Ithaca NY, Movement Publications 1978:52–59.

10. Prentice WE. Rehabilitation Techniques in Sports Medicine, 2nd ed. St. Louis: Mosby, 1994.

11. Prentice WE. Rehabilitation Techniques in Sports Medicine and Athletic Training, 4th ed. St. Louis: Mosby, 1998.

12. Starkey C. Therapeutic Modalities, 2nd ed. Philadelphia: FA Davis, 1993.

13. Tortora GJ, Grabowski SR. Principles of Anatomy and Physiology, 8th ed. New York: Biological Sciences Textbooks, Inc. of Harper-Collins Publishers, 1996.

14. Werner R. A Massage Therapist's Guide to Pathology, 3rd ed. Baltimore: Lippincott Williams & Wilkins, 2005.

15. Wilkerson GB. External compression for controlling traumatic edema. Physician and Sports Medicine 1985;13(6):97–106.

16. Woo SL-Y, Buckwalter JA, eds. Injury and repair of the musculoskeletal soft tissues. American Academy of Orthopedic Surgeons Symposium. 1987; Savannah, GA.

17. Zarins B. Soft tissue injury and repair: biomechanical aspects. Int J Sports Med 1982;3:9–11.

18. Hammer WI. Functional Soft Tissue Examination and Treatment by Manual Methods: The Extremities. Gaithersburg, MD: Aspen Publishers, 1991.

19. Lehto M, Jarvinen M, Nelimarkka O. Scar formation after skeletal muscle injury: A histological and autoradiographical study in rats. Archives of Orthopaedic and Traumatic Surgery 1986;104: 366–370.

20. Kottke FJ, Lehmann JF. Krusen's Handbook of Physical Medicine and Rehabilitation, 4th ed. Philadelphia: WB Saunders, 1990.

21. Hunter-Griffin LY. Chairman, Editorial Board. Athletic Training and Sports Medicine, 2nd ed. Park Ridge, IL: American Academy of Orthopaedic Surgeons, 1991.

Therapeutic Massage Techniques for Sports Health Care

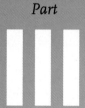

Lymphatic Facilitation Techniques

OBJECTIVES

After completing this chapter, the reader will be able to:

- Name three practical benefits of adding lymphatic facilitation (LF) techniques to common treatment practices for athletic injuries.
- Explain how each step of R.I.C.E. (rest, ice, compression, elevation) addresses acute-stage treatment goals.
- Explain the physiologic rationale that supports LF as a part of standard treatment protocols for athletic injuries.
- Name five absolute and four relative contraindications for LF techniques.
- Name six common attributes of all lymphatic strokes.
- Name and describe two types of LF strokes used in all massage treatments.
- Name the common sites for application of each LF stroke.
- Describe the differences in stroke mechanics between effleurage and the long strokes of LF.
- Name five key body mechanics or working strategies for licensed massage therapists when doing LF.
- Describe the three stages of all LF sequences for traumatic edema.
- Outline an appropriate LF sequence for traumatic edema in any region of the body.

The **lymphatic facilitation** (LF) strokes and treatment guidelines described in this chapter have been adapted and abbreviated for use in sports health care from various comprehensive manual lymph drainage techniques. Originally developed to manage true lymphedema, the effectiveness of these techniques has been well researched and documented for over 60 years by researchers in Europe and Australia[1–12] where the use of manual lymphatic techniques is commonplace in hospitals and physical therapy clinics. Although there is not as much research specifically focused on lymphatic techniques to treat the traumatic edemas common to athletes, it seems logical to project that techniques that are successful in treating true lymphedema should be just as successful, or more successful, when applied to athletes with healthy lymphatic and cardiovascular systems. Empirical and anecdotal evidence from the past decade strongly supports that the rate of healing and an athlete's recovery from exertion may be enhanced by improving edema uptake using manual lymphatic techniques.[1–3,13–16]

There are several practical benefits in adding LF to current management practices for athletic injuries (Box 7-1). First, lymphatic techniques do not require special equipment or supplies, so budgets are not affected. Second, the lymphatic techniques are the only massage strokes that can be safely and effectively used around the site of trauma during the acute phase of healing. In fact, not only are LF strokes safe for acute-stage care, but they also add a new dimension to standard care by stimulating the lymphatic system rather than simply managing cardiovascular changes in the area of trauma. Third, the techniques are simple enough to be taught to the athlete for self-care. By teaching the athlete to perform the basic strokes on themselves, acute-stage care is extended beyond the clinical environment, becoming an

BOX 7-1 BENEFITS OF LYMPHATIC FACILITATION FOR INJURY MANAGEMENT

- ↓ Secondary edema formation via protein removal
- Limit hematoma organization to damaged tissue
- ↓ Pain via gate control and reduced pressure on nociceptors

ongoing treatment for the time between appointments with the therapist. This serves the same purpose as teaching athletes to apply R.I.C.E. to any injury, which is the current standard for care with athletic injuries. If the athlete also includes lymphatic self-massage at home, the overall rate of resolution for the acute stage should be improved.

The Development of Lymphatic Massage

Doctors Emil and Estrid Vodder first coined the term "manual lymphatic drainage" in 1935, and they are universally accepted as the founders of modern manual lymphatic techniques. Their first publication in 1936 listed and described manual lymphatic strokes and the systemic application of those strokes required for reduction of edema. The Vodders originally described four types of strokes: (1) stationary circles, (2) pump techniques, (3) scoop technique, and (4) rotary strokes. Even today, with only a few modern variations on how to combine the four strokes, Vodder certified lymphatic therapists insist on strict adherence to the stroke techniques and treatment sequences as originally described. Doctor Vodder also first described the need for and use of compressive bandages in management of lymphedema.[1,2,4–6]

In the 1950s, a German doctor named Michael Foldi began using and researching the Vodder techniques. He demonstrated that slight modifications in the Vodder strokes and sequences are still effective and in some cases less burdensome for the therapist and patient. He founded an internationally renowned lymphedema treatment and training hospital in Germany, which is still educating therapists and providing care for lymphedema patients.[1,2,4,5,13,14] A third pioneer and innovator in lymphedema treatment is Dr. John Casley-Smith of Adelaide, Australia, whose work and studies in lymphedema treatment began in the 1970s. He was among the first practitioners to emphasize the use of long strokes in manual lymphatic techniques. In addition, Dr. Casley-Smith clarified the effectiveness and appropriate use of a group of drugs, the benzopyrones, for the treatment of lymphedema. His research and treatment protocols demonstrate that benzopyrones facilitate protein lysis that helps the lymphatic system with edema removal

and improves overall management of lymphedema.[1,2,4,5,13,14] More recently, French physician Bruno Chickly has modified and promoted his own blend of lymphatic techniques, thus bringing more visibility to the importance of this therapeutic intervention in the United States.

The strokes and treatment theories from all three schools of thought form the foundation for the LF techniques used in athletic environments. The LF techniques and procedures outlined in this chapter combine the two simplest lymphatic strokes—stationary circles and long strokes—and follow an abbreviated sequence based on the guidelines put forth by Vodder, Casley-Smith, and Foldi.[1–13,14]

Lymphatic Considerations for Standard Care of Injuries

The standard treatment protocol for acute-stage injury care has long been established as a combination of rest, ice, compression, and elevation (R.I.C.E.). There is sound physiologic rationale for each of these steps:

- Rest prevents further trauma and allows hematoma organization to begin.
- Ice reduces pain and spasm, causes vasoconstriction to help control primary edema, and lowers metabolic demand in the tissue to decrease hypoxic tissue death.
- Compression and elevation combine to slow hemorrhage and control primary edema formation.

The R.I.C.E. steps are indeed essential and effective, but they support only the cardiovascular side of acute-stage physiology and do nothing to engage the body's natural edema removal system, the lymphatic system. The exudate in damaged tissue is a protein-rich edema, and the presence of these proteins increases oncotic interstitial pressure, leading to secondary edema formation. To control secondary edema, the proteins must be removed from the interstitium since they cannot be reabsorbed by the capillaries, the only way to do so is to improve edema uptake through the lymphatic system. In 1990, Olszewaski and Engeset[17] demonstrated that external lymphatic massage is as effective as walking at increasing lymph flow. By adding LF to the standard R.I.C.E. measures, both primary and secondary edema formation are managed more effectively, which should limit hematoma organization and prevent proliferation of repair fibers into healthy tissues.

Moreover, the LF technique works with ice to reduce pain, which effectively interrupts the pain—spasm—pain cycle. The pain-reducing effect of LF can be explained by two factors: the gate control theory and reduction of edema. The light pressure and rhythmic movement of the tissue are soothing to the body as a whole and provide additional somatic stimulus (other than cold from the ice) to close the spinal gate to pain. By reducing edema, the LF technique also decreases fluid pressure on the nociceptors to further decrease pain. It is apparent that the addition of LF techniques to standard injury management measures could positively affect the rate of repair and resolution of injuries, thus hastening an athlete's return to activity.

From the Field

"We have found that the addition of lymphatic massage to our standard treatments is very valuable. Swelling is dramatically decreased in a short amount of time. We teach the athletes to do the technique on themselves several times a day, which effectively extends our treatment time during the early stages of injury."

Tara Lepp, ATC/R

Head Athletic Trainer and
Athletic Training Education Program Director
Linfield College, McMinnville, OR

As a separate consideration, therapists are reminded to use great care in their use of elastic wraps and/or compression pumps to control primary and secondary edema formation.

Even though external compression has been shown to be helpful in controlling primary edema, too much pressure in the interstitium—as little as 2 mmHg—can actually reduce edema uptake. In fact, use of elastic wraps and compression pumps without consideration of lymphatic physiology may exacerbate the problem by closing the initial lymphatic vessels and, in some cases, may push the edema away from the natural pattern of flow and the proper catchment.[9,18,19] In treatment of lymphedema, therapists use low-stretch/short-stretch compression wraps rather than the standard elastic bandages. The design of these special wraps and the rationale for their use are thoroughly described in Chapter 14.

Contraindications for Lymphatic Facilitation

As in all treatment modalities, the physiologic changes created by LF can be beneficial or problematic, depending on the status of the local tissue, the general health of the athlete, and the treatment goals for the treatment session (Table 7-1). There are a few *absolute* contraindications in which LF techniques should not be used at all, and some *relative* contraindications, meaning that either extra caution should be taken with LF applications or that specific body regions should be completely avoided.[1,2,4–6,9,10,13,14] In addition to these contraindications, therapists are reminded that the LF techniques described here are for use with traumatic edema only. Cases of circulatory edema and lymphedema must be identified and referred to a certified/licensed lymphedema therapist.

Body Mechanics and Other Considerations

The application of the LF strokes require therapists to stand and work with a more stagnant posture than other massage techniques; therefore, a few adjustments to body mechan-

TABLE 7-1	Contraindications for Lymphatic Facilitation Techniques	
Absolute	**Relative**
Current infection anywhere in the body	Malignant disease
Kidney dysfunction	Monitor closely if hypotensive
Active tuberculosis	Do not work over:
Current thrombosis, embolism, or phlebitis	Thyroid if hyperactive
Congestive heart failure	Sternum if asthmatic
	Open wounds

ics and general working strategies help decrease stress to the therapist but still maintain effectiveness of the technique (Box 7-2). For the therapist to avoid low back strain, the table height should be raised and the athlete positioned closer to the edge of the table than in other forms of massage. This position keeps the therapist from leaning and twisting the torso over the side of the table and allows maximum relaxation of the arms and shoulders. Therapists should use a slight flexion and extension movement in the knees during each stroke application, especially stationary circles, to help them maintain relaxed shoulders and hands. In addition, therapists are encouraged to change sides of the table frequently during the course of the treatment and occasionally to rest the front foot on a low stool to minimize back strain.[13,14]

Lymphatic Facilitation Strokes for Use With Traumatic Edema

To remain consistent with the terminology used in other therapeutic massage techniques, it is necessary to use the term "stroke" when discussing LF, even though the hands of the therapist do not glide over the tissue in most of the applications. To reduce traumatic edema, two physiologic processes must be stimulated: edema uptake and lymph flow. In other words, the LF strokes must open the initial lymph vessels to stimulate edema uptake and then move the fluid through the network of superficial and deep vessels for return to circulation. Only two of the standard manual lymphatic strokes are used in LF for traumatic edema: the stationary circle and a long stroke. As is true of all manual lymphatic strokes, the stationary circle and long stroke have several common attributes that allow them to create these effects.

First, LF strokes use very light pressure, which stretches the dermal layer of skin and must be applied in the general direction of lymph flow (toward the appropriate catchment). The light stretching of the dermis pulls on the anchor filaments of the initial vessels to fully open them for edema uptake. The amount of pressure commonly used in classic effleurage and pétrissage strokes to assist venous flow actu-

ally closes the lymphatic capillaries and can retard edema uptake. There are several different ways to approximate the amount of pressure used in the LF strokes. The weight of a 50-cent coin or eight #10 business envelopes are common examples of the appropriate amount of pressure. However, the best way to approximate the correct pressure is to experience it kinesthetically. Close your eyes, place a fingertip on one of your eyelids, and use the finger to manually move the eyelid over the eyeball. This amount of pressure is the same amount required for the LF strokes to stimulate edema uptake and facilitate lymph flow through the other superficial pathways, such as prelymphatic channels, collecting capillaries, and anastomoses. Second, for a LF stroke to be effective, the tissue must also be completely released and allowed to snap back to its original position. This release and recoil of the tissue closes the initial vessel with enough force to push the lymph into the collecting capillary, thereby reestablishing the negative pressure in the initial vessel to allow more uptake. The repeated opening and closing of the initial vessels create a pumping action at the distal end of the lymphatic network that facilitates edema uptake. In addition, improved edema uptake fills the lymphangia more completely and increases the contractile rate of the angions to further enhance lymph flow.[1,2,20]

Third, all manual lymphatic strokes are applied using a slow and rhythmic pace that approximates the normal autonomic contraction rate of angions. As edema uptake and superficial lymph flow are improved, this rhythm will improve flow within the lymphangia and gradually increase the autonomic contractile rate.[1,2,5,6,12,13,17] Finally, all lymphatic strokes must be applied over the same tissue area for 10 to 20 repetitions before the desired physiologic changes are achieved. Wittlinger[5] uses the analogy of a car stalled at the side of the road to illustrate the need for slow, rhythmic, and repeated strokes. To push the car to the gas station, one must apply slow, gradual pressure against the car that rocks it back and forth a little before getting it into a full rolling motion that pushes it along. This gradual and repeated application of force is much more effective than taking a running start and crashing into the car with a single burst of force. Even repeated applications of a sudden and crashing force moves the car only a few feet. The same is true of edema, requiring that slow rhythmic repetitions be applied to overcome the inertia of the stagnated fluid (Box 7-3).

BOX 7-2 BODY MECHANICS AND WORKING STRATEGIES FOR LF TECHNIQUE

- Raise the height of the table
- Position the athlete at the edge of the table
- Relax your shoulders and arms

- Gently flex and extend your knees during each stroke
- Change sides of the table as often as is appropriate

■ STATIONARY CIRCLES

The term "stationary circle" is a bit misleading because the action part of the stroke does not actually make a full circle. The hand(s) of the therapist do appear to move in a circle, but the tissue is not carried through the full circle. When the tissue is engaged, it is carried through more of an "L" pattern of stretch, then released and allowed to snap back into place, whereas the therapist's hands circle back to re-engage the tissue at the starting point of the stroke (Fig. 7-1). It is essential that the tissue is stretched in two vectors: first *across* the line of lymph flow and then *in line* with lymph flow. The stretch across lymph flow opens the initial vessels for edema uptake, and the stretch in line with lymph flow moves fluid through the superficial pathways toward the appropriate catchment.[1,2,4–6,9,13,14]

Therapists are reminded that the release of tissue after this L stretch is an essential part of the effectiveness of stationary circle strokes, and they must avoid carrying the tissue through the full circle.

To experience the correct pressure and tissue stretch of the stationary circle, practice by placing a hand lightly on the forearm that has your watch or a bracelet. Use the lightest pressure necessary to stretch the tissue horizontally across your forearm, making the watch move with tissue stretch. Now carry that stretch vertically up the length of your forearm, again observing the movement of your watch (see Fig. 7-1). Next, release the tissue completely, so that your watch snaps back into the original position. Stationary circles can be applied with the full hand, flat fingers, or fingertips, depending on the size and shape of the tissue area being worked. The catchments and specific

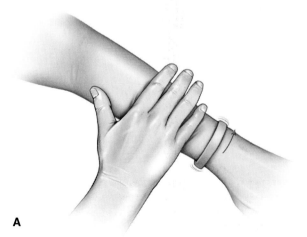
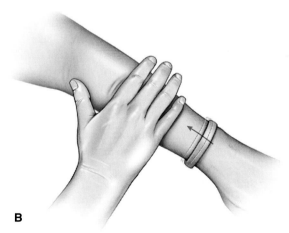

A   **B**

FIGURE 7-1 Practice the stationary circle stroke on your forearm that has a watch or bracelet. (A) First, stretch the skin across the forearm with just enough depth to make the watch move. **(B)** Second, stretch the skin vertically, making the watch move again. To finish the stationary stroke, release the skin completely so the watch returns to the starting position.

When an athlete dislocated her elbow, Dale Perry, a Licensed Massage Therapist and Certified Lymphatic Therapist was called in, and LF was initiated approximately 24 hours after the initial trauma. Before beginning the LF session, the elastic wrap used to hold the half splint in place was removed, and the athlete was seated with her arm comfortably abducted and resting on an adjacent table. The first two sessions consisted of 20 minutes of work in which the terminus and axilla were emptied bilaterally; then edema from the affected axilla was moved first to the back, then across the midsagittal watershed to the opposite axilla. Both axillas were emptied with stationary circles each time the therapist determined via palpation that they were full. When the half-splint was put back on at the end of the session, the standard elastic wrap was replaced by a short-stretch

wrap. The athlete reported that she did not have to loosen the wrap during the night and was able to get a full night's sleep. At her first follow-up with the orthopedist 2 days after the reduction, the doctor was shocked at the improvement in range of motion—now 50% of normal—and that the athlete reported she had not taken any of the prescribed pain medication because she felt just fine after the lymphatic treatments. When external indicators confirmed the injury to be in the subacute stage, long strokes from elbow to axilla and site-specific strokes were added to the daily treatment sessions that were still approximately 20 minutes in duration. The athlete regained 80% of active range of motion in the elbow within 10 days and returned to full activity 1½ weeks earlier than the orthopedist believed possible based on his examination of the initial injury.

areas of edema are the most common sites of application, and 10 to 15 repetitions of stationary circles are generally required to establish edema uptake and flow (see Figs. 7-7 through 7-12). Since the catchments offer 100 times more resistance to lymph flow than other areas of the system, more repetitions of the stationary circle strokes (15 to 20) may be necessary.[1]

■ LONG STROKES

Long strokes are applied by lightly sliding full hands or flat fingers over the surface of the skin. They are generally used in the extremities to stimulate lymph flow through the superficial lymphotomes toward the appropriate catchment. The stroke begins distally and slides in the direction of lymph flow toward the proximal catchment. Like the stationary circle, it is essential that the first part of the stroke stretches the skin to open the initial vessels. This tissue stretch must be maintained as the hands lightly slide over the tissue toward the appropriate catchment. To practice proper application of long strokes, place flat fingers on your forearm just proximal to your watch. Lightly stretch the tissue vertically until you observe the watch move and then slowly slide your hand up to the elbow while maintaining that stretch. When you reach the elbow, release the tissue completely so that your watch snaps back to the original position (Fig. 7-2).

Even though both light effleurage and lymphatic long strokes slide over the skin, they have very different stroke mechanics and create different effects. An effleurage stroke

begins with the therapist applying light to moderate pressure down into the tissue mass. The tissue is pushed proximally with enough pressure to maintain a slight roll of tissue in front of the therapist's hands. In contrast, the long stroke begins with only enough pressure to initiate a dermal stretch. The focus of the long stroke is to maintain the slight stretch in the tissue behind the therapist's hands as they slide proximally. This difference in stroke mechanics is guided by the different intentions of these strokes:

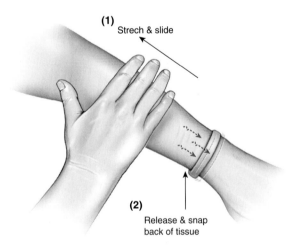

(1) Strech & slide

(2) Release & snap back of tissue

FIGURE 7-2 Practice long strokes in the same manner as stationary strokes. (1) Lightly stretch the skin vertically up the arm making the watch move, then slide over the surface maintaining the stretch up to the elbow before **(2)** releasing the tissue to return to normal position.

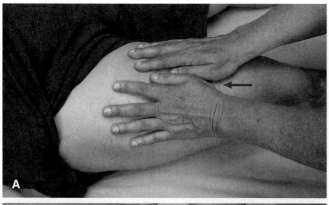

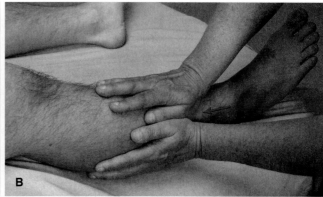

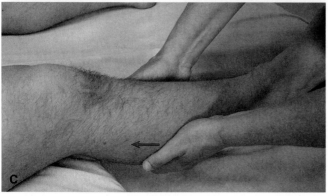

FIGURE 7-3 Long strokes for the lower extremity. (A) Long strokes over the thigh drain the superficial lymphotomes to the inguinal catchment. **(B)** Long strokes from ankle to knee in the anterior pathway stimulate flow to the inguinals. **(C)** Two hands over the posterior calf are used to drain lymphotomes to the popliteal catchment.

effleurage is intended to enhance venous flow, and long strokes are directed toward improving superficial lymph flow. Figure 7-3 shows a variety of long strokes used in the lower extremity. Long strokes for the upper extremity are depicted in Figure 7-4.

RESPIRATORY PUMP: EMPTYING THE DEEP LYMPHATIC STRUCTURES

As established in Chapter 3, compared with the superficial pathways, movement of lymph through the deep lymphatic trunks and ducts is more dependent on skeletal muscle contraction, the arterial pulse, and deep breathing. Because the arterial pulse is not easily increased when movement is limited from injury, the most effective way to enhance lymph flow through the deep structures is to use a specific pattern of hand positions and deep breathing exercises to stimulate the respiratory pump.[2,4,9–14,22]

When the diaphragm contracts and expands during deep breathing, two things happen that facilitate lymph flow. First, the negative pressure within the thoracic cavity decreases the resistance against the thoracic duct; second, the diaphragm mechanically squeezes the cisterna chyli to propel the lymph into the thoracic duct with a little more force. During the exhalation, pressure is taken off the cisterna allowing it to fully fill again. Deep breathing alone increases lymph flow through the thoracic duct by 50%.[4] Therapists can further increase the effectiveness of the respiratory pump by adding external pressure over the cisterna chyli during the inhalation and by releasing that pressure during the exhalation.

From the Field

"We use the Lymphatic Facilitation Techniques and edema tek® compression pads for all soft tissue injuries. It really makes a difference. I'm convinced that without the lymphatic techniques, Gary would not have been able to play in the NBA finals [1995]."

Frank Furtado

Head Athletic Trainer, Seattle Supersonics
Retired 2000

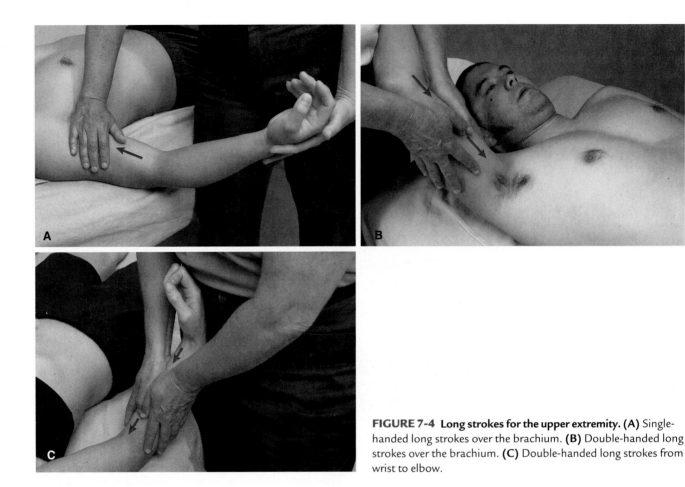

FIGURE 7-4 Long strokes for the upper extremity. (A) Single-handed long strokes over the brachium. **(B)** Double-handed long strokes over the brachium. **(C)** Double-handed long strokes from wrist to elbow.

The pattern of hand positions used in this technique also stimulates lymph flow through the lumbar trunks that carry lymph from the lower extremities into the cisterna chyli. The first hand position used to stimulate the respiratory pump is over the cisterna chyli. The palm of one hand is placed in the middle of the costal space at the base of the sternum with the fingers pointed toward the sternum to approximate the location of the cisterna chyli (Fig. 7-5A). The athlete is instructed to begin moderately deep and slow breathing focused on bringing the air into the bottom of the rib cage to lift the therapist's hand upward. During each inhale, the therapist applies slight manual resistance to the

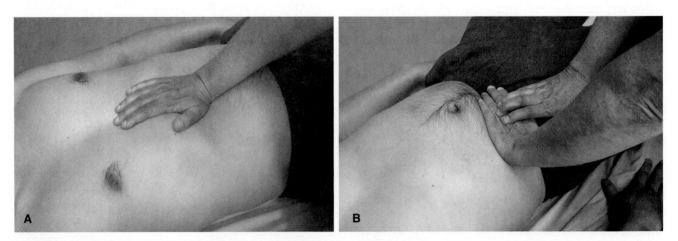

FIGURE 7-5 To stimulate the respiratory pump and empty the cisterna chili, therapists compress or resist expansion on the athlete's inhale and release the pressure on each exhale. (A) Compression over the cisterna. **(B)** Compression over one of the lumbar trunks.

expansion of the tissue, then completely releases that pressure when the athlete exhales. By resisting the tissue during the inhalation, the emptying of the cisterna chyli is enhanced, and the release of pressure during the exhalation allows it to fully fill again. This cycle is repeated for five breaths before the therapist moves his or her hand to one of the lumbar lymphatic trunk positions (Fig. 7-5B) and repeats the coordinated resist–release process for five more breaths. Step 3 in the sequence has the therapist move the hand back to position A to repeat the emptying of the cisterna chyli. Next, the opposite lumbar trunk is emptied in the same fashion as in step 2, and finally, the cisterna is revisited one last time to complete a 6-step inverted V pattern of application.

Athletes can stimulate the respiratory pump on their own by coordinating diaphragmatic deep breathing with a partial sit-up or crunch. To perform this *exhale–crunch* the athlete begins in a resting supine position and takes a deep breath that expands the belly during the inhale. At this point, the athlete forcibly exhales and simultaneously performs an abdominal crunch (Fig. 7-6). The combination of the forced exhale and crunch maneuver creates external compression over the cisterna chili, which empties the cisterna and boosts lymph flow up through the thoracic duct. For maximum effectiveness, this exhale–crunch should be performed five times only; any more than that could lead to hyperventilation. Therapists can assist the athlete in this exhale–crunch method of stimulating the respiratory pump by placing the hand over the athlete's cisterna to help ensure that the inhale expands the stomach and to add light manual compression to the crunch maneuver. The exhale–crunch technique is the recommended method of facilitating the respiratory pump when time is short, such as in event sports massage, and is a key component of an athlete's self-care program during treatment of injuries. However, the full five-step inverted-V pattern is the preferred method when therapists are using LF techniques to treat traumatic edema.[13,14]

Three General Stages of Lymphatic Facilitation Sequences

To improve both edema uptake at the site of trauma and lymph flow throughout the system, the same three-stage treatment procedure and specific stroke pattern are used. The most general description of the LF treatment sequence is that it follows a proximal-to-distal pattern that always begins in the neck, with all strokes being applied in line with lymph flow. This proximal-to-distal procedure is divided into three specific stages:

1. *Start the siphon* by increasing lymph flow back into the cardiovascular system.
2. *Clear the way* by emptying the catchments and superficial pathways proximal to the edema.
3. *Promote edema uptake and superficial flow* at the site of traumatic edema via specific LF strokes.

■ STARTING THE SIPHON

Edema uptake and overall lymph flow can be increased by improving the rate of emptying from the lymphatic ducts back into circulation.[1,2,5–7,13,14,21] When lymph is moved out of the lymphatic terminus into the subclavian veins, it creates a negative pressure inside the lymphatic network, which siphons more lymph through the vascular network of the entire lymph system. Therefore, all LF treatments start the siphon by *opening the neck* with a two-step process. There are two positioning options for this process: either the athlete is lying supine with the therapists at their side, or he or she is seated with the therapist standing behind. The first step is to *fill the terminus* by applying 10 to 15 stationary circles to the lateral neck nodes. The therapist places flat hands on the side of the athlete's neck with index fingers just under the earlobe of the athlete. The two stroke vectors are (1) perpendicular to the neck (either anterior or posterior tissue stretch), then (2) down the neck toward the clavicles (Fig. 7-7). Depending on the length of the athlete's neck and the size of the therapist's hands, lateral neck stationary circles may require one or two hand positions along the side of the neck.

The second step of opening the neck is to *empty the terminus* with 10 to 15 stationary circles at that location of the

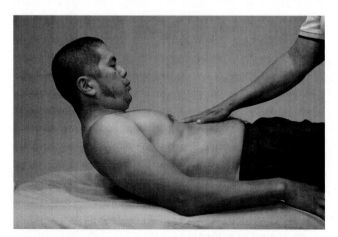

FIGURE 7-6 A faster method of stimulating the respiratory pump and emptying the cisterna is to have the athlete perform 5 exhale–crunches. The athlete performs an abdominal crunch simultaneously with each forced exhale.

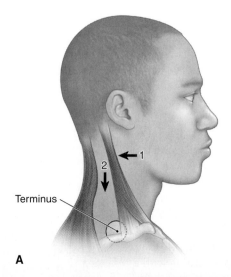

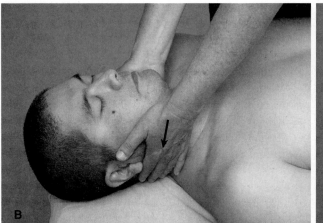

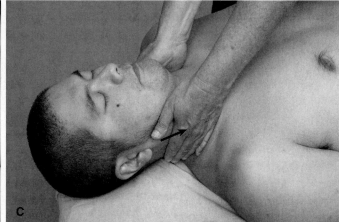

FIGURE 7-7 Filling the terminus. (A) Stationary circles at the lateral neck to fill the terminus. **(B)** Start of the stationary circles at lateral neck. **(C)** Finish of lateral neck with stationary circles.

terminus. The therapist places two or three fingers in the posterior triangle of the neck and first tests the amount of tissue stretch available at this location to determine the starting position for the terminus strokes. Establishing the "stretchy-ness" of the skin is important to ensure that the fingers finish this stationary stroke directly over the terminus. The first vector of tissue stretch pulls the skin down toward the clavicle, and the second vector stretches the skin medially toward the sternocleidomastoid muscle before releasing the tissue to begin the next stroke (Fig. 7-8). Again, approximately 10 to 15 stationary circles are necessary to empty the terminus and establish a strong siphoning effect. Because the siphon effect is such a vital part of improving lymph flow, the terminus strokes are repeated as the *last step* of any LF treatment to ensure that edema removal continues even after the treatment session is finished.

This two-step process of starting the siphon or opening the neck can be taught to the athlete for self-treatment at home. By continuing treatment at home, athletes are able to double the amount of actual treatment time for their injuries and perhaps improve the rate of resolution for the acute and subacute stages of healing. The self-treatment instructions given to athletes must emphasize the need for light touch and focus on the tissue stretch. Remind athletes that it is very difficult to be too light, but very easy to be too deep. The best hand positions for self-treatment of the neck strokes are depicted in Figure 7-9. When the athlete's traumatic edema is in the upper extremity or above the umbilical watershed on the torso, the two-step process of opening the neck is all that is necessary for at-home care. However, when the edema is in the lower extremities or below the umbilical watershed, athletes must add a third element to their self-treatment, the exhale-crunch, to effectively enhance edema uptake and systemic flow.

■ CLEARING THE WAY

Catchments receive lymph from several lymphotomes and create a natural resistance to lymph flow. Therefore, they

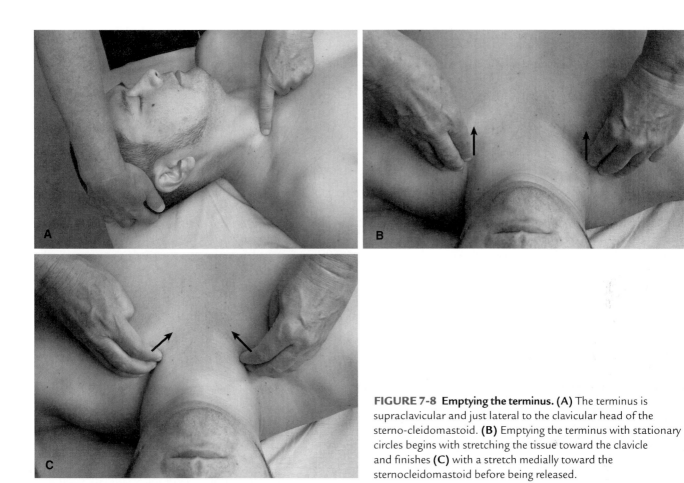

FIGURE 7-8 **Emptying the terminus. (A)** The terminus is supraclavicular and just lateral to the clavicular head of the sterno-cleidomastoid. **(B)** Emptying the terminus with stationary circles begins with stretching the tissue toward the clavicle and finishes **(C)** with a stretch medially toward the sternocleidomastoid before being released.

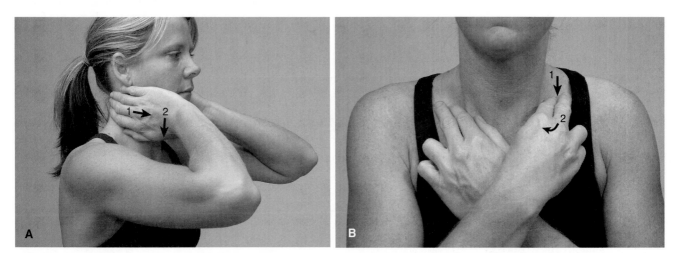

FIGURE 7-9 **Self-treatment of the neck. (A)** Self-treatment for stationary circles to lateral neck. **(B)** Self-treatment for the terminus.

must be cleared or emptied before more lymph can flow into and through them. The application of stationary strokes over a catchment requires two adjustments to the stroke mechanics. First, 15 to 20 stationary circles must be applied, and the amount of pressure used with stationary circles in other areas should be doubled over the catchment because of the depth of the lymph nodes in these areas. Second, the stroke vectors are different over catchments. The first vector for stationary circles in a catchment is simple compression down into the tissue, and the second vector stretches the skin in the line of lymph flow. Another consideration is that proximal catchments must be cleared first. For example, before the inguinal catchment can be effectively cleared, the deep thoracic duct and the cisterna chyli must be emptied via the respiratory pump, and the inguinal catchment should be cleared before the popliteal is treated. Figures 7-10 through 7-12 demonstrate the proper application of stationary circles for clearing of the catchments in both upper and lower extremities.

Once the catchments have been cleared, 5 to 10 long strokes are used to complete the clearing of the superficial pathways between the site of edema and the catchment.[1,13,14] For example, with a sprained wrist the axillary catchment is cleared first, then 10 long strokes are applied from the elbow to the axilla (see Fig. 7-3), and 10 from forearm to elbow (see Fig. 7-4). Although long strokes can be used over the full length of an arm or leg, it is difficult to maintain the necessary tissue stretch across the joint capsules of intervening joints. Therefore, it is better to use long strokes from joint to joint. By emptying the catchments and lymphotomes proximal to the edematous tissue, the siphon effect is intensified and lymph flow is increased. Foldi dramatically demonstrated the importance of clearing the catchments, and the powerful siphon effect that occurs when this is done. His experiments showed that the rate of edema removal was increased by 25% simply by emptying the groin and axillary catchments *on the opposite side* of the body from the target edema.[2,12] Because a significant increase in lymph flow can be stimulated without even working in the edematous limb, it seems logical that lymph flow would be further improved when the catchments and lymphotomes are cleared bilaterally, not just in the edematous extremity. This bilateral clearing of the catchments is a good treatment strategy to use when there is a significant amount of edema associated with a particular injury.

Stimulating lymph flow with contralateral work should also serve as a reminder to therapists that edema may be taken across a watershed from the area of injury into tissue with more open initial vessels and less congested lymphangia. Moving lymph across watersheds can be accomplished with either a series of stationary circles, or if working in the extremities, long strokes can be used. Presuming that athletes have healthy lymphotomes in all areas, moving edema across watersheds can dramatically speed up the reduction of swelling (see Case Study 7-1). Some specific treatment sequences that use this crossing the watershed strategy are described later in the treatment chapter.

■ EDEMA-SPECIFIC WORK

During the acute stage of injury, edema uptake at the site of trauma is sufficiently stimulated by the opening of the terminus and clearing of the catchments and lymphotomes. Once the hematoma is organized and the injury is in the subacute stage of healing, a series of stationary circles can be applied at the outer borders of the secondary edema to facilitate edema uptake at the site of trauma (Fig. 7-13). To begin direct work in an area of traumatic edema, the thera-

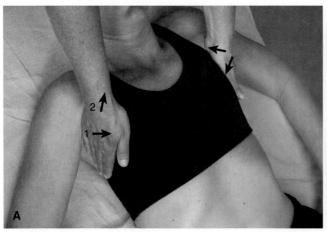
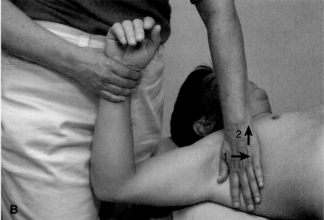

FIGURE 7-10 Clearing/emptying the axillary catchment. (A) Bilateral clearing/emptying of the axillary catchment. **(B)** Unilateral clearing. The hand is first flattened into the chest wall, then stretched on a slight angle toward the athlete's chin before being released (hand is relaxed or cupped).

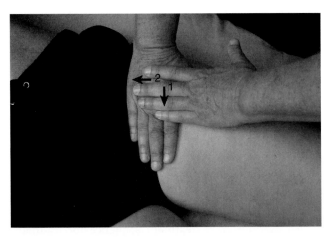

FIGURE 7-11 Clearing/emptying the inguinal catchment. Flat hand is pressed down into the tissue, then stretched on a slight angle toward the athlete's umbilicus before being released.

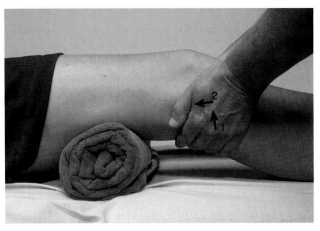

FIGURE 7-12 Clearing/emptying the popliteal catchment. The therapist cups both hands around the knee, so that fingers meet in the middle of the popliteal space. The first vector of stretch is simply up into the tissue, and the second slides the tissue vertically before being released.

pist must first visually inspect and palpate the area to establish the boundaries of the secondary and primary edema. The outer edge of the swelling is the beginning of the secondary edema, and light palpation to the middle of the edema will find a more rigid firm center with palpable boundaries. No lymphatic strokes should be applied over

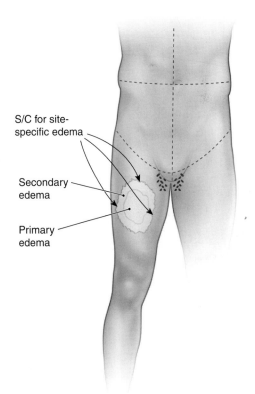

S/C for site-specific edema

Secondary edema

Primary edema

FIGURE 7-13 When performing stationary circles (S/C) specific to the site of edema, begin at the outermost and most proximal edge of the secondary edema. Fingertips or full hand may be used, whichever is most appropriate.

the primary edema, and even the strokes in the secondary edema must begin in the periphery. Edematous tissue is already stretched, so it feels firm to the touch and does not stretch easily at first, emphasizing the importance of stroke repetitions. As the secondary edema resolves, the outer boundary will recede toward the primary edema. However, strokes are still applied to the periphery even when finally addressing the primary edema. In chronic injury conditions that have little or no swelling, the stationary circles can be applied directly at the site of the lesion (the point tender area) to decrease pain and reduce the minute amount of swelling associated with the trauma.

Treatment Sequences for Traumatic Edema

Because there is only one direction of flow and one catchment (axillary) in the upper extremity, the same general sequence of strokes will be applied regardless of the exact location of the injury (Fig. 7-14). The following is an exam-

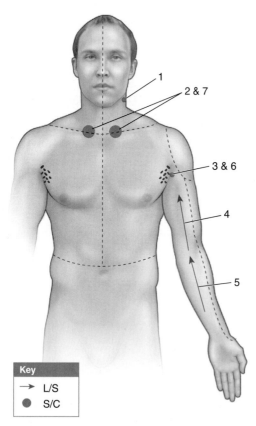

FIGURE 7-14 A step-by-step sequence of strokes for addressing traumatic edema in the upper extremity. L/S, long strokes; S/C, stationary circles.

ple of a treatment sequence for traumatic edema in the upper extremity.

1. Open the neck and empty the terminus (stationary circle).
2. Clear the catchments: axilla for upper extremity edemas.
3. Clear the lymphotomes between the edema and the catchment (long stroke).
4. Begin site-specific work in the periphery of the edema (stationary circle). In cases of large volumes of edema, move the fluid across the nearest watershed(s) to accelerate edema removal.

An example of a treatment sequence for traumatic edema in the lower extremity begins with the same first step, then shifts to focus on the catchments and lymphotomes specific to the legs (Fig. 7-15). Because the anterior watershed runs from the hip to the ankle, all traumatic edema can be routed to the inguinal catchment if desired. However, traumatic edema in the leg is resolved more quickly when the popliteal catchment is also utilized.

1. Open the neck and empty the terminus (stationary circle).
2. Respiratory pump to clear the cisterna chili.
3. Clear the catchments: inguinal and popliteal (stationary circle).
4. Clear the lymphotomes between the edema and the catchment (long stroke).
5. Begin site-specific work in the periphery of the edema (stationary circle). In cases of large volumes of edema, move the fluid across the nearest watershed(s) to accelerate edema removal.

When the edema/hematoma is located on the torso, such as in hip pointers and/or fractured ribs, the lymphatic sequences can follow either the upper or lower body protocols according to the watersheds and catchments most closely associated with the trauma. In these two examples, the hip pointer protocol would be most effective if the lower extremity sequence is used, and the fractured ribs treatment should follow the upper extremity sequence (Fig. 7-16).

Lymphatic Facilitation for Recovery from Exercise

During exercise the capillaries dilate and blood pressure is increased. This leads to a temporary increase in capillary filtration that can leave athletes with a sense of "full or heavy" extremities. It is not uncommon for recreational joggers to experience "puffy" hands after a long run, and competitive swimmers often express that their legs feel heavy on the

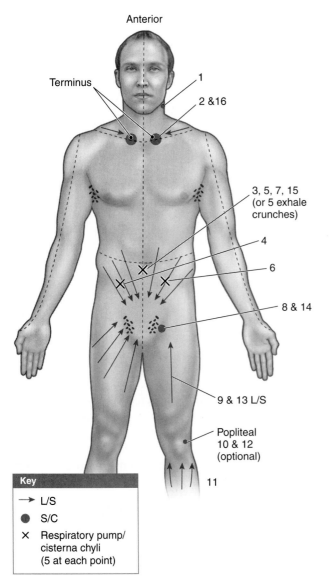

FIGURE 7-15 A step-by-step sequence of strokes for addressing traumatic edema in the lower extremity. L/S, long strokes; S/C, stationary circles.

increase of lymphatic flow gained by opening the neck and clearing the catchments. An important consideration when using LF for recovery from exercise is to evaluate the athlete's clothing/uniform for restrictive areas that block lymph flow. Female athletes must pull tight bathing suit or bra straps off the shoulders and below the axilla to avoid blocking lymph flow and negating the positive effect of the treatment. Of course, proper draping procedure is used in these cases.

■ RECOVERY FROM EXERCISE: UPPER BODY FOCUS

This sequence is most appropriate for swimmers, baseball/softball pitchers, and those in racket sports such as tennis.

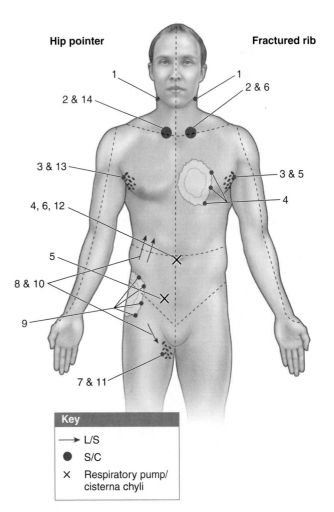

FIGURE 7-16 A step-by-step sequence of strokes for addressing traumatic edema in the torso. The left side of the figure outlines treatment for a fractured rib, and the right is for a hip pointer. Notice how both treatments take advantage of nearby watersheds to maximize the effectiveness of the treatment. L/S, long strokes; S/C, stationary circles.

third day of competition. Generally, the excess filtration that leads to this condition is rapidly relieved with no ill effects by the athlete's cool-down exercises. However, in sports such as swimming, track and field, and tennis in which several competitions occur on the same day and often over a period of several consecutive days, LF can be very helpful in speeding up this recovery process to help keep the athlete feeling as if he or she has "fresh" arms and legs during the course of the event. The sequence of strokes for recovery from exercise is an abbreviated form of the treatment sequences, plus the exhale–crunch technique for clearing the cisterna chyli to clear the lower extremity. When time is particularly short, therapists may also choose to eliminate the long strokes, focusing only on the 25%

CASE STUDY 7-2

The NCAA women's swimming and diving championships in 2000 presented some interesting anecdotal evidence regarding the positive impact of LF with these athletes. The Stanford team had only nine swimmers who were competing against teams of 18 to 20 swimmers, meaning that each of the nine swimmers had to compete in multiple individual events to get enough points to be in contention. Every day each swimmer received a brief LF recovery session of approximately 15 minutes between the morning and evening sessions and again after the evening competition. The championship came down to the last relay on the last day of competition, when Stanford lost the NCAA championships by only a few tenths of a second. The fact that so few swimmers were able to gather so many points over this 4-day competition was a testament both to the high caliber of athletes that these women were and to the value of LF for recovery from exercise.

Just as in the treatment sequence, begin with opening the neck, that is, filling the terminus with lateral neck strokes and emptying the terminus with stationary circles directly over it. Second, clear the axilla bilaterally, then the lateral aspect of the shoulders with a series of stationary circles with hands cupped on either side of the shoulder with the fingers steepled over the acromion. The stationary circles over the shoulder can be applied in a simultaneous fashion with both hands directing lymph flow toward the axilla, or with an alternating motion in which one hand directs fluid to the axilla and the other takes it over the clavicular watershed to drain to the terminus (Fig. 7-17). Next, a series of two to three stationary circles that begin at the midline and progress toward the axilla are applied over the upper back when prone and chest when supine (Fig. 7-18). Depending on the size of the athlete, two or three stationary circles are repeated to reach the axilla, and five sets of these stationary circle reps clear the torso most effectively. If time allows, 5 to 10 long strokes up the arm can be added when the athlete is supine before the axilla is cleared again, and the sequence is finished by clearing the terminus one last time.

1. Open the neck (15 stationary circles at lateral and terminus).
2. Clear the axilla (15 stationary circles).
3. Stationary circles (15) for shoulder with either hand position.
4. Clear the torso to the axilla with 5 sets of 2 to 3 stationary circles.
5. Long strokes (5 to 10) to the elbow to axilla, then wrist to elbow (optional).
6. Repeat axilla: 10 stationary circles.
7. Repeat terminus: 10 stationary circles

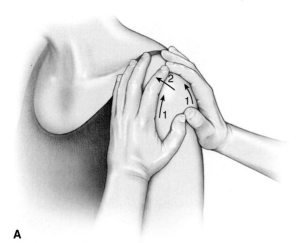

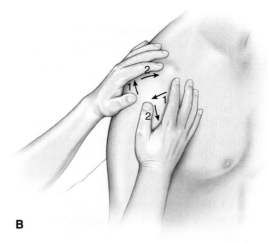

A

B

FIGURE 7-17 A brief lymphatic facilitation technique sequence for recovery from exertion for an upper body athlete should include stationary circles over the rotator cuff and deltoid. Therapists may choose to move all of the fluid toward the axillary catchment as depicted in **(A)** or alternate right hand–left hand stationary circles, as depicted in **(B)** to take some fluid over the clavicular watershed and the other to the axilla.

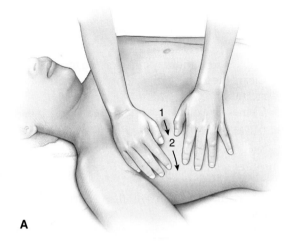

A

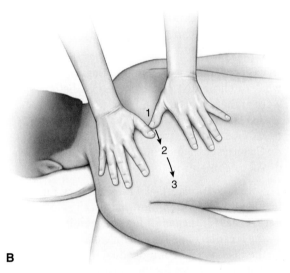

B

FIGURE 7-18 Five sets of three stationary circles performed in a medial-to-lateral pattern of hand placement encourages lymph flow from the torso muscles to the axillary catchment. **(A)** Hand positions over the chest. **(B)** Hand positions over the back.

■ RECOVERY FROM EXERCISE: LOWER BODY FOCUS

For athletes involved in lower body sports (eg, track, cross-country, basketball, swimming), the sequence again begins with stationary circles over the lateral neck then terminus. The second step is to stimulate the respiratory pump, and, for the sake of time, the athlete should perform the exhale-crunches. Next, clear the inguinal and popliteal catchments (see Figs. 7-11 and 7-12), and follow with 10 long strokes up the anterior thigh from knee to hip. Again if time allows, long strokes from ankle to knee with the hands cupped around the full calf will finish the clearing for the lower

extremity (see Fig. 7-3C). The therapist then works back up the limb by clearing the popliteal, then inguinal, catchments; skip the exhale–crunches, and finish with 10 stationary circles at the terminus.

1. Open the neck (15 stationary circles at lateral and terminus).
2. Five exhale–crunches.
3. Clear the inguinal catchment (15 stationary circles).
4. Clear the popliteal catchment (15 stationary circles).
5. Ten long strokes to anterior thigh from knee to inguinal.
6. Ten long strokes on ankle to knee with hands cupped around calf (optional).
7. Ten stationary circles to popliteal if the long strokes in #6 were used.
8. Ten stationary circles to inguinal.
9. Ten stationary circle to terminus.

SUMMARY

These abbreviated lymphatic facilitation (LF) sequences are efficient and effective ways to help athletes' recover physiologically and psychologically from the intense exertion of their sports. However, traumatic edema associated with a specific injury must be treated with the full LF sequence. To review the key points of this chapter:

• When classic/Swedish massage is used to facilitate edema removal, the lymphatic system has not been stimulated. The standard combination of petrissage and effleurage may help reduce swelling by shifting fluid into undamaged tissue areas, which increases the number of lymph and blood capillaries available for fluid reabsorption.
• Only two of the many different manual lymphatic strokes are needed for the LF sequences used in athletics: the stationary circle and long strokes.
• LF strokes must be light, slow, and repeated over the same tissue to be effective.
• All LF sequences can be divided into three distinct stages: starting the siphon effect of the lymphatic system, clearing the proximal catchments and lymphotomes, and addressing the actual site of edema last.
• Therapists can move fluid across watersheds into adjacent lymphotomes and catchments to enhance the resolution of edema at the site of trauma.
• Athletes can carry out effective self-treatment to continue LF therapy at home, which may reduce their recovery time.
• The use of LF technique after periods of prolonged or repeated bouts of exercise may enhance the athlete's recovery process, giving a sense of relief and preparedness for the next workout.

Review Questions

SHORT ANSWERS

1. Name three adjustments to normal massage mechanics and/or working habits that must be made to avoid stress to the therapist and a decrease in effectiveness of lymphatic facilitation (LF) techniques.

2. List the common attributes of all LF strokes and techniques.

3. Name five absolute contraindications for LF.

4. Explain three practical benefits to adding LF to standard acute-stage treatment procedures.

MULTIPLE CHOICE

5. What two vectors of tissue engagement must be used when applying the stationary circle LF strokes?
   a. Rotational and oblique lines across muscle fiber alignment
   b. In line and across the normal lines of lymph flow
   c. In line and across arterial flow lines
   d. Medial and lateral rotation that engages tissue in a full circle around venous flow

6. Which statement accurately describes the key distinction between a long stroke used in LF from an effleurage stroke used in classic massage?
   a. The long stroke uses a distal to proximal direction.
   b. Effleurage cannot move fluid across joint lines whereas long strokes can.
   c. The long stroke technique begins with a light stretch of the superficial tissue whereas effleurage begins with compression.
   d. Effleurage uses less pressure than the long stroke.

7. What type of LF stroke is used to start the siphon at the terminus and clear the catchments?
   a. Stationary circles
   b. Long strokes
   c. Alternating compression
   d. Rotary friction

8. What type of LF stroke is used to clear the lymphotomes in an extremity?
   a. Stationary circles
   b. Long strokes
   c. Alternating compression
   d. Rotary friction

9. Stimulating the respiratory pump to improve lymph flow through the thoracic duct is achieved by having the athlete do deep breathing while the therapist does what?
   a. Applies 10 stationary circles at the terminus
   b. Clears the thorax with 15 to 20 long strokes over the sternum
   c. Clears the axillary catchment
   d. Applies a compression–release over the cisterna chyli matched to the breathing cycle

10. The three general stages of all LF sequences are to first start the siphon,
   a. empty the cisterna chyli, then address the site of edema.
   b. address the site of edema, then push lymph up the vascular network.
   c. clear the lymphotomes and catchments, and address the site of edema last.
   d. empty all catchments of the body, and engage the respiratory pump.

11. In cases of traumatic edema in the upper extremity, what catchment(s) must be cleared before specific work at the site of edema?
   a. Axillary
   b. Cubital and axillary
   c. Cisterna chyli and cubital
   d. All catchments in the body

12. The three self-treatment LF techniques for athletes include teaching them how to start the siphon at the neck, exhale crunches for lower extremity edema, and
   a. the location of all the watersheds.
   b. the flow patterns of individual lymphotomes.
   c. stationary circles for the catchments.
   d. the location and function of anastomoses.

13. The *relative* contraindications for LF include malignant disease, hypotension, and
   a. kidney dysfunction.
   b. varicose veins.
   c. no work over hyperactive thyroid.
   d. systemic lupus erythematosus.

14. The proper amount of pressure used in the LF stroke is approximately equal to the
   a. weight of a 10-cent coin.
   b. weight of a ream of paper.
   c. pressure required to palpate the ischial tuberosity.
   d. pressure required to slide the eyelid over the eye.

15. To overcome the fluid inertia of edema, LF strokes must be slow, light, and
   a. repeated over the same tissue zone.
   b. applied with no more than three strokes to each area treated.
   c. continuously applied for several hours.
   d. applied with abrupt thrusting strokes.

16. The exhale–crunch technique used to empty the cisterna chyli is best described by which of these statements?
    a. Athletes exhale as the therapist bunches up the skin over the terminus.
    b. The athlete performs a half sit-up that hinges at the lower rib cage in conjunction with a forceful exhale.
    c. The therapist exhales to moderate their pressure over the athlete's belly while the athlete performs a full sit-up.
    d. The athlete performs a long, slow exhale that allows the therapist enough access to manually crunch the cisterna chyli.

17. What two steps are involved in starting the siphon of the lymphatic system?
    a. Deep breathing and trunk flexion
    b. Long strokes over the sternum plus exhale-crunches
    c. Stationary circles over the lateral neck and terminus
    d. Deep breathing and clearing all catchments

18. What physiologic process in the acute stage of healing is most affected by the addition of LF strokes?
    a. Amount of primary edema
    b. Level of inflammation
    c. Rate of hematoma organization
    d. Amount of secondary edema

19. When should therapists begin edema-specific LF strokes in the area of trauma?
    a. Immediately in the acute stage
    b. Early in the subacute stage
    c. Late in the subacute stage
    d. Not until the maturation stage

20. After opening the neck and emptying the terminus, what sequences of strokes must precede specific work for traumatic edema in the thigh?
    a. Clear the cisterna chyli, clear the inguinal catchment, long strokes from the area proximal to the edema to the inguinal catchment.
    b. Clear the inguinal catchment, long strokes from the area proximal to the edema to the inguinal catchment, and exhale–crunches.
    c. Long strokes over the sternum, exhale–crunches to clear the cisterna chyli, then clear the inguinal catchment.
    d. Long strokes between the edema and inguinal catchment, clear the inguinal catchment, and clear the cisterna chyli.

REFERENCES

1. Casley-Smith JR. Modern Treatment of Lymphoedema. Adelaide, Australia: Henry Thomas Laboratory, Lymphoedema Association of Australia, 1994.
2. Foldi E, Foldi M. Textbook of Foldi School. Austria: self-published, English translation by Heida Brenneke, 1999.
3. Badger C. Treating lymphoedema. Nursing Times 1996;92(11):84–88.
4. Chagnon SE. Carpal Tunnel Massage Program for Yourself and Others. Course workbook. Chagnon Health Institute, Glen Falls, NY, 1999.
5. Wittlinger H., Wittlinger G. Textbook of Dr. Vodder's Manual Lymph Drainage, vol. 1: Basic Course. 6th English translation revised and edited by Robert H. Harris. Heidelburg, Germany: Karl F. Haug Publishers, 1998.
6. Kasseroller R. Compendium of Dr. Vodder's Manual Lymph Drainage. Heidelburg, Germany: Karl F. Haug Publishers, 1998.
7. Chikly B. Lymph Drainage Therapy: Study Guide for Level 1. France: UI and self-published, 1996, revised 1999.
8. Slade G. (secretary) The lymphedema association of Australia, Inc. newsletter, 1997.
9. Eliska O, Eliskova M. Are peripheral lymphatics damaged by high pressure manual massage? Lymphology 1995;28:21–30.
10. Kurz I. Textbook of Dr. Vodder's Manual Lymph Drainage, vol. 2: Therapy, 3rd ed. Heidelburg, Germany: Karl F. Haug Publishers, 1986.
11. Kurz I. Textbook of Dr. Vodder's Manual Lymphatic Drainage, vol. 3: Treatment Manual. Heidelburg, Germany: Karl F. Haug Publishers, 1986.
12. Foldi M. Treatment of lymphedema. In: Nishi M, Uchino S, Yabuki S. Progress in Lymphology–XII, 1990;95–97.
13. Perry DE, Hanlon H. Lymphatic Techniques for Injury Rehabilitation, vol. 1: Upper Extremities. Course Workbook. Koru Seminars, 2000.
14. Perry DE, Hanlon H. Lymphatic Techniques for Injury Rehabilitation, vol. 2: Lower Body. Course Workbook. Koru Seminars, 2000.
15. Petlund CF. The complex decongestive therapy in lymphedema. In: Nishi M, Uchino S, Yabuki S. Progress in Lymphology–XII 1990;91–94.
16. Kolb P, Denegar C. Traumatic edema and the lymphatic system. Athletic Training 1983:Winter:339–341.
17. Schmid-Schonbein GW. What causes initial lymphatics to expand and compress to form lymph fluid? Fan historic perspective. In: Nishi M, Uchino S, Yabuki S. Progress in Lymphology–XII 1990;205–208.
18. Hooker DN. Intermittent compression devices (Chapter 14). In: Prentice WE, ed. Therapeutic Modalities for Physical Therapists, 2nd ed. New York, McGraw-Hill, 2002.
19. Boris M, Weindorf S, Lasinski BB. The risk of genital edema after external pump compression for lower limb lymphedema. Lymphology 1998;31:15–20.
20. Wallace E et al. Lymphatic system: Lymphatic manipulative techniques. In: Ward RC, ed. Foundations for osteopathic medicine. Baltimore: Williams & Wilkins, 1997.
21. Olszewski WL, Engeset A. Peripheral lymph dynamics. In: Nishi M, Uchino S, Yabuki S. Progress in Lymphology–XII 1990;213–222.
22. Mortimer PS. Managing lymphoedema. Clinical and Experimental Dermatology 1995;20:98–106.

8

Neuromuscular Techniques

After completing this chapter, the reader will be able to:

- **Define neuromuscular release and list at least five names of specific styles of this technique.**
- **Name and define the three major categories of neuromuscular release.**
- **Describe the clinical characteristics of trigger points.**
- **Describe the clinical characteristics of tender points, and distinguish these from trigger point characteristics.**
- **Name at least four proprioceptive neuromuscular release methods, and describe the neuromuscular physiology behind each of them.**
- **Describe the application guidelines for trigger point, tender point, and proprioceptive techniques.**
- **Demonstrate proper trigger point release techniques for selected major muscles.**
- **Demonstrate proper tender point/positional release techniques for selected major muscles.**
- **Demonstrate the proper use of contract-relax, reciprocal inhibition, and passive stimulation of proprioceptors with specific massage.**

One of the most common complaints from athletes is tight and sore muscles that limit either their ability to train or to compete at their highest level. To improve performance, athletes push their bodies to constantly adapt to higher and higher stress loads. These increased demands must be balanced with sufficient recovery time and regular soft tissue treatments to avoid causing injury. However, even if true injury is avoided, occasional delayed-onset muscle soreness, cramps, and tight spots remain an everyday part of athletics that contribute to muscle fatigue, loss of power, poor biomechanics, and painful or limited range of motion.[1–6] All these factors have a negative impact on the athlete's performance potential and ability to recover from intense workouts. The neuromuscular release techniques outlined in this chapter are based on physiologic principles and are effective and efficient methods of relieving the acute and chronic muscle tension/pain conditions so common in ath-

letes. Regular use of neuromuscular release can help to identify tight spots, low-grade tension, and slight movement restrictions before overt injury occurs and to give immediate relief to specific tight spots that crop up during intense workouts and competition to help keep athletes training and performing at their best.

What Is Neuromuscular Release?

Neuromuscular release (NMR) includes any technique that is directed at reducing muscle tension and spasm that restricts range of motion and/or makes that movement painful. Different neuromuscular techniques accomplish this by using several different theories of muscle physiology and reflex activity. Although many different names and styles of work are included under the NMR umbrella (Appendix A), all techniques can be grouped into three major categories based on their shared physiologic rationale. The techniques within each category can easily be incorporated into standard treatment protocols and are supported by adequate clinical data and/or research to indicate that they are effective without significant adverse performance effects when properly administered.[1-6] The three major categories of NMR techniques are:

1. Trigger point
2. Positional release
3. Proprioceptive techniques

Although each style of NMR explains how abnormal muscle tension and focal points of tenderness and spasm might occur by using different terminology and physiologic rationale, each also recognizes the others as effective techniques based on sound physiologic principles. The fact that each style of NMR can claim a high success rate in relieving muscle pain and tension provides strong support for the concept that no single method is correct with the others being wrong. Clearly, many physiologic processes are involved in the development of general tension, pain, and hypersensitive points within muscles. Therefore, it makes sense that multiple therapeutic interventions can be used to address the problem. Perhaps the best approach would be to combine some of the various NMR techniques.

Indications and Contraindications for Neuromuscular Release

Changes in skeletal muscle tension can modify balance, create poor biomechanics in sport specific movements, alter blood chemistry by restricting breathing, and cause stress to the articular surface of bones.[1-6] Because inappropriate muscle tension has such profound and widespread effects, one can logically say that NMR is indicated any time that an athlete has limited and/or painful movement. This should not be interpreted to mean that NMR is either the *only* therapy effective in relieving complaints of limited, painful movement or that NMR *by itself* solves all musculoskeletal problems. NMR is simply a quick and effective means of normalizing muscle tone, and as such is indicated as a primary modality for treating muscular pain.

Contraindications to the use of NMR are relatively few. During the acute stage of a musculoskeletal injury, the muscles surrounding the trauma site go into a protective spasm called **splinting.** This reflex muscle response is designed to avoid more extensive tissue damage by decreasing the movement around the damaged tissue. Therefore, neuromuscular techniques should not be applied directly to muscles involved in the splinting process of the acute stage or over areas of acute swelling/inflammation, open wounds or sutures, local infection, acute rheumatoid arthritis, or malignancy. It is possible that NMR could interfere with the protective muscle splinting, leaving the area unstable and vulnerable to further trauma. NMR may be applied to other body areas that respond to the splinting with general increase in muscle tension, but are in areas not directly traumatized. For example, in an inversion ankle sprain the peroneal muscles specifically, and all other muscles of the lower leg, should not be treated with NMR techniques during the acute phase. However, when an athlete limps or uses crutches during the acute stage, the hamstrings and quadriceps become stressed in new ways. These muscle groups should be investigated for excess tension and/or tender spots and treated with NMR as needed. Early intervention in these and other compensating and supporting muscles minimizes the impact of the trauma on the athlete's body as a whole.[1,7-9]

Proprioceptive Techniques

The techniques in this category of NMR are some of the most available, effective, and easiest to apply of all of therapeutic massage methods. Using active muscle contraction, these techniques reduce muscle tension by stimulating specific neuromuscular reflexes that control muscle tone. This category of NMR includes contract–relax (proprioceptive neuromuscular facilitation), post-isometric relaxation, muscle energy techniques, reciprocal inhibition, and the contract–relax antagonist contract (CRAC) methods. Although each style of proprioceptive technique was developed independently, there is some shared history. In the 1940s, Kabat, Knott, and Voss[10] pioneered a technique they called **proprioceptive neuromuscular facilitation (PNF).** During this same period, Fred Mitchell, Sr, Fred Mitchell, Jr, and Karl Lewit were innovators and proponents of a similar type of bodywork they called **muscle energy techniques (MET).** Travell and Simons[7] credit Lewit with presenting the concepts of **post-isometric relaxation (PIR),** although Mitchell, Sr, originally discussed the concept.[11] Post-isometric relaxation is a technique that has only a few variations from the PNF contract–relax method. With PIR techniques, Lewit added controlled breathing and specific eye movements during the contraction and relaxation phases to improve the effectiveness of the release.[11]

From the Field

"I have regularly worked the finish line of the Chicago marathon with hundreds of my students and faculty since 1984. Both the elite runners and thousands of slower finishers have greatly benefited from the therapeutic sports massage [we provided]. Over the years I have noticed a consistent tightening and spasm of the lumbar erectors among marathon runners, especially the slower finishers, whose tendency is to fall into torso flexion toward the end of the race. I get excellent results from slow compression and fascial lengthening over the lumbar region combined with gentle hip flexor stretches, which are usually performed in a side-lying position."

Robert King, LMT

Founder Chicago School of Massage Therapy, and Sports Massage Specialist

■ GOALS AND CHARACTERISTICS OF PROPRIOCEPTIVE TECHNIQUES

Regardless of the name, all proprioceptive techniques have similar goals: (1) to inhibit muscle spasm that restricts range of motion and causes pain and (2) to enhance the effectiveness of trigger point and positional release techniques. The second goal is in keeping with the idea that a comprehensive treatment for myofascial pain and dysfunction should include all three varieties of NMR as well as other therapeutic massage techniques.

Stimulation of the Golgi tendon organ (GTO) inhibits muscle tension. Stimulation can be achieved through an active process, most commonly isometric contraction, or through a passive process, such as static stretching or tissue compression. Most proprioceptive techniques have common roots with the PNF technique called **contract–relax**. In this technique, the tight muscle, or **target muscle**, is engaged in an isometric contraction and then relaxed.

The contraction phase of this technique decreases muscle tone through stimulation of the GTO, whereas the relaxation, or stop-contracting signal, creates a lag time that allows therapists to lengthen the muscle with less resistance. Because the technique relies on an active contraction of the muscle by the client, Mitchell began calling this same work muscle energy technique, and because the range of motion increase occurs during the relaxation phase that follows the isometric contraction, Lewit termed this same process post-isometric relaxation. A similar proprioceptive neuromuscular facilitation method involving active muscle contraction is called hold–relax. There is a slight technical difference between these two proprioceptive neuromuscular facilitation techniques, specifically whether the athlete or the therapist initiates the movement that signals the active contraction. However, this difference is of little or no consequence if therapists focus their attention on making sure the contraction is isometric and that athletes are clear that the intention is to slowly engage the muscle in less than 25% of a full-strength contraction.

Another proprioceptive neuromuscular facilitation technique, called **reciprocal inhibition** is based on the physiologic principle of reciprocal innervation (Chapter 4). Reciprocal inhibition engages the *antagonist* of the target muscle in isometric contraction to inhibit spasm and tension in the target muscle. This inhibition of the target muscle can be magnified by first engaging the target muscle (contract–relax), then immediately engaging the antagonist (reciprocal inhibition); a technique termed CRAC for the mnemonic of the two steps, contract–relax antagonist contract (Table 8-1).[5,12,13]

Passive stimulation of the GTO involves the application of manual pressure directly to the musculotendinous junction (high-density area for GTOs). Pressing firmly into the musculotendinous junction creates tension in the tendon without muscle contraction and without taking the muscle through a full stretch. To help visualize this, stretch a rubber band between your thumb and index finger. The rubber band represents a muscle tendon, and your thumb is the musculotendinous junction. Now take the fingers of the other hand and press firmly down into the rubber band close to the thumb. The pressure creates a local stretch in the tendon (rubber band) that if sufficient will stimulate the GTOs and inhibit muscle tension.

■ APPLICATION GUIDELINES FOR PROPRIOCEPTIVE TECHNIQUES

All applications of proprioceptive techniques require the athlete to be relaxed and well supported throughout the procedure. The therapist must also be comfortable, stable, and appropriately positioned to resist without strain. All techniques, with the exception of reciprocal inhibition, begin

TABLE 8–1	Proprioceptive Techniques
Contract–relax	**Target Muscles: Hamstrings** Therapist resists athlete's isometric hip extension for approximately 10 seconds, then passively flexes the hip on the relaxation. 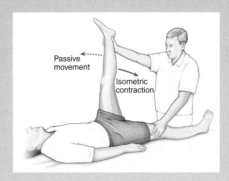
Reciprocal inhibition	**Target Muscle: Gastrocnemius** Therapist engages isometric dorsiflexion for approximately 10 seconds, then passively stretches into plantarflexion. 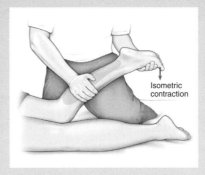
Contract–relax Antagonist–contract	**Target Muscles: Hamstrings** Therapist resists athlete's hip extension approximately 10 seconds. Athlete actively flexes the hip after the isometric contraction. 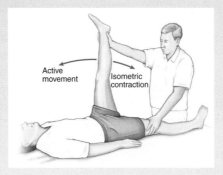

with the assessment of passive range of motion or muscle length tests. During these tests, therapists must assess all the myofascial elements in the region for palpable tension and/or **movement barriers.** Movement barriers can be related to several factors such as muscle tension, fascial restrictions, the structural integrity of joints, edema, or pain. The proprioceptive techniques are designed to reduce movement barriers related to muscle and fascial tension only. Specific evaluation methods to identify fascial restrictions are detailed in Chapter 9.

A 17-year-old top-seeded female tennis player had been complaining of shoulder pain, especially with her serve, for several weeks. A full battery of medical tests ruled out overt muscle or labrum tears, impingement syndrome, and articular cartilage damage. Her physicians referred her to a licensed massage therapist for soft tissue assessment and massage as needed. During subjective information gathering, the athlete reported that the problem had come on gradually and now bothered her every day with a constant ache in her shoulder rated as a 2 to 3 out of 10. The pain became sharp and severe when she contacted the ball on her serve, and it felt as if it went through her whole arm and chest on that side. Objective findings were moderate stretch-pain in the chest at the end of neck extension and shoulder hyperflexion. Resisted medial shoulder rotation showed some mild weakness, and her shoulder pain increased to a 5 by the end of testing. The therapist found active trigger points in the right latissimus and teres major, the clavicular head of the pectoralis major, and the subscapularis in addition to latent points bilaterally along the sternocostal border and upper trapezius. General hypertonicity was evident throughout the upper quadrant.

In the first session, the massage therapist released the active trigger points, followed each release with muscle-specific stretches, and completed the session with general massage on the athlete's back, neck, chest, and both arms. The athlete was instructed in contract–relax stretching for all shoulder and neck motions, which were assigned as homework for the next several days. After 1 week, the athlete had no sharp pain with serving and the aching was only occasional. With continued weekly treatments for the next month, she was able to compete over the 4-day state tournament without any flare-ups and finished higher than she ever had done before.

Contract–Relax

Because the contract–relax proprioceptive technique is the primary component of both muscle energy techniques and post-isometric relaxation, only this procedure is detailed in this section.

1. The tight muscle (target muscle) is passively lengthened within its pain-free range of motion by the therapist until he or she senses the slight tissue resistance that denotes a movement barrier and backs off that point just slightly. Backing off the stretch barrier before the contraction reduces the risk of stimulating the stretch reflex and causing a cramp.
2. The therapist engages the target muscle in a gentle isometric contraction that is just enough to feel the muscle work: 25% or less of maximum. The therapist must carefully match the amount of resistance to the force of the contraction to make this an isometric contraction.
3. The position and contraction are held for 10 to 15 seconds. The therapist counts the seconds out loud and at 10 asks the athlete to take a deep breath and slowly exhale.
4. As the athlete exhales, the therapist must verbally cue the athlete to relax and stop contracting. The therapist continues to hold the initial position until sensing the complete relaxation of the muscle. At that time, the therapist deepens the stretch (follows the tissue release) to the new movement barrier.
5. Repeat steps 2 to 4 until no further improvement in range of motion occurs—approximately three sets.

Reciprocal Inhibition

The procedure for reciprocal inhibition is the same as that outlined for contract–relax but with one key distinction. The muscle engaged in the isometric contraction is the *antagonist* to the tight muscle.[1,13] This technique is useful to use during a massage to soften the tissue for deeper manipulation. For example, during a back massage, work over the rhomboids and mid-trapezius may be enhanced by engaging the shoulder in resisted protraction.

1. The tight muscle (target muscle) is passively lengthened within its pain-free range of motion by the therapist until he or she senses the slight tissue resistance that denotes a movement barrier and backs off that point slightly.
2. The therapist engages the antagonist of the target muscle in a gentle isometric contraction.
3. Repeat steps 3 through 5 from the contract–relax procedure.

Contract–Relax Antagonist Contract (CRAC)

This combination procedure follows the same general outline as the contract–relax technique, but with the athlete engaging in an *active movement* during the relax phase to activate reciprocal inhibition.

1. The tight muscle (target muscle) is passively lengthened within its pain-free range of motion by the therapist until he or she senses the slight tissue resistance that denotes a movement barrier and backs off that point slightly.
2. The therapist engages the target muscle in a gentle isometric contraction for 7 to 10 seconds, counting the seconds out loud. At 8 or 9 seconds, the therapist asks the athlete to take a deep breath and release the contraction while slowly exhaling.
3. The therapist verbally cues the athlete to actively move the limb to a new movement barrier. This engages the antagonist of the target muscle, thus magnifying the inhibition of the target through reciprocal inhibition.
4. Repeat steps 2 through 4 from the contract–relax procedure until no further improvement in range of motion occurs—approximately three sets.[12,13]

Trigger Point Techniques

Trigger points are fibrous nodules within taut bands of tissue that are painful and give rise to a predictable pattern of pain when compressed.[8] Although identified as early as 1915, it wasn't until 1942 that Dr. Janet Travell called these palpable nodules "trigger points" because pressure to them triggered a pattern of referred pain.[7] She substantiated electromyographic activity in the trigger areas and mapped 32 common points and their pain patterns. In 1983, Travell together with Simons published *Myofascial Pain Dysfunction: The Trigger Point Manual*, vol. 1, which became the preeminent resource among manual therapists for trigger point techniques. It remains so to this day. The text also identified the existence of nonmuscular trigger points that can occur in cutaneous, ligamentous, fascial, and periosteal tissue, noting that these points may display some, but not all of the defining characteristics of myofascial trigger points.[7,8] Trigger points are the root cause of a multitude of chronic pain complaints that had previously been labeled as psychosomatic or as other vague conditions such as lumbago and fibrositis. Today, the term **myofascial pain syndrome** is more often applied to these types of regional pain conditions to better describe the composite effect trigger points can have on the entire locomotor system.[7,8,14]

The second volume of *Myofascial Pain and Dysfunction* was published in 1992, and studies by Simons in 1996 and 1997 further clarified the scientific rationale for the pathogenesis of trigger points. Finally, the publication of the second edition of *Myofascial Pain and Dysfunction*, vol. 1, in 1998, offered the most comprehensive understanding of trigger point pathophysiology and a thorough explanation of a number of trigger point release techniques.[1,7] Leon Chaitow and Judith Walker DeLany published *Clinical Application of Neuromuscular Techniques*, vol. 1, in 2000. This text is like an encyclopedia of neuromuscular techniques, providing a source for the theoretical principles and practical applications of the many and varied neuromuscular techniques currently being practiced. What began as a palpation technique for assessment of fibrosity, local spasm, and general muscle tension has now shifted to a primary treatment technique for these conditions (trigger point therapy) simply by shifting the therapist's focus from just locating the tight band and nodule, to treating it by increasing the depth and duration of their pressure over the point.

■ CLINICAL CHARACTERISTICS OF TRIGGER POINTS

When active, trigger points are common sources of an athlete's complaint of regional pain by itself or in association with muscle tension. In some instances, athletes have already located a focal point for the pain and are able to guide the therapist to the trigger point. However, it is more common that athletes are aware only of the muscle tension and general area of pain. Muscles with active or latent trigger points have decreased active and passive range of motion and are resistant to stretch, which helps therapists identify muscles that require further examination with palpation. The muscle harboring the point has a taut band of tissue running in line with the muscle fibers. The first step in identifying this taut band is the application of a sweeping cross-fiber movement over the muscle believed to hold the trigger point (Fig. 8-1). Once this taut band is located, a gliding stroke along the length of the band or a sifting and rolling motion through the muscle fibers with a loose pincer grip leads to the trigger point (Fig. 8-2).

A trigger point is considered active when it is the one currently producing the myofascial pain and limitation, and athletes are generally aware of this dysfunction. However, when athletes describe the area of pain, therapists must remember that they may be indicating the referral pattern for a specific trigger point and the muscle housing the point can be in another area. For example, an athlete complaining of a stress headache and rubbing over the temporal area above the ears is describing the referral zone for a trigger

Taut (palpable) bands in muscle

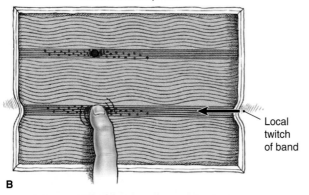

Taut
bands

Relaxed
muscle
fibers

A

Local twitch response

Local
twitch
of band

B

FIGURE 8-1 **Locating trigger points in taut bands. (A)** Palpation
across the muscle fibers identifies the taut band of tissue within
the normal loose fibers. **(B)** Snapping the taut band causes a
twitch response in the skin, and sliding along the band locates the
most tender point. The twitch response may also be elicited with
the therapeutic pressure over the point.

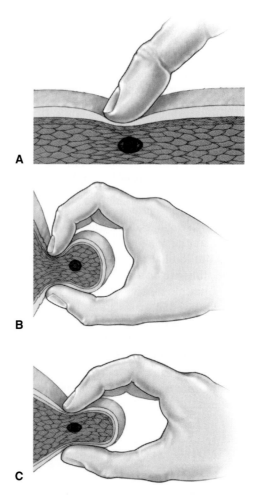

A

B

C

FIGURE 8-2 **Flat palpation of a taut band. (A)** In flat muscle
areas. the tender point is located with superficial pressure.
(B and C) To locate a tender point in muscles with the pincer
grip, use a rolling, sifting motion through the fibers.

point in the suboccipital muscles. Therefore, both the temporal and suboccipital areas must be palpated to determine
the primary source of pain. When compressed, active trigger points reproduce pain recognized by the athlete as part
of their problem and often create a **local twitch response** (see
Fig. 8-1), which is a visible or palpable transient contraction
of fibers within the taut band.[7] At times, this local twitch
response is erroneously referred to as a jump response, a
term now more correctly identified with tender points. The
irritability and sensitivity of trigger points increase in direct
relation to the amount of overload, repetitive use, and/or
overuse of muscles.

Myofascial trigger points share a group of well-defined
characteristics that help therapists distinguish these points
from other tight and/or tender areas in the musculature
(Table 8-2). As previously established, trigger points always
occur in a taut band of tissue, although this band may be
difficult to discern with some deep trigger points and those
located in the attachment areas of muscles.

A trigger point has a distinct feel to it, described as a
thick or fibrous nodule. Normal pressure into this point
causes both sharp local pain and a predictable pattern of
pain specific to the muscle housing the trigger point. This
radiating pattern of pain is not confined to a specific dermatome or myotome, which is consistent with the concept
that trigger points are not caused or mediated by nervous
system lesions. Left untreated, trigger points spread tension and pain throughout the myofascial chain, leading to
measurable motor dysfunction that manifests as restricted
and/or painful movement, reflex cutaneous and/or visceral dysfunction, and persistent pain.[1,7,15]

Travell and Simons[7] go into great detail to distinguish
six distinct types of trigger points based mostly on the location of the point and its sensitivity to pressure. Knowledge
of the different kinds trigger points helps therapists make
appropriate decisions on treatment sequence and may
clarify the need to reassess an area or change the focus of

TABLE 8–2	Identifying Characteristics of Latent and Active Trigger Points[7]
Essential criteria Present in all active and latent trigger points	1. Palpable taut band 2. Nodular feel to the point 3. Exquisite point tenderness to moderate compression 4. Athlete recognizes the pain elicited by compression 5. The pain radiates in a predictable pattern with active trigger points 6. The muscle housing the trigger point has a painful limit to full stretch
Common observations Provide confirmation but may not always be present in trigger points	1. Visual or tactile local twitch response 2. Altered sensation in the muscle housing the trigger point within the typical pain pattern for that trigger point 3. Altered autonomic and/or somatic sensitivity throughout the associated spinal segment

the treatment. For example, if the therapist treats only associated or satellite trigger points, the patient may experience some temporary relief of pain, but the problem of painful and limited motion returns quickly because the key or dominant trigger point has not been removed. In this situation, therapists must reassess the area of complaint to locate the key or dominant trigger point and focus the treatment on relieving this point.

- *Associated*—a trigger point in one muscle that occurs concurrently with a trigger point in another. Often, one trigger point has induced the other, or both may have developed in response to the same mechanical or neurologic dysfunction.
- *Attachment*—a trigger point located at the musculotendinous or tenoperiosteal junction of the muscle at the ends of the taut band of tissue. This trigger point is often the result of the constant strain produced by the central trigger point.
- *Central*—a myofascial trigger point located near the center of a muscle and is associated with the motor end plate for that muscle.
- *Key*—the trigger point responsible for activating one or more satellite trigger points. Inactivation of this trigger point also inactivates several surrounding trigger points.
- *Satellite*—a central trigger point that develops in response to a key trigger point. (This relationship is often not identified until inactivation of the key trigger point also inactivates the satellite.) The satellite trigger point can develop in the synergist or antagonist of the muscle harboring the key trigger point, the referral zone of the key, or in a muscle with shared innervation.
- *Latent*—painful only when palpated, with the individual often unaware of this tender area until pressure is applied. Compression of latent trigger points does not reproduce the pattern of pain associated with the athlete's current complaint, but may create a familiar aching sensation that can be associated with past trauma.[7]

The associated, attachment, central, or satellite trigger points may be active or latent points, and they shift between these two levels of activity as muscular activity and/or therapeutic intervention alters the myofascial environment. Figure 8-3 depicts several common trigger points from the paraspinal muscles and the pattern of pain associated with each point.

■ APPLICATION GUIDELINES

After assessment confirms the presence of a trigger point, therapists have several trigger point–specific techniques to choose from for relief of the point, all based on understanding the physiologic processes of trigger point development (Chapter 4). Deactivation or release of trigger points can be accomplished in a variety of ways, including injection of a local anesthesia, dry needling (acupuncture), application of a spray coolant followed by stretch, or through manual soft tissue techniques. Injections must be performed by a physician, and dry needling may be used by a physician or licensed acupuncturist. Generally, the spray and stretch techniques are also outside the scope of practice for massage therapists, so the manual soft tissue techniques are the best therapeutic choice for most therapists. One of the most common manual techniques for trigger point deactivation is general massage focused on deep kneading, deep long strokes, and stretching of the muscle. However, the application of specific trigger point release techniques has proved to be the most effective manual soft tissue technique.[1,7,8]

The key principle of trigger point release is to create a *mechanical barrier* to the actin–myosin bonding that forms the contraction knot.[1,7,15] To do this, therapists use their fingers, thumbs, and/or elbows to apply specific pressure into the hypersensitive nodule (trigger point) to push the contracted sarcomeres apart (Fig. 8-4) and wait for the knot to

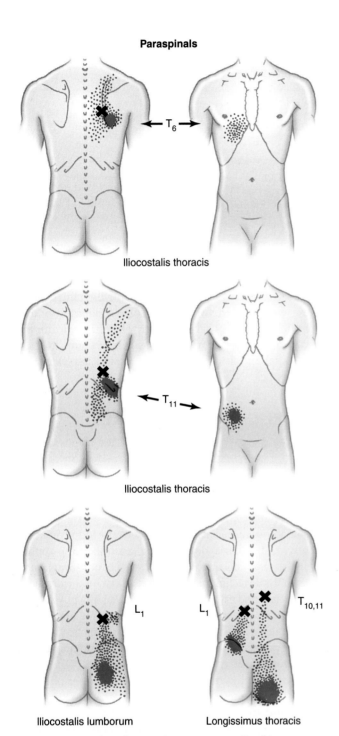

FIGURE 8-3 Active trigger points create a predictable pattern of pain when compressed that is specific to the muscle housing the point. The X marks the location of the point, and the stippling indicates the pattern of pain associated with that trigger point. The dense coloration in the stippling indicates the area of most intense pain.

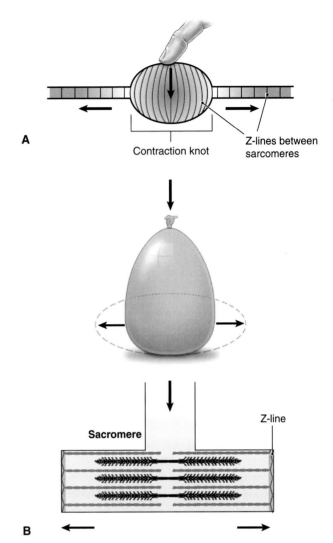

FIGURE 8-4 Trigger points are relieved by creating a mechanical barrier to the contraction knot in the sarcomeres. (A) Therapeutic pressure over the tender nodule separates sarcomeres, **(B)** similar to the way pushing down on a balloon causes its sides to expand and move farther apart.

gently release. In the past, the amount of pressure used for trigger point release has been improperly described as ischemic pressure, which seems to call for deep compression that creates pain. The amount of pressure applied over the point may create discomfort for the athlete, but should *not* create a sharp increase in the athlete's pain. On a pain scale of 1 to 10, with 1 being barely noticeable and 10 being excruciating, the proper **therapeutic pressure** for trigger point release should be described as a 5 or 6 by the athlete. Usually, therapists feel light tissue resistance at this pain level. However, therapists must regulate their pressure according to the athlete's level of pain regardless of their own sense of the tissue. This therapeutic pressure must be held until the muscle tension is felt to completely release, generally 30 to 90 seconds.[7,8,15]

The sensation of a trigger point release can sometimes feel sudden, like a rubber band snapping, but more often it feels like a slow melting of the tissue. Therapists should follow the melting tissue by gradually increasing their pressure to meet each new tissue barrier as it occurs.

Although trigger points can be relieved in only 15 to 30 seconds, this method requires a more aggressive application of pressure that elicits a 7 or 8 pain response, which is not recommended. Recent research seems to indicate that this short and aggressive style of trigger point deactivation may actually damage the muscle, as demonstrated by high levels of hemoglobin in the area immediately after the technique has been applied.[15] A step-by-step outline of a trigger point release treatment that is not specific to any particular muscle looks like this:

1. Palpate the athlete's indicated area of pain and limitation *and* the muscles that could create that area of pain with an active trigger point.

2. Once the key trigger point is located (recreates the athlete's pain), position the muscle housing the trigger point for the best access into the point that also keeps the athlete stable and relaxed.

3. Apply a moderate amount of pressure over the point with fingers, thumb, or elbow until you sense resistance, constantly checking in with the athlete to avoid going beyond the 5 to 6 pain level.

4. Hold the point for approximately 90 seconds and gradually increase pressure into the point, taking up the slack created by the layer-by-layer release of the point.

5. At the end of this time frame, gradually lift out of the tissue and apply a light stretch to the area for 15 to 30 seconds to further encourage release of the contraction knot.

Once the key trigger point has been deactivated, therapists should proceed with the evaluation to locate and deactivate any attachment or latent trigger points. Myofascial pain syndromes caused by trigger points are rarely fully relieved if only one or two trigger points are deactivated.[1,4,5,7,16,17] Trigger points that have developed in response to acute overload or overuse seem to respond more readily to the trigger point release procedure than those related to long-term overuse syndromes, especially if a significant amount of tissue fibrosis has developed.

The over-use, mis-use, or abuse patterns that activated the point must be identified and changed for complete resolution of these chronic syndromes. Several *perpetuating factors* that may cause the trigger point to reactivate include incomplete initial treatment, poor nutrition, occupational stresses, hypometabolic disease, structural imbalances, and psychological or emotional distress.[1,7,8]

■ TRIGGER POINT DEACTIVATION FOR SELECTED MUSCLES

Persistent and chronic pain syndromes may have many trigger points in many muscles, requiring a series of treatment sessions over an extended period of time (Figs 8-5 through 8-9). When this kind of extensive trigger point therapy is needed, athletes commonly experience some general discomfort after their session. Research has established that approximately 30% of patients who receive extensive trigger point treatment sessions report general muscle soreness similar to an overexercised feeling or flu-like symptoms for 24 to 48 hours after the sessions. The incidence and intensity of this side effect can be reduced by limiting the total number of points treated in a single session to six or eight and by treating no more than three of four trigger points in the same muscle.

In addition, therapists should encourage the athlete to drink 6 to 8 glasses of water during the 8 to 12 hours after treatment to help rehydrate the tissue and restore proper lubrication and spacing between collagen and muscle fibers.[1,7,8,17] Because it is far more common for athletes to seek relief from the pain and restriction in acute overload or overuse strain trigger points, therapists often only need to treat three or four trigger points to provide full relief. However, after the trigger points have been released, it is essential for the affected muscle to be stretched to prevent re-irritation of the point, and the activating/perpetuating factors must be discovered and eliminated.

Positional Release Techniques

The use of body positioning to relieve pain and to achieve physical and mental balance can be traced back thousands of years through practices such as yoga. Modern positional release techniques date back to the late 1940s, when Hoover introduced a technique he called *functional technique.*[18] This technique relied on placing the body in a position of *dynamic reciprocal balance* for relief of movement dysfunctions.[5] Hoover's method did not rely on locating specific tender spots, but on assessing movement restrictions through palpation and range-of-motion testing and then moving the patient toward the position of least resistance to reduce muscle tension and allow the body to resolve the problem spontaneously rather than movement into the barrier for stretch. At this same time, Denslow and Korr proposed the theory of facilitated spinal segments.[4] Their research indicated that the hypersensitive myofascial points found in muscle were indicators of facilitated or hypersensitive spinal segments. The facilitated segment theory provided the physiologic explanation for the common clin-

Suboccipitals

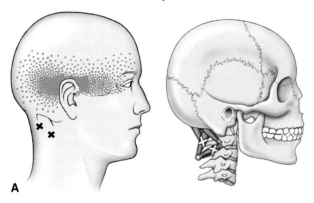

A

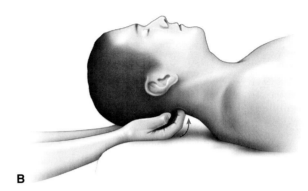

B

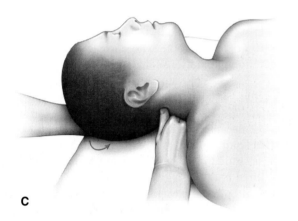

C

FIGURE 8-5 Trigger points in the suboccipitals create "stress headache" pain across the temporal region from the occipital to frontal bones. Common activating/perpetuating factors include emotional stress and active trigger points in the trapezius. Suboccipital trigger points are not common sources of neck *pain,* but may contribute to *limited rotation* of the neck. **(A)** Location. **(B)** Method of release for across the full muscle group: Fingers are curled up and under the occiput. **(C)** Single trigger point release is accomplished by placing one thumb over the point, then extending and rotating the head over the point pressure.

ical findings of restriction and dysfunction in muscles and organs other than those harboring the hypersensitive point, and how decreasing the sensitivity of the point also tends to resolve other somatovisceral problems.[1,2,4,5,7,8,17,19–23]

Although no single researcher or clinician can be credited with the development of the positional release techniques, the man widely credited as being the most influential is Dr. Lawrence Jones, DO. In 1954, Jones found that he could correlate findings of a specific tender spot in muscles with a specific movement dysfunction within the facilitated segment, and he began mapping these points. He initially called these trigger points, based on his reading of Travell's work, but later changed the term to tender point because he found that the points he was mapping did not meet the criteria set forth to be called a trigger point. Specifically, his points were hypersensitive to pressure, but did not refer pain, were often in the antagonists of muscles that the patient perceived as being tight, and did not always have a distinctive fibrous or nodular feel to them to indicate that the point itself was a site of pathology. Jones found that passively moving the patient to the position of comfort was the key to reducing the sensitivity of these tender points, which then relieved the movement dysfunction. He called his method of NMR *Strain Counterstrain* and first published his assessment and treat-

ment methods in 1964.[4,5,19] Several clinicians and researchers through the 1980s and 1990s modified Jones's work slightly[1–4,24] and named the technique *positional release* as a more accurate descriptor for the method of treatment.

■ CLINICAL CHARACTERISTICS OF TENDER POINTS

A tender point (TeP) is a small zone of tense and exquisitely tender myofascial tissue that represents a facilitated segment of the spinal cord. Although it may feel mildly edematous and/or slightly firmer than surrounding tissue, it does not have the distinct nodular and fibrous feel of a trigger point nor does it radiate pain when pressure is applied.[1,2,4,5,25] Tender points commonly occur at muscle attachments and are often located in the antagonist of a muscle that is perceived as tight by the athlete. In fact, Jones claims that 50% of the dysfunction that produces pain on the posterior side of the body is represented on the anterior aspect of the body as tender points.[25] Another distinction between TePs and TrPs is that compression palpation over a tender point does not elicit a

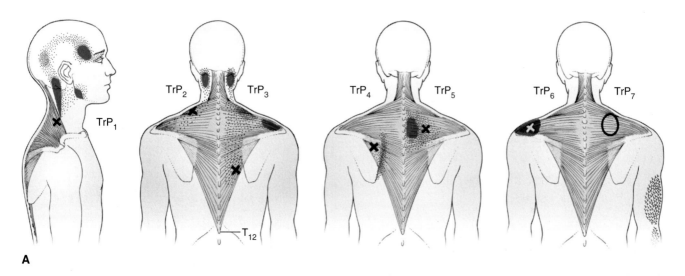

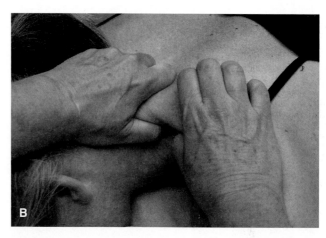

FIGURE 8-6　Trigger points (TrP) in the trapezius. (A) Location of TrPs in the trapezius and the associated pain patterns. Activating/perpetuating factors for these points include tension in the pectoral muscles, such as occurs in the upper crossed postural dysfunction. TrPs in the trapezius can cause satellite points in the temporalis and occipital muscles and can mimic tension headaches. **(B)** Deactivation of the TrP with direct therapeutic compression.

local twitch response. Instead, the athlete tends to flinch and/or pull away from the point pressure—a **jump response.** Because there is no taut band or nodular feel to tender points, this jump response is considered a key indicator for confirming the presence of a tender point. It is also common for dominant tender points, like dominant trigger points, to create satellite points in surrounding areas. Pressure over a satellite tender point does not elicit the jump response, but it is more sensitive than the surrounding tissue. Because tender points do not radiate pain, but are hypersensitive and restrict movement, it has been speculated that tender points may actually be latent trigger points. However, there is no clear evidence to prove or disprove this idea other than the high correlation between point locations.

There is a significant difference between the pathophysiology of how a contracture knot of a trigger point develops and the development of the localized spasm associated with a tender point. The contracture knot in a trigger point is a localized sarcomere contraction due to

tearing of the sarcoplasmic reticulum or motor end plate of a sarcomere. In contrast, the local spasm associated with a tender point is of *neuromuscular origin,* because it occurs in response to a stretch reflex signal from the muscle spindle.[1,2,4,5,16,24–27] Another distinction is that unlike trigger points, tender points are not thought of as the actual site of pathology (contraction knot). Instead, tender points are considered *diagnostic points* that indicate stress and strain in that muscle and/or joint owing to a facilitated (hypersensitive) spinal segment. Specifically, the point indicates hypersensitive muscle spindles in the muscle housing the tender point and that a false stretch reflex contraction has been signaled. By deactivating the tender point, the hypersensitivity of the spinal segment is also diminished and seemingly unrelated pathologies and dysfunctions are eased. In addition, dominant tender points may stimulate the development of satellite points (Figures 8-10 through 8-13 are examples of tender point releases for several common points among athletes).

Quadratus Lumborum

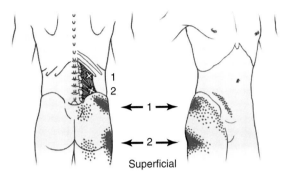

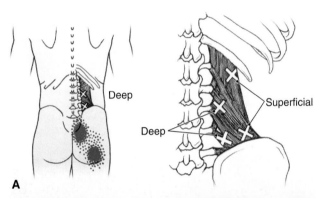

A

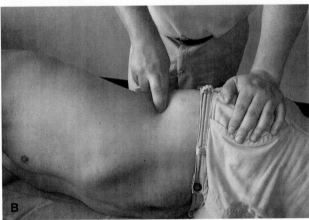

B

FIGURE 8-7 Trigger points in the quadratus lumborum. Trigger points in the quadratus lumborum muscle can mimic sciatica, sacroiliac dysfunction, and trochanteric bursitis and often contribute to pelvic tilt. Common activating/perpetuating factors include leg length differences, weak gluteal muscles, poor lifting mechanics, and running on uneven surfaces. **(A)** Locations of the points. **(B)** Deactivation of trigger point in the quadratus lumborum.

■ APPLICATION GUIDELINES

Because tender points develop via the gamma gain process, release of these points requires an interruption, or reversal, of the neuromuscular message from the muscle spindle causing the localized spasm. In fact, tender points

cannot be relieved through either simple direct pressure or stretching. Positional release techniques use passive positioning of the body to quiet the excitability of the muscle spindle and relieve the muscle spasm marked by the tender points. With positional release, the body is moved away from the restriction and toward a **position of ease**, which is generally a shortened position for the muscle harboring the point. For example, tender points located on the anterior side of the body are generally treated with flexion, and posterior tender points with extension. Although tender points on or near the midline of the body can be effectively treated with flexion and extension only, points more lateral to the midline require more rotations and side-bending.

Wrist / Hand Extensors

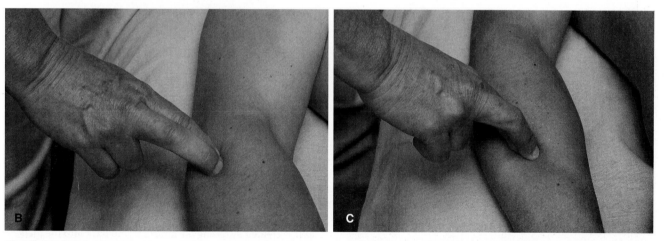

Extensor
carpi ulnaris

A

Extensor carpi
radialis brevis

FIGURE 8-8 **Trigger points in the extensor carpi radialis.** Trigger points in the extensor carpi radialis muscles are more common than in the extensor ulnaris muscle. The most common activating/perpetuating factor is repetitive stressful gripping and twisting motions of the hand/wrist. **(A)** Location of the points. **(B)** Deactivating extensor carpi radialis longus trigger point. **(C)** Deactivation of extensor carpi radialis brevis trigger point.

The position of ease, and therefore release of the tender point, is rarely the fully shortened position for the muscle. Rather, it is more common for the point of release to be somewhere in the mid range of the concentric action of that muscle.[9,25] To sense this position of ease for the muscle, the therapist holds one or two fingers directly over the point with only enough pressure to stay over it during the movement. Somewhere in the mid range of the movement, therapists feel the tissue fully soften and find that further movement in any direction seems to increase tension in the tissue. At this

point, a slow and deep pressure into the point is applied, and the athlete is asked about the level of tenderness. The position of ease should lead to an immediate decrease in tenderness, approximately 70%. If tenderness has decreased by only 50%, the position requires a little more fine tuning, which should start with increasing the flexion or extension followed by slight adjustments with rotations and side bends.[9,25] The position of ease must be held for 90 seconds for full reversal of the gamma gain process and release of the tender point. After 90 seconds, therapists should apply firm

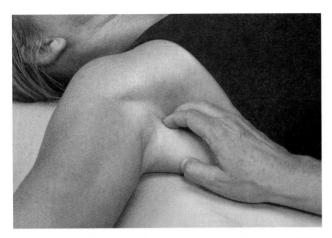

FIGURE 8-9 Deactivation of trigger point in the subscapularis. After the point is released general friction can also be applied in this position.

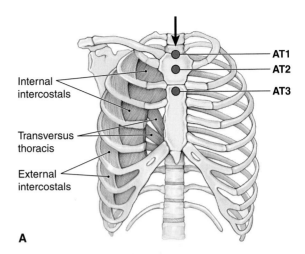

A

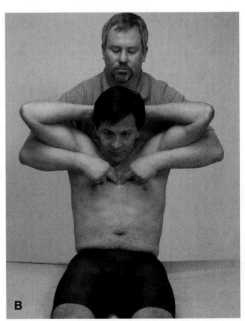

B

FIGURE 8-10 Tender points in the sternalis. (A) Location of tender points along the sternalis muscle. **(B)** The position of ease is created by having the athlete slump back into the therapist's knee/thigh with arms raised and resting on top of the head. The arms overhead give slight elevation and rotation to the ribs, and the slump puts more slack on the sternalis.

From the Field

"Athletes come to me all the time with complaints of aching pain and tight muscles and always ask if I know any good stretches for that particular area. I just smile and say 'let's see what else we can do to help.' I almost always find several trigger points or tender areas that the athlete is completely unaware of. I combine general massage with my own version of trigger point and positional release, which has been very successful for me. I also teach the athlete how to use light pressure and some basic positional release on their own as an adjunct to their stretching routines."

Martha Stevenson, LMT, NCTMB

Massage Therapist and Sports Massage Specialist
Fairbanks, AK

■ POSITIONAL RELEASE FOR SELECTED MUSCLES

When multiple tender points are present, the treatment sequence of the points is of great importance (Box 8-1). The most sensitive or dominant tender point should always be treated first because release of this point also relieves satellite points. Therefore, a full-body, or at least regional, assessment that maps all tender points should be carried out to guide the treatment procedure. Some athletes may have a dense cluster of smaller points rather than a single dominant point. In this case, the most central point in the cluster is addressed first, and the treatment continues from there. The

pressure into the point to confirm that it is no longer tender and that the point has been released before slowly moving the muscle and body part back to neutral. To avoid reactivation of the point, it is essential for the athlete to be completely passive during this return to the neutral position.

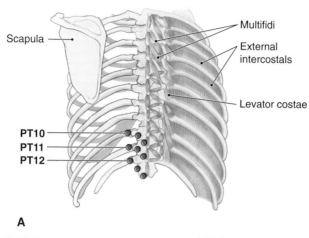

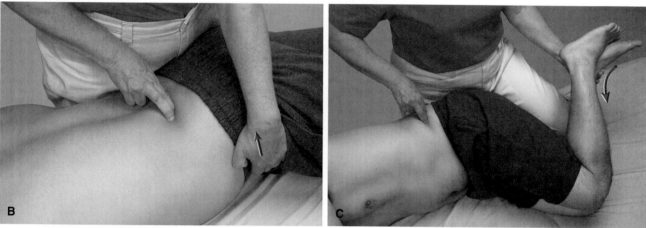

FIGURE 8-11 Tender points in the quadratus lumborum. (A) The quadratus lumborum muscle commonly has multiple tender points. **(B)** The position of ease/release for these points begins by first positioning the athlete in hip flexion and slight external rotation. The therapist lifts the athlete's hip from the table and holds each point for 90 seconds. **(C)** Alternate method of deactivation of tender points in quadratus lumborum with the therapist creating the hip elevation and rotation from behind the athlete.

general procedure is to work from larger joints and muscle groups to the smaller ones—first in a proximal to distal pattern, then medial to lateral. (See Figures 8-12 and 8-13 for illustrations of positional release in the tensor fascia lata and thoracic area.) When multiple tender points occur in a single row, the middle point should be treated first. The step-by-step protocol for tender point release is as follows[1,2,4,5,22,25,28]:

1. Confirm the location of the point by applying brief firm pressure into the point. Release the pressure, but keep the finger in that spot with light "monitoring" pressure.

2. Move to the position of ease, generally a shortened position of the muscle. Without consideration for a specific muscle, the position of ease is achieved by folding tissue and body parts into and around the point.

3. Monitor the tissue under the finger for softening. The position of greatest comfort for the patient/athlete should correspond to the feeling of complete relaxation of the tissue under the monitoring finger. This point is called the "mobile point" by Jones because movement in any direction adds tension to the tissue under the finger.[25]

4. Apply brief firm pressure into the point to confirm that this is the position of maximum comfort. The patient/athlete should report at least a 70% reduction of tenderness. Continue to fine-tune the position with small movements to reach and maintain this reduction of pain.

5. Maintain the position for 90 seconds. Apply brief firm pressure into the point several times during the 90 seconds—approximately every 30 seconds.

6. Slowly and passively move the part back to the neutral position. Give verbal instructions that make it clear that the patient/athlete must remain completely passive and allow the therapist to move the part. If the patient athlete assists in the motion, the tender point may be reactivated.

7. Apply brief firm pressure into the point to confirm that it is no longer sensitive.

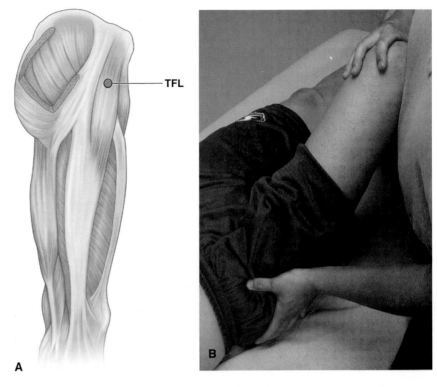

FIGURE 8-12 Tender point in the tensor fasciae latae (TFL). (A) The common tender point for the tensor fasciae latae is in the same general location as the trigger point for this muscle. **(B)** The primary movement toward the position of ease is hip flexion, and internal rotation/abduction are the fine-tuning movements.

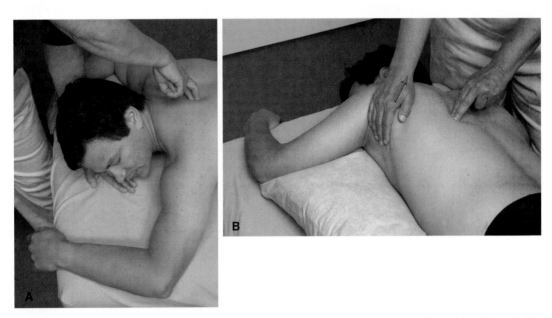

FIGURE 8-13 Tender point release for common thoracic points. (A) Upper thoracic points. The athlete is positioned with the head rotated to the same side as the point and resting on the therapist's hand so that the head is also in slight lateral flexion. The athlete's arm position also helps create the release for these points. **(B)** Middle–lower thoracic points. The athlete's position is the same as in **(A)** except that the pillow underneath his chest and shoulder adds slight torso rotation. Therapist adds scapular retraction while monitoring the point for full release.

BOX 8-1 GENERAL TREATMENT GUIDELINES FOR POSITIONAL RELEASE

- Perform full evaluation and mapping of dominant points.
- Treat the most sensitive tender points first.
- Treat proximal to distal and medial to distal.
- Evaluate and treat larger joints and muscles before smaller ones.

- When a cluster of points occurs, treat the center of the cluster.
- When multiple tender points occur in a row, treat the middle point first.

Guidelines for Combining Proprioceptive Techniques

The common factors among the various NMR techniques easily outweigh their differences. Whether called trigger or tender points, many occur at origins, insertions, and the anatomic motor points of the muscles.[1,28,29] A comparison of charts of common trigger points, tender points, and anatomic motor points shows a remarkable number of common locations (Fig. 8-14). In addition, a 1977 study by Melzack et al.[29] compared the location of acupuncture points for pain (Ah Shi) with Travell's trigger point chart and demonstrated a 70% correlation between the two.[11] The high correlation among all these points supports the probability that more than one physiologic explanation is valid regarding how muscle tension and painful points develop.

The bottom line is that any technique that returns a muscle's full-stretch and length and stimulates circulation is an effective neuromuscular technique,[1,21,28] and the proponents for each of the three categories of NMR readily acknowledge that the other techniques are valid and effective. When muscle tension and multiple tender points are identified as primary or contributing factors in painful and restricted movement, any one or all of the above methods, when properly applied, is helpful. However, for complete relief of pain and dysfunction, a combination of the techniques may be more effective than choosing one method over the other. It is more important for the therapist to understand the nature of the muscle tension and the physiologic principle that applies than it is to have the correct name for the technique or to rigidly follow only one neuromuscular application procedure. Remember that the body does not know whether Shiatsu, trigger point, strain counterstrain, or positional release is being used; it simply responds according to the stimulus.

Of the three categories of NMR, both trigger point and proprioceptive techniques are considered *direct* treatment approaches. Trigger point applies direct pressure into identified trigger points in a tight muscle, and the proprioceptive techniques move directly into the movement barrier or stretched position of the muscle. In other words, both confront the pain and tension with some type of opposing force or reverse soft tissue manipulation. Positional release techniques are considered *indirect* treatment approaches. The tender points associated with these techniques are not viewed as a site of pathology to be treated, but as a diagnostic and monitoring point for treatment of the entire muscle and spinal segment. Unlike trigger point and proprioceptive techniques, the treatment method for positional release is to move away from the restriction and into a position of comfort, making it indirect.

Based on the athlete's individual response, therapists may choose to address muscle tension through any combination of NMR techniques by alternating between them. In general, the proprioceptive techniques should be applied before any point-specific work because they are more general and address the entire myofascial network. Moreover, the use of proprioceptive techniques after trigger/tender point release may reactivate the points because muscles are engaged in active contraction. The following is an example of how the techniques can be combined into an effective protocol for point deactivation and reduction of muscle tension. The general concept is to follow the trigger point protocol when evaluation clearly identifies those characteristics and to follow positional release when the evaluation is less clear or confirms a tender point.

1. Locate the point through visual inspection and palpation. The athlete may come in with a clear complaint about a painful and/or restricted motion or even be aware of one particular tender spot. In either case, the therapist should specifically palpate for points in the origins and insertions of the muscles under most demand for that athlete, as well as his or her antagonists.
2. Apply general massage to the entire region using extra petrissage and linear friction strokes.
3. Apply a contract–relax stretching protocol to the target muscle containing the identified point(s).
4. Gradually press into the point to reach a 5 on the discomfort scale until the tissue begins to melt under the

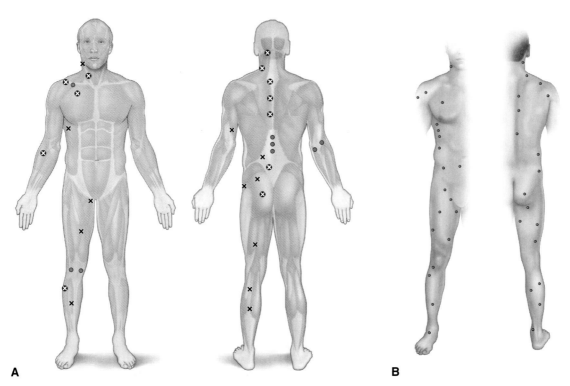

FIGURE 8-14 Comparison of trigger, tender, and anatomic motor point locations. (A) There is a high correlation between the location of trigger and tender points. Black X, trigger point; 0, tender point location; white X, common point. **(B)** The anatomic motor points of muscles (where the nerve enters) also have a strong correlation to these points.

palpating finger(s) and the pain decreases. If this pressure elicits the predictable pattern of pain associated with trigger points, continue pressure for 90 seconds until the point deactivates and continue to step 7.

5. If the initial pressure does not elicit referred pain or if the pain does not diminish within 30 seconds, decrease pressure into the point and slowly move the muscle toward a shortened position to deactivate the point through positional release.

6. Monitor the point and maintain the position of ease for 90 seconds, adjusting the position as needed to keep the tissue soft.

7. When deactivation/release is complete, slowly release the pressure, but maintain the treatment position for a few seconds. Slowly return the body part to the starting/neutral position, making sure the athlete remains passive during the movement.

8. Finish with a slow static stretch of the muscle.

Neuromuscular Release for Specific Muscles

It is beyond the scope of this text to show specific releases for all muscles. More comprehensive illustrations of the individual NMR techniques can be found in the textbooks for each specific technique. A broad sampling of NMR releases for muscles commonly involved in athletic injuries is shown in Figures 8-15 through 17. Additional neuromuscular releases are included in Chapter 13 as part of the treatments for specific injuries.

SUMMARY

Any technique that is directed toward reducing muscle tension should be considered a neuromuscular technique, and these techniques can be divided into three basic categories: Trigger point, positional release, and proprioceptive. The key concepts for application of the neuromuscular techniques are the following:

• All of these techniques are based on sound physiologic rationale and have been shown to be effective. Therefore, no single one of them is correct and the others incorrect. Therapists are encouraged to understand the principles of application for each technique and to choose the most appropriate approach for that athlete in a case-by-case approach.

• When common trigger, tender, motor, and acupressure points are mapped and compared, there is a significant correlation among all of them. Therefore, it is likely that

A 42-year-old avid jogger was suffering from severe plantar fasciitis and really wanted to get back to his regular running routine. The massage therapist found severe fascial restriction throughout his legs and several tight and tender points in the posterior compartment muscles and the medial longitudinal arch of the foot. The session began with deep Swedish massage over the back of both legs, and when the therapist was working over the affected foot, positional release was used to address two tender points along the medial arch and one at the medial base of the calcaneous, as depicted in this figure. General back massage that included skin rolling over the lumbosacral aponeurosis finished the session. The athlete was surprised to find that his pain with walking had been significantly reduced and was excited to continue massage with this therapist. After 6 weeks of weekly sessions, he was running without pain.

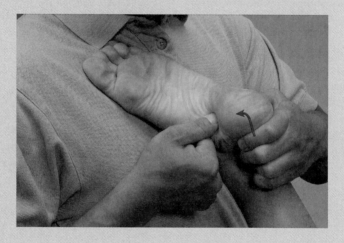

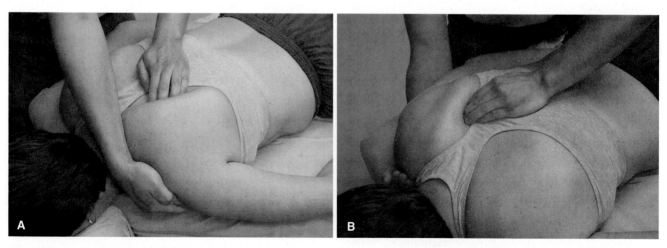

FIGURE 8-15 Combination releases for neuromuscular tension and spasm of the rhomboids and middle trapezius. (A) Therapist stands on the opposite side of the table. **(B)** Scapular retraction is engaged with the therapist standing on the same side of the table.

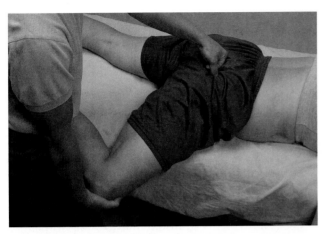

FIGURE 8-16 Combination release of the piriformis uses hip abduction and external rotation to reduce tension and local points.

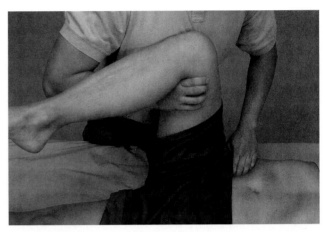

FIGURE 8-17 Combination release for iliopsoas. Therapists can access the psoas muscle by supporting the athlete's hip in 90-degree flexion and by fine-tuning with abduction/adduction and rotation of the hip. Therapists may also choose this position for a deep fascial release of the psoas.

more than one physiologic process is involved in creating and relieving the points.
- Because trigger points are believed to be caused by a localized contraction knot that is *not signaled by motor neurons,* the therapeutic approach is simple application of sustained pressure to mechanically spread the sarcomeres apart and block further actin and myosin bonding.
- Because tender points are believed to be caused by an abhorrent stretch reflex signal from the muscle spindle, a contraction that *is signaled by the motor neurons,* the therapeutic approach is to reverse the signal for contraction by repositioning the muscle, generally a shortened position.
- The proprioceptive neuromuscular techniques use normal muscle physiology, specifically the reflex actions caused by the muscle spindle, Golgi tendon organ, and the reciprocal innervation of agonist and antagonist to manipulate muscle tension.

- Therapists may choose to use any of these techniques exclusively or combine the techniques for added flexibility in their therapeutic interventions.
- If athletes are complaining of a specific pain pattern and if pressure over a specific tender nodule recreates this pain, trigger point protocols are more likely to be effective than the other two techniques.
- If therapists locate a tender and tight area in the tissue (during the assessment or massage) that causes sharp pain without a radiating pattern and elicits a jump response in the athlete when it is pressed, tender point protocols are more likely to be effective than the other two.
- When multiple trigger points or tender points are present, the sequence of treatment is of great importance.
- Neuromuscular techniques should be combined with appropriate myofascial techniques to achieve the best treatment results.

Review Questions

SHORT ANSWERS

1. List five specific styles of massage/bodywork included under the neuromuscular release (NMR) definition.

2. Name and define the three major categories of NMR.

3. List the six characteristics that are present in all active and latent trigger points.

4. List the four most commonly used proprioceptive neuromuscular techniques.

MULTIPLE CHOICE

5. Which of the following best defines NMR techniques?
    a. All techniques that are based trigger point theories
    b. Any technique that uses passive positioning to reduces muscle tension
    c. Any technique directed at reducing muscle tension
    d. Techniques that manipulate muscle physiology

6. What is the general position of release for a tender point?

a. At the beginning of the range of motion
b. Mid-range of the concentric movement
c. The fully shortened position
d. The stretched position

7. How long should a trigger point be held for complete release of the point?
   a. 15 to 30 seconds
   b. 0 to 10 seconds
   c. 30 to 90 seconds
   d. 1 to 3 minutes

8. If the rhomboids are tight, which of these muscles should be engaged in an isometric contraction to inhibit it?
   a. Levator scapulae
   b. Rectus abdominis
   c. Subscapularis
   d. Pectoralis minor

9. What muscle is the target muscle when contract–relax techniques are used?
   a. The tight muscle
   b. Antagonist to the tight muscle
   c. The closest synergist to the tight muscle
   d. The muscle proximal to the trigger point

10. The clinical characteristics for tender points include being hypersensitive to moderate pressure, and

    _____.
    a. having a distinct nodular feel
    b. eliciting a local twitch response in the muscle
    c. eliciting a jump response from the athlete
    d. creating a recognized pain for the athlete

11. What is the primary movement used to find the position of ease for a tender point on the posterior side of the body?
    a. Flexion
    b. Extension
    c. Lateral flexion
    d. Rotation

12. How long should the position of ease be held for full release of a tender point?
    a. 15 seconds
    b. 30 seconds
    c. 60 seconds
    d. 90 seconds

13. Therapists know they have reached the position of ease when the tissue under the monitoring finger is fully relaxed and the athlete reports that tenderness of the point has decreased by _____.
    a. 30%
    b. 50%
    c. 70%
    d. 100%

14. What is the best method of muscle palpation for a therapist to use when attempting to locate a trigger point?
    a. A moderately deep sweep across the fibers of the muscle
    b. A series of deep presses beginning in the middle of the muscle
    c. A light stroking movement in line with the muscle fibers
    d. Probing with the elbow from the muscle belly toward the attachments

15. What is a local twitch response?
    a. The recoil from pain movement commonly associated with trigger points
    b. Repeated local muscle cramps that occur in hypertonic muscles
    c. The essential characteristic displayed by tender points when palpated
    d. A brief muscle spasm in the taut band of muscle associated with trigger points

16. The proper therapeutic intervention to relieve a trigger point is to _____.
    a. repeatedly strum across the taut band of tissue housing the point
    b. press directly into the point with moderate pressure
    c. apply light pressure with one finger and slowly shorten the muscle housing the point
    d. press firmly into the point until the athlete reports a pain rated 7 out of 10

17. Approximately how long should the contraction used in proprioceptive techniques be held?
    a. 30 seconds
    b. 60 seconds
    c. 10 seconds
    d. 5 seconds

18. Trigger points that develop in response to another trigger point are called what?
    a. Associated trigger point
    b. Satellite trigger point
    c. Latent trigger point
    d. Attachment trigger point

19. What is the term used to describe a trigger point that the athlete is unaware of until pressed?
    a. Hidden
    b. Inactive
    c. Latent
    d. Passive

20. An athlete's tension headache that has pain over the temporalis area is commonly caused by a

    _____.
    a. trapezius
    b. occipitals
    c. scalenes
    d. teres major

REFERENCES

1. Chaitow L, DeLany JW. Clinical Application of Neuromuscular Techniques, vols. 1 and 2: The Upper Body. Edinburgh: Churchill Livingstone, 2000.

2. Chaitow L. Positional Release Techniques. New York: Churchill Livingstone, 1996.

3. Chaitow L. Muscle Energy Techniques. New York: Churchill Livingstone, 1996.

4. D'Ambrogio KJ, Roth GB. Positional Release Therapy: Assessment and Treatment of Musculoskeletal Dysfunction. St. Louis: Mosby, 1997.

5. Glover JC, Yates HA. Strain Counterstrain Techniques. In: Ward RC, ed. Foundations of Osteopathic Medicine. Baltimore: Williams & Wilkins, 1997.

6. Goodridge JP. Muscle Energy Technique Procedures. In: Ward RC, ed. Foundations of Osteopathic Medicine. Baltimore: Williams & Wilkins, 1997.

7. Simons DG, Travell JG, Simons LS. Myofascial Pain and Dysfunction: The Trigger Point Manual, 2nd ed. vol. 1: Upper Half of Body. Philadelphia: Lippincott Williams & Wilkins, 1999.

8. Smolders JJ. Myofascial Pain and Dysfunction: Myofascial Trigger Points. In: Hammer WI, ed. Functional Soft Tissue Examination and Treatment by Manual Methods: The Extremities. Gaithersburg, MD: Aspen Publishers, 1991.

9. Speicher T. Positional release therapy techniques: Un-kinking the chain. Workshop, June 2005; NATA Annual Meeting.

10. Knott M, Voss DE. Proprioceptive Neuromuscular Facilitation: Patterns and Techniques, 2nd ed. New York: Harper & Row, 1968.

11. Lewit K. Manipulative Therapy in Rehabilitation of the Locomotor System, 3rd ed. Oxford: Butterworth Heinemann, 1999.

12. Latey P. Feelings, muscles and movement. Journal of Bodywork and Movement Therapies 1996;1(1):44–52.

13. McAtee RE. Facilitated Stretching. Champaign, IL: Human Kinetics, 1993.

14. Travell JG, Rinzler S. The myofascial genesis of pain. Postgraduate Medicine 1952;11:425–434.

15. McLeod I, Mistry D, Archer P et al. Massage therapy utilization and application in the treatment of myofascial trigger points. Advanced track seminar, June 2005; NATA Annual Meeting.

16. Juhan D. Job's Body: A Handbook for Bodywork, expanded edition. Barrytown, NY: Station Hill, 1998.

17. Kuchera ML, McPartland JM. Myofascial Trigger Points. In: Ward RC, ed. Foundations of Osteopathic Medicine. Baltimore: Williams & Wilkins, 1997.

18. Ward RC, ed. Foundations for Osteopathic Medicine. Baltimore: Williams & Wilkins. 1997.

19. Johansson H, Sojka P. Pathophysiological mechanisms involved in genesis and spread of muscular tension in occupational muscle pain and in chronic musculoskeletal pain syndromes: A hypothesis. Medical Hypotheses 1991;35(3):196–203.

20. Korr IM. Somatic dysfunction, osteopathic manipulative treatment, and the nervous system: a few facts, some theories, many questions. JAOA 1986;86(2):109–114.

21. Patriquin DA. Chapman's Reflexes. In: Ward RC, ed. Foundations of Osteopathic Medicine. Baltimore: Williams & Wilkins, 1997.

22. Roth GB. Positional release therapy. Reprint from webpage: WellnessSystems.com. July 2003.

23. Schaible HG, Grubb BD. Afferent and spinal mechanisms of joint pain. Pain 1993;55: 5–54.

24. Schiowitz S. Facilitated Positional Release. In: Ward RC, ed. Foundations of Osteopathic Medicine. Baltimore: Williams & Wilkins, 1997.

25. Kusunose RS. Strain and Counterstrain for the Upper Quarter; course syllabus, 1990.

26. Korr IM. Proprioceptors and somatic dysfunction. JAOA 1975;74 (March):638–650.

27. Mense S. Peripheral mechanisms of muscle nociception and local muscle pain. Journal of Musculoskeletal Pain 1993;1:133–170.

28. Rosomoff HL et. al. Physical findings in patients with chronic intractable benign pain of the neck and/or back. Pain 1989;37: 279–287.

29. Melzack R, Stillwell DM, Fox E. Trigger points and acupuncture points for pain: Correlations and implications. Pain 1977;3:3–23.

Myofascial Techniques

OBJECTIVES

After completing this chapter, the reader will be able to:

- Define myofascial technique, and name four to five different names for this form of massage.
- List at least 10 absolute contraindications for the use of myofascial techniques, and discuss why they are contraindications.
- List at least five regional contraindications for the use of myofascial techniques, and discuss why they are contraindicated.
- Name and describe four methods of assessing myofascial restrictions.
- Describe the key differences between site-specific and broad plane myofascial techniques, and give three examples of strokes within each category.
- List and explain six criteria that are the keys to effectiveness for deep transverse friction (DTF).
- Outline the six-step general treatment formula for DTF.
- Describe the rationale and general application guidelines for broad plane myofascial releases.
- Demonstrate proper application of DTF at several sites, including extensor pollicis tendon; hamstring tendons; cervical ligaments; insertion of the subscapularis and supraspinatus; humeral epicondyles and supracondylar ridges; and the medial, lateral, and inferior edges of the patella.
- Name five muscles or myofascial regions that are most suited for muscle rolling.
- Define and give examples of direct and indirect myofascial techniques.
- Demonstrate the proper application of broad plane pin-and-stretch, linear shift, horizontal plane, and traction–release methods of myofascial release.

The fascial system is the one consistent element of an athlete's locomotor system connecting each muscle fiber to the other, muscle to muscle, muscle to bone, bone to bone, and skin to muscle. There are direct myofascial connections between different body regions, making it clear that injury in one area creates strain and compensation in far-away structures. If this far-away strain goes undetected and untreated, the common result is a chronic strain, or persistent pain syndrome that can nag an athlete for months or even years with untold effects on performance and training.[1–6]

Although it is recognized among sports health care professionals that general movement and specific soft tissue mobilization such as deep transverse friction is often a vital part of any treatment protocol, the complexity and all-encompassing nature of connective tissue in our bodies requires that therapists open their view to a wider array of myofascial techniques. Because fascia directs and moderates the power of muscles, unique therapeutic tools that address this body-wide system to facilitate healing, enhance the athlete's performance potential, and decrease his or her risk of injury are beneficial.

Less measurable, but of equal importance to athletes is the sense of "feeling loose." This is most often a subconscious awareness, but it is difficult to quantify or predict its effect on performance. However, owing to the intense proprioceptive function of fascia, it is logical to attribute a good portion of this "sense of ease" to healthy and mobile connective tissue. The converse is also true. Restricted, adhered, and/or dehydrated connective tissue creates a sense of tight and restricted movement even when joint range of motion and muscle tone are assessed as within normal range. The myofascial techniques described here offer sports health care therapists simple tools that are easily integrated into current preventive, treatment, and rehabilitation protocols.

The Myofascial Techniques

Whether superficial or deep, site-specific or broad plane, any technique directed toward stretching, broadening, and/or loosening fascia is a myofascial technique. Therefore, even the general frictions described in basic sports massage and friction strokes applied with an emollient in Swedish massage are superficial myofascial techniques. Like the neuromuscular techniques described in Chapter 8, a number of different names are used to distinguish one myofascial technique from another (see Appendix A). However, regardless of the name of the technique or the differences in the methods of application, all these techniques have the goal of maintaining or restoring the functional capacity of the integrated myofascial network. For learning purposes, it is helpful to make some broad distinctions among the multiple forms of myofascial techniques. By dividing myofascial techniques into only two categories—those that address the broad fascial zones and horizontal planes and those that address specific structures or lesions—therapists are encouraged to choose the method of application based on the structural dysfunctions rather than the name of the technique.

From the Field

"Every injury I treat has a fascial component. To ignore this will limit the results from treatment. The use of massage, myofascial release, and strain-counterstrain combined with appropriate modalities, mobilizations and progressive exercise has allowed for earlier return to functional levels and less recurrence of problems for the athletes I treat."

Thomas Burton, PT, EMT

Supervisor of Outpatient Services
Providence—Holy Cross Medical Center
Mission Hills, CA

Indications and Contraindications

As with most massage techniques, body-wide or systemic diseases or conditions are generally considered absolute contraindications for myofascial techniques, and localized injuries or conditions may be considered as regional contraindications (Table 9-1). When the condition is listed as an *absolute contraindication,* none of the broad plane myofascial techniques should be used anywhere in the body, although a site-specific technique may be applied to a specific adhesion or restriction. In conditions listed as *regional con-*

TABLE 9-1	Contraindications to Myofascial Techniques
Absolute Contraindications	**Regional Contraindications**
Malignancy	Severe hematoma
Cellulites	Local infection
Fever	Traumatic edema
Systemic infections	Open wounds or fractures
Aneurysm	Degenerative joint disease (eg, osteoarthritis, chondromalacia, gout)
Lymphedema	
Acute rheumatoid arthritis	
Advanced osteoporosis	
Advanced diabetes	
Hemophilia or anticoagulant therapy	
Hyperesthesia/hypersensitivity of skin	

traindications, both site-specific and broad plane techniques may be applied with caution in uninvolved areas.[2,3,5]

The indications for myofascial work are too numerous to list as individual injuries or conditions, but they can be described in general as any injury or condition that impairs and/or alters normal musculoskeletal function and is not part of a specific disease process.[2] Because athletes stress and strain their musculoskeletal systems daily, myofascial techniques are indicated for all athletic injuries and conditions not on the absolute contraindications list. Specifically, myofascial techniques are indicated when athletes experience any of the following:

- Restricted range of motion with or without specific injury
- Decreased power or strength
- Visible scars in the area of complaint or the myofascial chain
- Painful movement (passive or active) with or without specific injury
- Tenderness in muscles or fascial zones without specific injury
- Palpable thick, adhered, and/or fibrous fascia anywhere in the body.

Assessing Myofascial Restrictions

Many of the assessment techniques and special tests used by sports health care therapists evaluate a specific joint, ligament, or muscle and are used only when an athlete has suffered an injury. When testing identifies a specific joint restriction or muscle weakness and/or recreates pain both athlete and therapist are able to recognize a particular structure as part of a problem. The tendency for an inexperienced therapist is to stop the evaluation there. However, because fascia extends three-dimensionally throughout the body to functionally join all muscles, joints, nerves, and blood vessels, it is more appropriate to evaluate entire myofascial chains and recognize that such diverse complaints as tingling, numbing, and general aching sensations may indicate fascial restrictions rather than trauma to a single joint or muscle. If only the joint structures or muscles in the area of complaint are assessed, we may end up treating and relieving symptoms rather than identifying *the source* of the pain and restriction. By assessing the full myofascial chain, therapists can identify *all* points of strain and compression, whether local or in areas other than the site of complaint. This comprehensive assessment provides key information for the creation of comprehensive and effective treatment and rehabilitation programs[2-5,7] There are four general methods used to assess myofascial health: (1) a postural assessment and visual inspection of tissue; (2) general palpation, tissue excursion, and skin rolling; (3) passive range of motion and general movement assessments; and (4) contract–relax neuromuscular techniques.

■ POSTURAL ASSESSMENT AND VISUAL INSPECTION

A simple and comprehensive way of evaluating myofascial restrictions and/or imbalances is to do a full body postural analysis. Imbalances and restrictions in myofascial chains are seen as rotations, elevations, protractions, and retractions in the alignment of the body. Although it is *not* the most important element of an acute injury evaluation, a thorough postural analysis is essential to proper assessment of chronic and persistent pain syndromes. Postural adaptations such as a high ilium, anterior/posterior pelvic tilt, protracted head, and the upper- and lower-crossed syndromes detailed in Chapter 4 are apparent in most chronic and persistent pain syndromes. The challenge to the therapist is to see these adaptations not just as individual problems, but to "connect the dots" between each of these body regions, viewing them as a pattern of myofascial dysfunction that must be balanced at all points for the full benefit of the athlete. That being said, it may not be wise to attempt wholesale postural changes in the midst of the athlete's competitive season because it could negatively affect the athlete's biomechanics and performance. In such cases, therapists should address only a few key areas of fascial restriction to relieve some specific strain or limitation for the athlete, and avoid making major shifts in his/her postural alignment. Finding postural asymmetry should direct the therapists to specific areas that need further evaluation with palpation, range of motion, and/or strength testing. A visual assessment of the soft tissues may also reveal myofascial restrictions in the horizontal bands, seen as flat or pulled-in tissue, or the classic spiral line of restrictions. These areas should also be palpated and included in range-of-motion testing to determine the best combination of myofascial techniques (Box 9-1).

■ PALPATION: TISSUE EXCURSION AND SKIN ROLLING

Palpation for myofascial restrictions involves more than simply confirming that the area of the athlete's complaint is tight. Therapists must specifically evaluate the *thixotropic* status of the fascia—specifically its tenderness, mobility, texture, and adherence to itself or surrounding tissue. Assessing these qualities in the fascia requires a much lighter touch than the pressure used to identify bone landmarks or specific muscle tears, and it takes a good deal of practice to develop the proper touch. Remember that the

BOX 9-1 PRIMARY METHODS OF ASSESSING MYOFASCIAL TISSUE

- Postural assessment and visual inspection of the soft tissue
- General palpation, tissue excursion, and skin rolling
- Muscle length tests
- Contract–relax neuromuscular techniques

superficial fascia is just under the skin, so tune your senses to this level of the tissue first and gradually increase your depth and perception of the tissue.

During palpation, it is common to find that the attachment zone of the horizontal bands and broad fascial sheets, that is, iliotibial band and lumbosacral aponeurosis, are tender to specific palpation even when an athlete is unaware of specific pain or tension at that site. For example, an athlete complaining of tight hamstrings may be point tender around the greater trochanter and along the posterior edge of the iliotibial band. This tenderness is indicative of tight and restricted fascia in need of release. However, fascia may be adhered and stiff even when it is not tender. When the postural assessment shows the drawn-in tissue associated with the horizontal bands, palpation at the spinal attachment of the band generally finds a thick and adhered knot of tissue around the spinous processes.

Tissue excursion is a special form of palpation used to assess the mobility of broad areas of superficial fascia such as the lumbosacral aponeurosis and iliotibial band. These broad sheets of fascia have multiple layers, and each layer should easily slide over the other in any direction. To assess this, one or both hands are used to gently compress the tissue and stretch it to its limit in all directions. It is important that the superficial tissue is moved as one unit with the hands, rather than letting the hands slide over the surface of the skin. With tissue excursion, therapists may sense more tension and resistance to movement, and/or a firmer end-feel to the stretch in one or more directions (Fig. 9-1). This tension or resistance generally indicates a fascial restriction that may be due to a variety of problems such as dehydration, ischemia, fibrous build-up, or stagnation of the ground substance in the fascia leading to inappropriate cross-links between collagen fibers.[2–6,8]

Skin rolling is a specific type of palpation that serves as both an evaluation and a treatment tool (Fig.9-2). In skin rolling, the therapist applies a loose pincer grip to the skin, creating a roll of tissue between thumb and fingers. If the superficial fascia is free of adhesions, the roll of tissue pops up easily on its own and can be gently rolled back and forth (like rolling a pencil between your fingers) with minimal discomfort to the athlete. If the tissue is adhered and restricted, it will not pop up between the thumb and fingers without being forced. It may also be resistant to

rolling and feels crunchy and fibrous, crackling as it is rolled. The most appropriate fascial areas to assess with skin rolling are the lumbosacral and abdominal aponeuroses, iliotibial band, fascial compartments of the leg and forearm, and the full erector spinae. As in the fascial excursion tests, skin rolling must be multidirectional to fully assess and relieve restrictions and adhesions.

When skin rolling is used as a broad plane release for thick and adhered superficial fascia, therapists must recognize that it is uncomfortable for the athlete and slow the rolling to a tolerable pace. When the fascia is severely adhered and resistant to rolling, therapists must limit the duration of the technique and amount of tissue that is rolled.

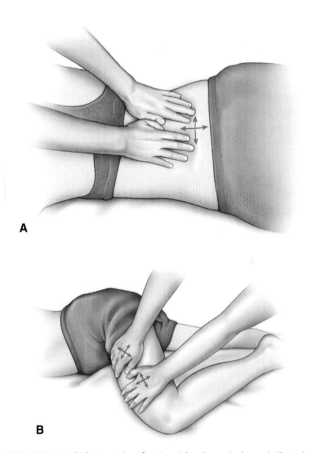

A

B

FIGURE 9-1 **(A)** Assessing fascia with a broad plane shift in the lumbar fascia, and iliotibial band **(B)**.

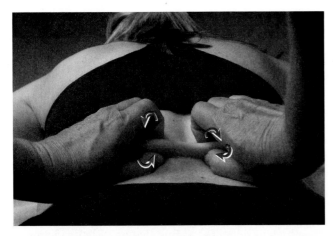

FIGURE 9-2 Skin rolling for assessment and release in the lumbosacral fascia.

MUSCLE LENGTH TESTS

Sports health care therapists commonly use active, passive, and resisted range-of-motion tests to identify specific joint and muscle problems, and Chapter 12 fully describes the use of these tests. It is also common practice to use muscle length tests like a sit-and-reach, or straight-leg raise test to evaluate muscle tension in the hamstrings and low back muscles.[2,9–11] Because muscle and fascia are anatomically and functionally inseparable, tension and limitations in these and other muscle length tests can also be caused by fascial restrictions. Furthermore, the deeper fascial elements in joints, that is, joint capsule and ligaments, can also restrict mobility and create pain. In other words, a muscle length test provides more than simple information about muscle tension: it assesses the extensibility of all myofascial elements in that area. For example, a positive Ober's test (see Fig. 12-5B) result can indicate hypertonicity in the tensor fasciae latae, gluteus maximus, or quadratus lumborum or a thick and adhered iliotibial band. To distinguish one condition from the other, the therapist must ask the athlete where he or she feels the most tension; palpate each of the muscles for tender points; and evaluate the tissue excursion over the iliotibial band, hamstrings, and quadriceps and lumbosacral aponeurosis. Another example of limited and painful movement is frozen shoulder syndrome. In this condition, the limited shoulder flexion and external rotation are more related to adhesions and restrictions in the deeper fascial structures, specifically the joint capsule, than to muscle tension in the extensor or internal rotator muscles. Recognizing the differences between these conditions can help direct therapeutic choices.

CONTRACT–RELAX TECHNIQUES

Muscle length test results that identify a restricted range of motion can be due to either muscle tension/spasm or fascial tension/compression. A simple and efficient way to determine which of these tissues is the major problem is to perform a contract–relax, or post-isometric relaxation technique (Chapter 8). If the limited range of motion improves dramatically after the contract–relax, the primary cause of the movement restriction was most likely due to neuromuscular dysfunction. If the limited range of motion stays the same or has very little improvement, fascial restrictions are more likely to be involved in limiting the movement.[11]

Because muscle and fascia are integrally linked, it is extremely rare to have only neuromuscular or only myofascial involvement in movement dysfunctions, especially in the repetitive stressful motion conditions common to athletes. Therefore, therapists must fully evaluate the athlete's complaint using more than just the myofascial assessment tools described here and must integrate their findings to determine the specific combination of therapeutic massage techniques to apply in each situation.

Site-Specific Myofascial Techniques

Whenever a therapist focuses a myofascial technique over a specific structure or small region of muscle or fascia, it is considered a site specific technique. These techniques are commonly used over the smaller structural elements of the fascial network such as ligaments, tendons, musculotendinous junctions, or specific points along a myofascial division between muscles, and are also used to address existing scars or localized lesions during healing. The site-specific techniques can be classified as direct or indirect. **Direct myofascial techniques** are applied in the area of complaint and over the site of restriction, whereas **indirect myofascial techniques** are applied in an area outside the area of complaint. Therapists may use both direct and indirect site-specific techniques as a regular part of preventive massage, either to address a known area of scarring or adhesion, or to address sites where bind and strain often occur.

DEEP TRANSVERSE FRICTION

Deep transverse friction (DTF), sometimes called deep cross-fiber friction, is a site-specific technique applied to connective tissue lesions during the subacute and maturation phases of healing. Most therapists are familiar with this technique through the writings of Dr. James Cyriax,[12] an early advocate for the inclusion of DTF during healing. The first repair fibers at the site of trauma are disorganized, and movement is necessary to indicate the normal lines of stress and establish an organized alignment of

A sprinter in his last week of training before the state high school championship meet complains that both of his hamstrings are feeling tight, a condition that has been developing for a few weeks, and he just cannot seem to get them "loosened up." He has been religious about completing his full warm-up and stretching routine before and after each workout and has even added some additional hamstring stretches to the routine. He has been using analgesic cream during workouts and icing afterward, and this combination seems to have kept the tightness from getting worse. But the sense of tension remains during practice, and he is concerned that his performance will be affected, or even worse, that he will sustain a muscle strain during this week's workouts and be unable to compete in the championships.

His therapist locates extremely tender points in the middle of the gluteals and at the medial and lateral mus-

culotendinous junctions of the hamstring tendons. The therapist uses neuromuscular release to rid the musculature of these tender points, explaining to the athlete that stretching does not help a muscle decrease tension or facilitate the other mechanical action of a muscle, which is to broaden. The therapist assesses the iliotibial band and lumbosacral aponeurosis and uses broad plane release and skin rolling to reduce restriction when they are found. The therapist then asks the athlete to perform his regular leg-stretch routine, and the athlete is delighted to find that he feels less hamstring tension during the stretches and excitedly heads out to practice. This session is repeated daily, allowing the athlete to practice fully all week long, and he entered the championship competition as one of the favorites to win.

these fibers. DTF introduces tissue movement across the normal lines of stress to prevent the formation of any fibers that would literally be at cross-purposes to the intended fiber alignment. In addition, DTF causes mast cells to release histamines that create a local hyperemia and increased capillary permeability enhancing the normal healing process.[12–14]

Stroke Mechanics

Deep transverse friction is commonly applied with either a braced fingertip or thumb(s) pressed deep enough into the tissue to engage the lesion. The appropriate amount of pressure is variable from athlete to athlete, with pain and tissue resistance serving as the primary guidelines. The tissue is moved as one unit with the fingers/thumbs to the "stretch point" without sliding over the skin. The initial direction of tissue stretch should be perpendicular to the fiber alignment of the muscle, ligament, or tendon containing the lesion. It is this stretch across the normal fiber alignment that breaks apart the unwanted cross-links and disorganized repair fibers. In other words, the stretch across the normal lines of stress makes DTF effective, not the depth of tissue engagement. For this technique to be effective, its application should be[12–14]:

- Preceded by thorough warming and preparation of the tissue, either through general massage or brief heat applications
- Applied without an emollient to avoid sliding over the skin.

- Applied with a broad enough stroke to stretch and separate fibers.
- Performed with the muscle or tendon in a *relaxed* position, except for sheathed tendons (wrists and ankles), which should be treated in a *stretched* position. By stretching the sheathed tendons for DTF, the sheath is moved and stretched separate from the tendon breaking apart adhesions between the two structures (Fig. 9-3).
- Perpendicular to the fibers initially, then adjusted as necessary to address the multiple directions of restriction caused by connective tissue adhesion.
- Applied frequently enough to affect permanent change in the tissue.

Treatment Formula for Deep Transverse Friction

The treatment goals of the subacute and maturation stages of the healing cycle include facilitating the proper alignment of the repair fibers, which is the primary purpose of deep transverse friction. Because the initial repair fibers that appear in the subacute stage are fragile, very little pressure is required to break apart the cross-links, and great care must be taken to not re-irritate the tissue and cause more inflammation and swelling. To be effective but still avoid overworking the tissue, the first several treatments of DTF must follow a cautious formula. No treatment should ever elicit sharp pain or pain that is rated above a 5- on a 10-point severity scale. DTF should never be used directly over edematous tissue, but once the swelling is gone in the area of lesion, it can be initiated using the following guidelines for application.[12–14]

1. Warm up the tissue with a short heat application or general massage without emollient such as dry pétrissage and/or rhythmic compressions (approximately 5 minutes).
2. Begin DTF at right angles to the fiber run of the muscle, using only enough pressure to engage the tissue and keep the discomfort rating for the athlete at a 5 on a 10-point scale.
3. After 1 minute of DTF, check in with the athlete regarding the discomfort rating. If it has decreased, the treatment can continue, and the therapist may or may not choose to increase the pressure of the stroke to bring the discomfort rating back up to 5. If the discomfort rating has not decreased at the 1-minute mark, the direct DTF treatment stops for that session.
4. When the DTF treatment continues past 1 minute, the therapist must continue to check in with the athlete at 1-minute intervals to ensure that discomfort continues to decrease and must stop the treatment if it does not. Three minutes is the recommended maximum duration for the first DTF treatment.
5. Whenever DTF is stopped, passively move the muscle housing the lesion into a shortened position, then have the athlete perform a minimum of five isometric contractions in this position against the manual resistance from the therapist. These isometric contractions serve to enhance the normal muscle-broadening aspect of the injured area. In some cases, therapists may choose to introduce isometric contractions from a shortened position during the later part of the acute stage before DTF can be used.
6. Follow isometric resistives with light stretching, then ice the site of direct DTF and apply 5 to 10 minutes of

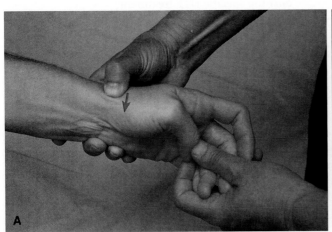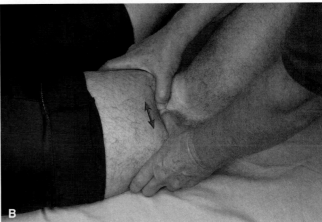

FIGURE 9-3 Deep transverse friction (DTF) to sheathed and nonsheathed tendons. (A) DTF to the extensor pollicis tendons. Sheathed tendons must be stretched for DTF. Stabilize the flexed thumb of the patient and add ulnar deviation to the wrist. **(B)** Nonsheathed tendons such as the hamstrings are shortened for DTF.

general massage (with or without emollient) to the surrounding muscles and antagonists. If practical, the icing and massage may be simultaneous, or general massage may precede the ice application.

This treatment formula is repeated *daily* until the full 3 minutes of DTF is tolerated without residual soreness the following day. Once this goal is achieved, the duration of DTF is increased by 1 to 2 minutes per session, again using decreased discomfort as the guideline for stopping or continuing until 5 minutes is well tolerated. The number of isometric contractions and the amount of time for general massage also increases over this time frame. Therapists may choose to continue increasing the duration of the DTF up to 10 minutes or shift to using a second repetition of 5 minutes after the general massage because frequency of treatment is more important than the duration of the session. In either case, it is recommended that no more than 10 minutes of DTF be applied in a single treatment session. Once the injury has progressed well into the maturation stage of healing, daily treatment sessions and icing after the DTF may no longer be necessary, but the isometric contractions and general massage should be continued.[2–12]

When DTF is used in cases of chronic injury lesions and/or well established, thick and matted scars, the application formula can be more aggressive than described in the acute injury formula. The heat application in step 1 may be increased to 10 minutes to fully soften collagen prior to DTF. In some cases, heat applications of more than 10 minutes can cause the tissue to feel edematous and make it difficult to palpate the specific landmarks necessary for precise application of DTF. The first DTF application may also be increased to 5 minutes rather than 3 minutes when treating these chronic injury lesions.

In conditions such as tendonitis/tendinosis, the repair process is not directed toward mending a specific tear and the entire tendon can be irritated. Repetitive stress causes a constant inflammation and proliferation of frayed and disorganized repair fibers that restricts and irritates the tendon leading to further inflammation. Therefore, the first step in a DTF treatment for active tendonitis may be to ice the area for 5 minutes to reduce pain and inflammation. This allows the therapist to engage the tissue on a deeper level and to extend the duration of the treatment to the full 3 minutes in the first session. The rest of the formula remains the same. However, it is still important to watch for and avoid residual soreness and increased swelling.

Following is an example of proper DTF (chronic Achilles tendonitis):

1. Ice massage over the Achilles tendon for 7 minutes or until the area is red and numb.
2. Place the foot/ankle into neutral or slight dorsiflexion, and begin DTF across the tendon using a pressure of a 5 on a 10-point discomfort scale as rated by the athlete (Fig. 9-4).
3. After 1 minute of DTF, check-in with the athlete regarding the discomfort rating. If the discomfort has decreased, the therapist increases the pressure of the stroke to bring the discomfort rating back up to 5 and continues the treatment for another 2 minutes. If not, DTF should not be continued.
4. Place the foot/ankle into full plantarflexion and have the athlete perform five isometric contractions against manual resistance.
5. Passively stretch the Achilles tendon to the point of first resistance and hold for 10 seconds; then release for 10 seconds. Repeat this hold–release stretch five times.
6. Secure an ice pack over the tendon, and apply general massage to the full leg that includes appropriate neuromuscular techniques to reduce any tender points found in the lower extremity musculature. Note that therapists may choose to use more general and superficial fascial releases such as the leg pull or broad plane release in hamstrings and posterior calf *before or after* the specific DTF treatment.

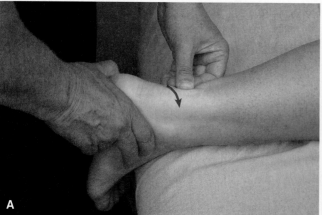
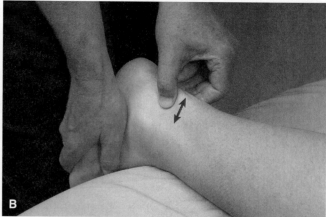

FIGURE 9-4 Deep transverse friction to the Achilles tendon. (A) Superficial over the top of the tendon. **(B)** More three-dimensional.

Common Sites for Deep Transverse Friction

Muscle attachments, musculotendinous junctions, and superficial ligaments and tendons are the most common sites of strain and tearing. Therefore, they are also the common sites for DTF application. The following series of figures depict the proper positioning and direction of application for DTF at sites commonly associated with athletic injuries (Fig. 9-5 through 9-10).

■ REVERSE-J STROKE, S STROKE, AND BRACED FINGERS AND THUMBS

Several site-specific myofascial techniques can be used to address a small connective tissue zone or structure even when an injury is not present. These connective tissue sites, like the common origin of the hamstrings or the hip flexor tendons, are subject to repeated strain during training and treatment of these structures can be an important element of maintenance massage for athletes. The first two techniques—reverse-J stroke and S stroke—are very similar to each other. Their names describe the direction of tension/ stretch applied to the specific anatomical site being treated.

The reverse-J stroke engages tissue with the thumb pad or braced fingers and then stretches it in an upside-down "J" pattern: that is, first a vertical stretch, then a horizontal stretch (see Fig. 2-6B). The reverse-J is the same stroke described in Chapter 2 as one of the basic sports massage strokes; however, when used as a site-specific myofascial

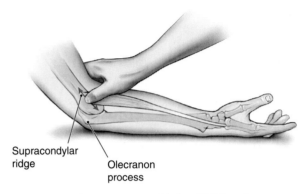

Supracondylar ridge

Olecranon process

FIGURE 9-6 Deep transverse friction (DTF) to the extensor carpi radialis longus. DTF at the supracondylar ridges of the humerus is applied parallel with the humerus.

stroke, the reverse-J stroke is applied without an emollient to engage the tissue on a deeper level and affect greater release (Fig. 9-11). Although it is perfectly acceptable to not reverse the J, the therapist is pulling the tissue rather than pushing it, which may result in less pressure and stretch being applied. The effectiveness of the reverse-J stroke may be improved by first applying a broad plane release to the larger tissue area before addressing the specific point of restriction. This is particularly effective in muscles such as the erector spinae and quadriceps, or in a larger fascial zone such as the posterior edge of the iliotibial band. Common sites of application for the reverse-J stroke include specific sites of adhesion along the erector spinae, and iliotibial band, and in fascial septa within or between muscles.[3-5,8]

In the S stroke, tissue is engaged and stretched with the thumb pads. Both thumbs are positioned on opposite sides of the specific tendon or site of restriction to be released. When pushed together, the thumbs create an oppositional stretch, forming an "S" pattern in the tissue (Fig. 9-12). S strokes can be used in the same areas as J strokes, but

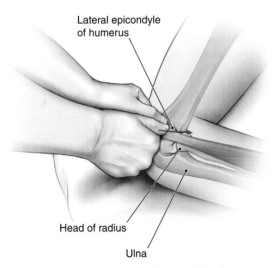

Lateral epicondyle of humerus

Head of radius

Ulna

FIGURE 9-5 Deep transverse friction (DTF) to the extensor carpi radialis brevis. DTF is applied perpendicular to the radius and ulna using a stronger pushing motion, which applies more tissue stretch and release than a pulling motion.

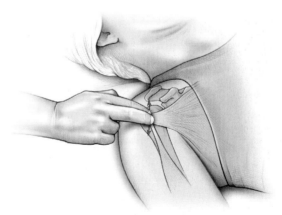

FIGURE 9-7 Deep transverse friction (DTF) at the insertion of the subscapularis. Externally rotate the humerus until the lesser tubercle is palpated, and apply DTF parallel with the humerus.

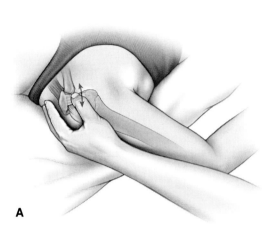

A

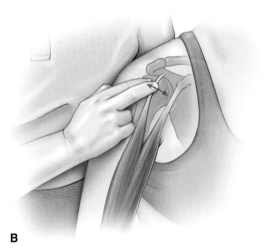

B

FIGURE 9-8 **Deep transverse friction (DTF) to the tendons of the supraspinatus and biceps. (A)** To access the insertion of the supraspinatus for DTF, extend the humerus to expose the expose the tendon and apply DTF parallel with the anterior-lateral edge of the acromion. **(B)** DTF to the biceps tendon also requires the shoulder to be extended, treating it like a sheathed tendon *as it runs intracapsularly.*

they are particularly appropriate for fascial release around the patella (as depicted in Chapter 10) and specific adhesions in the erector spinae.

For musculotendinous junctions and fascial septa between muscles, site-specific techniques using braced fingers or a braced thumb are particularly effective (Fig. 9-13). These techniques mechanically loosen the connective tissue, and when applied to the musculotendinous junction, stimulate the Golgi tendon organs to reflexively reduce tension. In these strokes, the bottom hand is the instrument or tool used for tissue engagement, and the top hand provides the power and pressure for the stroke. The therapist engages the connective tissue site by *scooping it into mild*

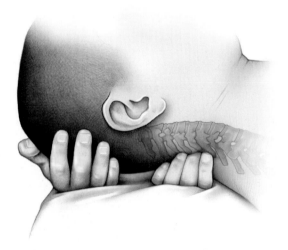

FIGURE 9-9 **Deep transverse friction to supraspinous and/or interspinous ligament in the neck is applied perpendicular to the processes.**

stretch (not pressing straight down into the tissue) with the pads of several fingers or the thumb pad of one hand. The palm or heel of the other hand is then pressed over the top of the fingers or thumb of the "down" hand to add more pressure and depth to the stroke. This top hand supplies the movement and pressure across the fibers to stretch and broaden the tissue. By bracing the thumb or fingers with the top hand, therapists provide the athlete with a sense of full hand pressure that disguises the intensity of the site specific work. These techniques also move a larger amount of tissue than the other site-specific strokes.

▓ MUSCLE ROLLING

Muscle rolling is a deeper and more three-dimensional form of skin rolling (Figs. 9-14 through 9-16). It is used in specific anatomic areas that allow the therapist to loosely grip an entire section of a muscle or muscle group and roll it between their fingers, mechanically sifting through the fibers to break apart adherent tissue. For maximum depth and effectiveness, the muscle must be passively shortened so that it is soft and easily lifted for rolling. The intention is to work the muscle in a three-dimensional manner, gently sifting through the fibers to identify tight or restricted areas. This creates a thixotropic change in the muscle that ensures independent fiber movement, supporting the natural broadening action of the muscle during contraction.[2–5,9,15] Muscle rolling may also be helpful in locating trigger points that can then be treated by an appropriate neuromuscular technique. Appropriate sites for muscle rolling include:

- Upper trapezius
- Posterior cervicals
- Sternocleidomastoid

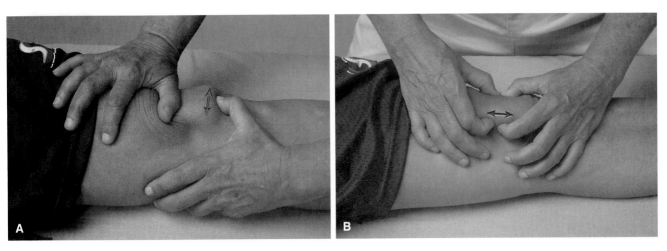

FIGURE 9-10 **Deep transverse friction around the patella requires the therapist to tip up the edge to be frictioned and stabilize it to access the underneath edge of the tendon as it envelopes the patella. (A)** The most common point of irritation is the inferior pole. **(B)** The medial superior pole is also commonly irritated.

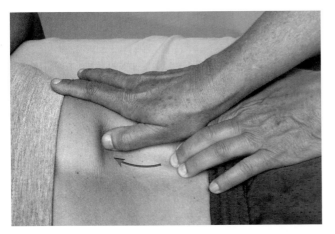

FIGURE 9-11 **Reverse-J stroke with opposition stretch for stabilization.**

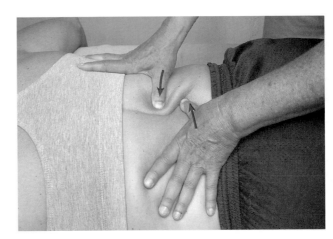

FIGURE 9-12 **S strokes in the erector spinae.**

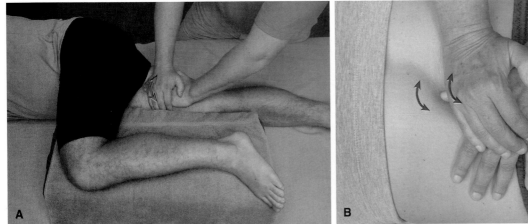

FIGURE 9-13 **(A)** Braced fingers for site-specific myofascial releases of the origins of the adductors. **(B)** Braced thumb friction through the laminar groove.

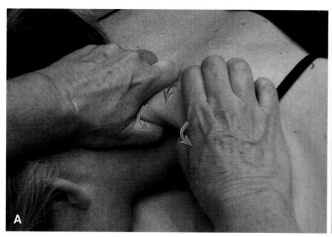
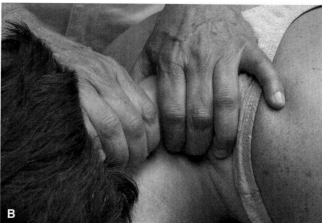

FIGURE 9-14 Muscle rolling. (A) The upper trapezius and levator scapula. **(B)** Posterior cervicals.

- Wrist/hand flexor and extensor groups
- Biceps brachii
- Triceps brachii
- Latissimus dorsi and teres major junction
- Pectoralis major and minor
- Pes anserine group

■ RELEASING SCARS

Whenever an athlete has a visible scar, surgical or otherwise, it is a likely site of fascial restriction. If the tissue has not been properly mobilized during healing, the scar acts like a knot in a sweater; it holds fibers together for repair, but creates pulling and strain throughout the garment. In fascial terms, the knot is a thick, matted scar that leads to restricted movement, tissue strain, and pain anywhere in the fascial chain. If DTF is properly applied during healing, the negative effects of scar tissue can be minimized. However, when faced with a well-established scar, therapists must aggressively treat it using a combination of site-specific myofascial techniques. Visual inspection and specific tissue excursion are generally used to assess and identify specific points of pain and/or restriction in the scar, whereas any combination of the site-specific techniques discussed above can be used for treatment. A good general approach is to begin with broad plane releases for the area housing the scar and to follow with reverse-J strokes or small linear stretches directly over the scar. Skin rolling and muscle rolling, both in line and across the scar, are also important techniques to include.[3–5,8]

CASE STUDY 9-2

A right-handed pitcher on the local college baseball team is complaining of chronic shoulder pain in his pitching arm. The team physician and Certified Athletic Trainer have thoroughly assessed the athlete, and no specific structural problem can be identified. Therefore, he is being treated for chronic strain using hydrotherapy, anti-inflammatory medication, and strength and flexibility exercises. The athlete reports that he is "OK" and continues to practice and compete, but never feels completely symptom-free. In mid-season, he is referred to a sports massage specialist. On review of the health history, the therapist notices that the athlete had an inguinal hernia repair on his left hip just a year ago. Postural assessment confirms a visible spiral line restriction from the left posterior neck, through the right rhomboids/mid-trapezius, and obliquely across the torso from the right serratus and left abdominal obliques to the left hip. Based on these findings, the therapist begins the session with broad plane pin-and-stretch across the left hip and a variety of site-specific myofascial strokes over the inguinal scar. Next, the therapist does skin rolling over the abdomen and linear shifts from ilium to axilla on the right side of the athlete's torso. The massage is finished with general massage to both arms and to the chest and neck. The athlete is surprised to find that his shoulder is symptom-free for the next few days, and both he and his coach are convinced that the continuing weekly treatment sessions with the sports massage therapist are helping him remain injury-free.

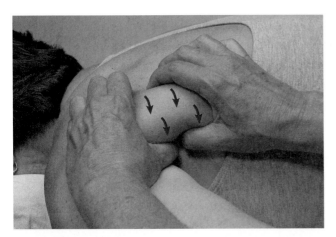

FIGURE 9-15 Muscle rolling of the latissimus dorsi and teres major. The tissue is gently squeezed between the thumbs and fingers, then rolled back and forth as if it is a pencil.

Broad Plane Myofascial Techniques

Broad plane techniques are used to address fascial tension and restriction in the large sheets of fascia plus the deep fascial layers within and surrounding each muscle. They are highly effective for treating areas such as the lumbosacral and abdominal aponeuroses, the iliotibial band, the four horizontal planes, and the hinge areas of the body, that is, anterior hip, shoulder, and neck. Like the site-specific techniques, broad plane myofascial releases can be categorized as direct or indirect. **Direct broad plane techniques** are those that are applied in an area of complaint or that push the tissue in the same direction as the restricted fascial excursion (Table 9-2). An **indirect broad plane technique** is applied in an area outside of an area of complaint or one that shifts toward the restricted tissue creating slack.[2–5,8]

■ BROAD PLANE PIN-AND-STRETCH

Two strokes—pin-and-stretch and active assistive releases—have already been described in Chapter 2 but are included here as broad plane myofascial strokes because they affect both the superficial and deep fascia of a full muscle group or body area. When being used for broad plane myofascial release, these strokes must be applied without an emollient to maximize the stretching and broadening effects to the muscle. In addition, the speed of movement used in both of these strokes is slowed, and the duration of the application is increased to 3 to 5 minutes to achieve full release of the tissue. The anterior aspect of the neck, shoulders, and hips, are three anatomic sites where broad plane pin-and-stretch releases are most often needed. These three sites have at least one horizontal band running through them, plus they are common flexion hinges in the body where contractile stress is often concentrated. When the anterior tissues at these sites have adapted to a short and tight position, the posterior tissues in the neck, back, and hips are under tensile stress, and it is these posterior areas that are generally identified by the athletes as feeling tight and painful.

Before performing the anterior neck release, or any technique that fully extends or rotates an athlete's neck, therapists must check for the possibility of cervical artery compression. For this test, the athlete is supine with the head resting at the top of the massage table. First, the therapist passively rotates the athlete's head as far as it will go and holds this position for 60 to 90 seconds. The second position to hold and evaluate is full extension of the cervical spine (Fig. 9-17). If the athlete experiences any dizziness, visual disturbance, or nausea or if the therapist notices changes in the pupils of the athlete's eyes, there is a strong possibility that the cervical arteries are being compressed or overstretched, and the broad plane release is contraindicated.

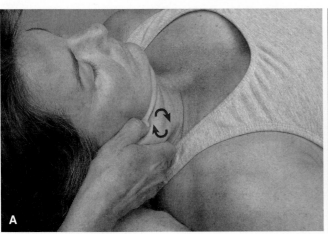

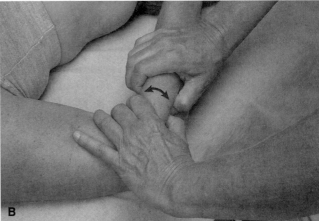

FIGURE 9-16 Muscle rolling. (A) The sternocleidomastoid. **(B)** Wrist extensors.

TABLE 9-2	Direct and Indirect Myofascial Techniques	
	Direct	**Indirect**

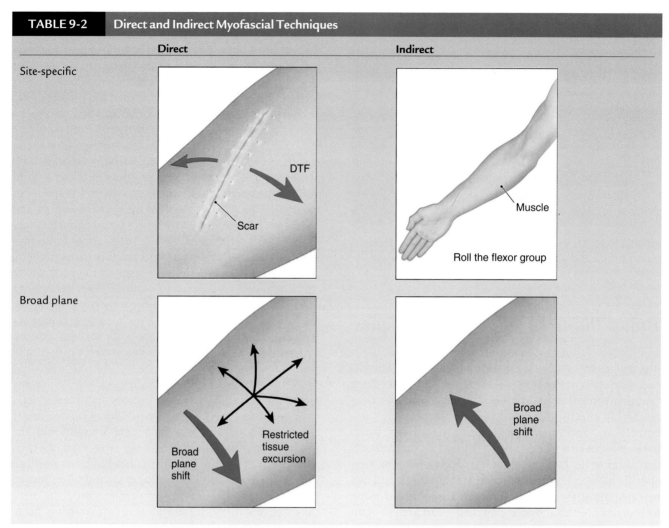

DTF, deep transverse friction.
Site specific fascial releases are direct when applied over the lesion or adhesion and indirect when applied in other areas associated with the problem (same myofascial chain). Broad plane releases are direct when a fascial shift release is applied over the restricted tissue and in the same direction as the restriction. Indirect broad plane releases do not specifically engage the restricted tissue and generally shift tissue into the restricted area to create slack.

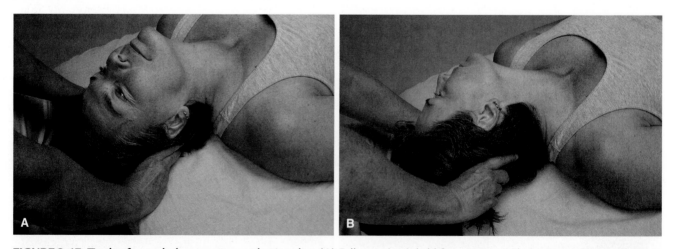

FIGURE 9-17 Testing for cervical artery compression/tension. (A) Full extension is held for approximately 1 minute while monitoring the athlete's pupils and verbally checking in about nausea and/or pain. **(B)** Rotation is added to the extension and held for a minimum of 30 seconds to complete the test.

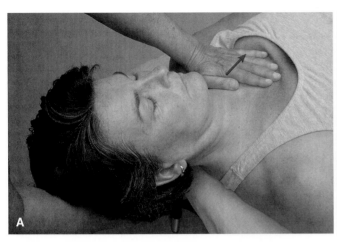
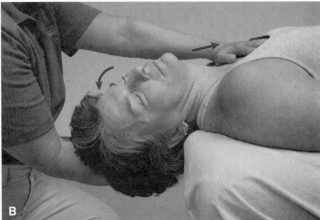

FIGURE 9-18 **Broad plane pin-and-stretch to fascia of the anterior neck. (A)** Start position. **(B)** Finish position.

The broad plane pin-and-stretch technique used to release the fascia on the anterior neck, positions the athlete supine on the treatment table, with the head slightly flexed and passively resting in the therapist's hand off the end of the table (Fig. 9-18A). The therapist scoops the anterior fascia of the neck toward the clavicle, creating a mild tension stretch in this tissue. While maintaining this tension in the anterior fascia, the therapist slowly extends the athlete's head until a movement barrier is sensed. This position is held until the resistance in the tissue decreases, indicating a fascial release. The therapist then extends the head farther to find the next movement barrier and repeats the hold–release–re-engage process until all movement barriers have been eliminated (Fig. 9-18B). If the athlete describes a burn-ing sensation in the fascia, indicating that the stretch is too intense or the movement is too fast, proper adjustments must be made. In addition, when other restrictions are sensed, small rotation and lateral flexion movements can be used during extension of the athlete's head to engage more tissue in the release. Finally, when the last barrier has released, the therapist must slowly release the tissue stretch before returning the athlete's head to the starting position.

The broad plane pin-and-stretches for the anterior shoulder (Fig. 9-19) and thigh (Fig. 9-20) are done in the same fashion as the anterior neck, with the therapist first engaging the anterior fascia in a mild stretch across the joint line, then slowly extending the joint through the movement barriers while maintaining that light tissue tension.

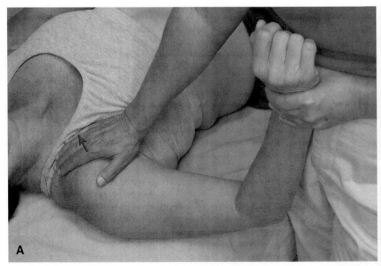
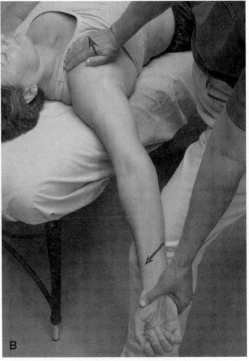

FIGURE 9-19 **Broad plane pin-and-stretch of the anterior shoulder.** **(A)** Start position. **(B)** Finish position.

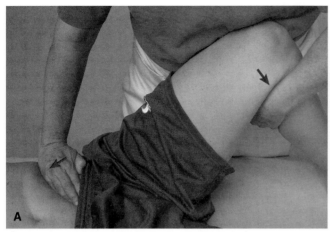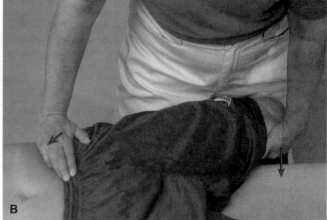

FIGURE 9-20 Broad plane pin-and-stretch of the anterior hip. (A) Start position. **(B)** Finish position.

The posterior wall of the axilla, formed by the layering of the latissimus dorsi, teres major, serratus anterior and subscapularis muscles, is another fascial area that can become restricted in athletes. The broad plane pin-and-stretch for this area is performed with the athlete in supine, and the therapist standing at the head of the table with their inside hand holding the athlete's adducted arm in 90 degrees of flexion (Fig. 9-21). The therapist pins the posterior tissue of the axilla into the subscapular fossa using the palm of the outside hand, then gently stretches the tissue toward the foot of the table. Once the tissue is pinned, the shoulder can be slowly moved through to full flexion pausing as necessary to release the movement barriers.

■ LINEAR SHIFTS

The superficial layer of fascia begins at the junction of epidermis and dermis and is contiguous with the deep invest-

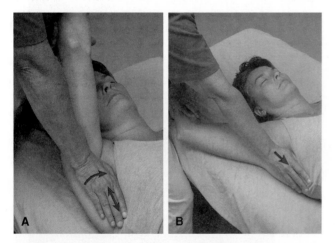

FIGURE 9-21 Broad plane pin-and-stretch for latissimus dorsi and teres major. (A) Start position. **(B)** Finish position.

ing fascia that winds throughout the musculoskeletal system. Therefore, a shift and stretch in the skin will be transmitted to the deeper layers, making the superficial fascia a "handle" for the therapist to affect deeper fascial release.[2–6,8,16–21] Linear shifts require the use of one or both hands to apply a slight stretch to the superficial fascia by sliding the skin to its point of tension or resistance, generally referred to as a *movement barrier*. The hands should not slide over the skin, but should hold the tissue at the movement barrier until a shift or release occurs. These strokes are appropriate and effective for all body regions, especially the multilayered fascial zones such as the lumbosacral aponeurosis, iliotibial band, or large body regions such as the full anterior thigh.

This broad plane stroke applies the same tissue excursion to the fascia as described in the assessment section of this chapter (see Fig. 9-1). However, it becomes a *release* when the tissue stretch is held at the movement barrier until crosslinks and restrictions between fascial layers are mechanically broken and the tissue shifts. In addition to these mechanical changes, the heat and pressure from the therapist's hands create *thixotropic* changes in the tissue, making it more fluid and soft. This stretching and softening of the fascia, described by therapists as "melting away," "creeping," or "letting go," may take several minutes to occur. Once complete, therapists must remember to gradually reduce the stretch and pressure in the tissue before removing their hands, so that the benefit of the release is maintained.[2–6,8,16–21]

■ HORIZONTAL PLANE RELEASES

The myofascial techniques used to reduce restrictions in the horizontal planes of the body require a great deal of practice, patience, and palpatory sensitivity on the part of the therapist. Although the hand placement is specific to each different plane, all the release techniques are essentially the same. Therapists always position their nondominant hand under the torso and the dominant hand on the anterior torso over the horizontal plane to be released. The release begins with the therapist applying a gently compression into the anterior tissue while the bottom hand stabilizes the area with a slight lift into the torso. This translates into a light stretch of the deep transverse planes of fascia. Think of holding a balloon with one hand on either side and gently pressing your hands together. The air in the balloon creates resistance to complete compression while the sides of the balloon stretch outward. When the hands are positioned on opposite sides of a torso and compression is applied, a stretch occurs in the horizontal planes similar to the sides of the balloon. This three-dimensional stretch releases any tension or restriction in these deeper fascial structures. The compression–stretch must be maintained for 30 to 60 seconds before the fascia begins to shift and release. As with other myofascial techniques, the hands must not slide over the skin but move together with the tissue. As tissue resistance melts and releases, the therapist "takes up the slack" by gradually adding more compression and stretch to the tissue until no further movement barriers are sensed. For

complete release of the horizontal planes, this process must be continued for approximately 3 to 5 minutes.[2–6]

Thoracic Inlet Release

The purpose of the thoracic inlet release is to relax the myofascial elements of the upper thorax to improve respiration, reduce compressive or tension forces over the neurovascular bundle in the upper quadrant, and decrease strain in the face, head, cervical, and upper back muscles.[2–5] The athlete lies supine on the table with legs fully extended, and the therapist sits at the head of the table. With fingers pointing toward the athlete's feet, the therapist slides the nondominant hand under the athlete's upper back and positions it directly over the spine with the heel of the hand over or just inferior to the spinous process of C7 (Fig. 9-22A). The dominant hand of the therapist is then placed flat over the sternum with the fingers pointing toward the feet and the heel of the hand over the manubrium, just inferior to the sternal notch (Fig. 9-22B). The bottom hand stabilizes the upper rib cage by lightly lifting up into the torso as the top hand first compresses then adds a very slight stretch of the anterior tissue toward the feet. The compression–stretch is held at the first point of tissue resistance—the movement barrier—until resistance decreases and tissue release is sensed by the therapist. This light compression–stretch process is repeated as each successive movement barrier is found and released. The therapist then slowly reduces first the stretch and then the compression before gently lifting the hands from the tissue.[2–5] If the hands are removed too quickly and without gradually decreasing the stretch and compression, a fascial rebound occurs that decreases the effectiveness of the release.

A second phase of the thoracic inlet release is similar to the first, but this time the anterior hand of the therapist is placed horizontally across the midsternum (see Fig. 9-22C), and once the compression barrier is sensed, the tissue is placed in a light traction stretch toward the chin. Again, the compression-stretch is sustained until all movement barriers have been released.[5]

Diaphragm Release

When postural assessment reveals protracted shoulders, head, and/or kyphosis, a diaphragm release is indicated and necessary to relieve pain and strain in the posterior neck and upper and mid-back. In addition, releasing the diaphragm should also improve the athlete's breathing and general organ functions because the diaphragm effectively engages all tissue from the pharynx to the perineum when it moves.[11] The athlete is once again lying in a supine position, but this time the therapist sits at the side of the table. The therapist slides the nondominant hand hori-

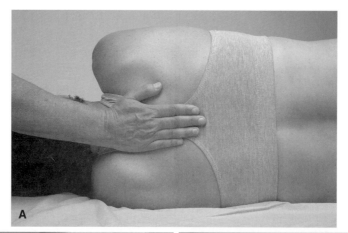

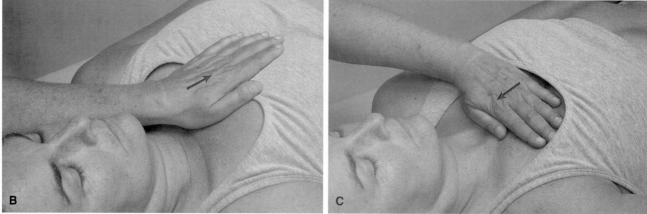

FIGURE 9-22 Horizontal plane release for the thoracic inlet. (A) Position the posterior hand at the cervicothoracic junction. **(B)** Position the anterior hand over the sternum with the heel at the manubrium. Note: The finger should be inside, underneath clothing for skin-to-skin contact for full therapeutic effect. **(C)** Alternate/second hand position for the anterior hand, across mid-sternum. Light tissue stretch is applied toward the chin.

zontally under the torso to the thoracolumbar junction of the spine, resting the spinous processes in the palm of the flat hand (Fig. 9-23A). The therapist's dominant hand is positioned on the anterior side of the athlete's torso just inferior to the xyphoid process so that the heel of that hand

rests in the apex of the lower rib cage (Fig. 9-23B). The bottom hand of the therapist stabilizes the thorax with a slight lift while the top hand applies gentle pressure until the compression barrier is felt. Then a light traction stretch toward the feet is applied. The compression–stretch over

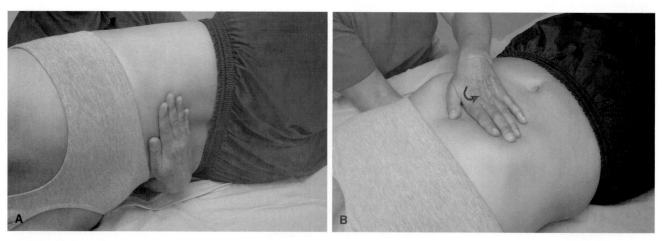

FIGURE 9-23 Diaphragm release. **(A)** Position the posterior hand at the thoracolumbar junction. **(B)** Position the anterior hand across the apex of the rib cage opening.

the diaphragm is sustained and adjusted until all barriers have been released.[2-5]

Pelvic Floor Release

This transverse plane release is helpful in relieving chronic low back and hip pain. As with the diaphragm release, the therapist's posterior hand placement is horizontal across the athlete's torso, but this time at the lumbosacral junction of the spine (Fig. 9-24A). The anterior hand of the therapist is placed across the pelvic cavity with the ulnar border of the hand resting just superior to the pubic bone (Fig. 9-24B). After the first compression barrier has released, the therapist applies slight traction to the tissue, stretching it toward the head. Again, this compression–stretch is maintained until all movement barriers have been released.[2-5]

▪ TRACTION RELEASES

Manual traction, over-the-door pulleys, and traction tables are common clinical modalities used by sport health care therapists. The intention of these methods is to decompress a specific joint or vertebral zone such as the cervical or lumbar spine to relieve tension and pain. Instead of isolating a single joint, the full-limb traction releases described here are broad plane fascial releases. Their intention is to engage the three-dimensional fascial cylinder of an extremity to gently stretch and release the full myofascial chain. Theoretically, by engaging all fascial elements of the limb, any and all points of fascial restriction in the limb will be released, not just those directly under the hands of the therapist. This is in contrast to single-joint traction methods that engage only the capsule, ligaments, and tendons of a single joint.

Traction Release for the Arm

To perform the full arm traction release, the athlete lies supine on the table with arm adducted and hand in the handshake position. To reduce stress to the therapist's body and provide the optimal stretch for the athlete, the table height should be adjusted so that the therapist can hold the athlete's arm with his or her own arms fully relaxed and extended. Standing at the athlete's side facing the head of the table, the therapist grasps the heel of the athlete's hand, "sandwiching" it between the palms of the hands. The therapist begins the release by shifting his or her body weight to the back foot to apply gentle traction to the extremity in line with the muscle fibers of the deltoid and biceps and holds this position until all traction barriers are released. At this point, the therapist begins to slowly abduct and externally rotate the athlete's arm (traction still maintained) until a new movement barrier is sensed. Again, the position is held until the barrier releases, and the process is repeated through the full arc of shoulder movement until the athlete's arm is in the overhead position, fully flexed and externally rotated (Fig. 9-25). Constant visual and verbal monitoring of the athlete's response is necessary to ensure that the movement never exceeds pain-free range of motion. The therapist can focus the release to a particular joint or tissue segment of the arm by moving one hand up to the target area and intensifying the stretch of that tissue (Fig. 9-26). If the athlete has a hand, wrist, or elbow injury, the release can be adapted by changing the therapist's hand placement to just proximal of the effected joints(s) before the traction-tension is applied.[2-5]

In some cases, it may be necessary to apply a second traction release for the upper extremity through the horizontal adduction plane of the shoulder. For this release, the athlete's starting arm position is again fully adducted except that 90 degrees of shoulder flexion is added. With one hand at the athlete's wrist and the other under the

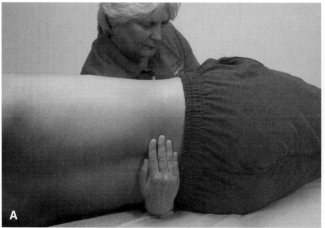
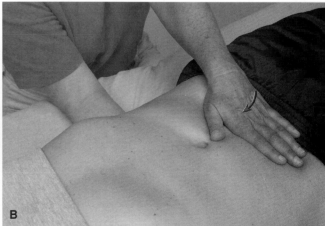

FIGURE 9-24 Horizontal plane release of the pelvic floor. (A) Position the posterior hand at the lumbosacral junction. **(B)** Position the anterior hand across the lower pelvic cavity just superior to the pubic bone.

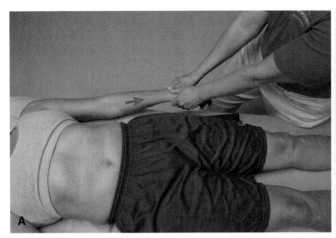

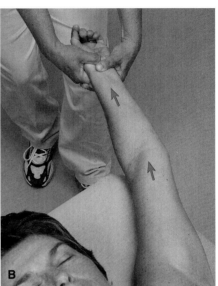

FIGURE 9-25 Traction release for the upper extremity. (A) Start position requires the therapist to apply light traction by gently leaning back. (B) Finish position.

scapula or at mid-brachium, the therapist applies a gently traction-stretch to the full arm by lifting it toward the ceiling, then moving it slowly through horizontal adduction, releasing movement barriers (Fig. 9-27A). As traction is maintained through horizontal adduction, the shoulder will lift off the table as the arm crosses the midline. At this point, the therapist's lower hand position shifts from the brachium to under the scapula (Fig. 9-27B), and additional traction-tension is added to the release by gently sliding the scapula into protraction while full arm traction is maintained.[6,12]

Traction Release for the Leg

To perform this broad plane myofascial technique, the athlete is supine on the table and the legs are adducted. From the foot of the table, the therapist cups the athlete's poste-

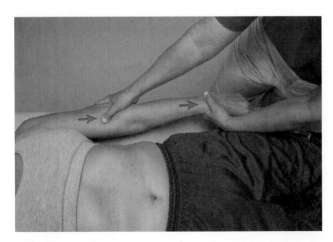

FIGURE 9-26 Alternate hand positions for traction release of the arm.

rior calcaneus in the palm of one hand and dorsiflexes the athlete's foot with the other hand. The first phase of the release begins with the therapist slowly shifting their body weight to the back foot to establish traction to the full leg. Similar to the traction release of the arm, movement barriers are released through the full arc of abduction and external rotation allowed by the leg while traction-tension is maintained (Fig. 9-28). Again, if the athlete has foot, ankle, or knee injuries, the therapist's hand position can be adjusted to avoid traction of the affected joint as depicted in Figure 9-28C.[5]

In the second phase of this release, the hand positions and leg traction are similar, but this time the ankle is in slight plantarflexion. The release begins with the therapist lifting the athlete's leg into slight hip flexion before establishing the traction-stretch on the full extremity. The leg is moved through internal rotation and hyperadduction until the leg crosses the midline, releasing the successive movement barriers as they are sensed by the therapist (Fig. 9-29). At the end point of this hyperadduction and internal rotation, the athlete's hip will lift up from the table causing slight torso rotation to release the sacroiliac and lumbosacral areas.[3-5]

Often it is more difficult to maintain traction on the full release while moving through the full range of motion. Therefore, therapists may choose to segment the lower extremity and apply traction–stretch releases to each segment separately.[3-5]

SUMMARY

The myofascial techniques can and should be combined and modified by therapists to address the changing and variable needs of the athletes in their care. The key concepts for application of the myofascial techniques are:

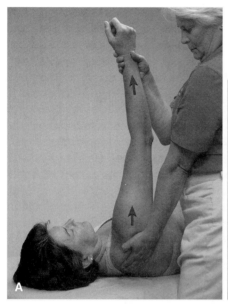
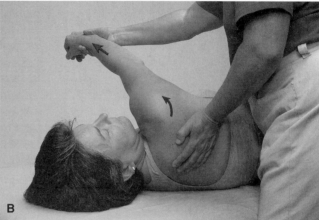

FIGURE 9-27 Horizontal traction release for the upper extremity. (A) Traction release. **(B)** Finish this release with focused stretch of the scapula.

- The intention of all myofascial strokes is to separate adherent fibers and layers of connective tissue that may restrict and/or add stress to the athlete's movement.
- By relieving myofascial restrictions, compressive and tensile stress to nerves, blood and lymph vessels is decreased to help reduce pain and improve circulation and lymph flow.

- Therapists should assess the full body and specific myofascial chains related to an athlete's complaint of pain and tension in order to choose the appropriate combination of techniques to relieve the athlete's complaint. This is true especially with chronic and persistent pain syndromes.
- For maximum effectiveness, myofascial techniques must be applied without an emollient.

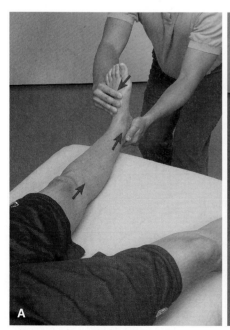
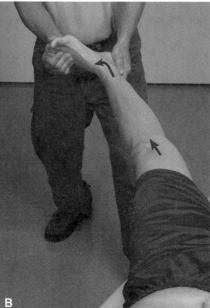
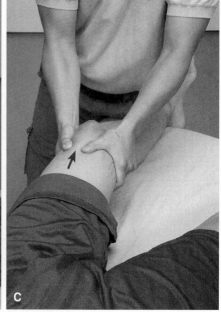

FIGURE 9-28 Traction release for the full lower extremity. (A) Start position requires the therapist to first stabilize the heel and dorsiflex the ankle, then apply light traction by gently leaning back. **(B)** Finish position. **(C)** Alternate hand position for isolation of the myofascial elements in the hip and thigh.

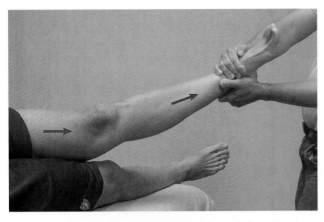

FIGURE 9-29 Traction release of the leg through the adduction–internal rotation range of motion.

- Whether the technique is site-specific or broad plane, the superficial fascia and the therapist's hands/fingers/thumbs move as one unit.
- Use the site-specific techniques to address a specific anatomic structure, lesion, or small restricted zone.
- Use the broad plane techniques to address full myofascial chains and fascial zones. These strokes serve as good preparatory strokes before site-specific work and may also be used as finishing strokes.
- No myofascial technique should cause sharp pain or muscle guarding (DTF and skin rolling are uncomfortable, but not painful).
- Myofascial techniques should be combined with appropriate neuromuscular techniques to achieve the best treatment results.

Review Questions

SHORT ANSWERS

1. Define the term myofascial technique, and name four specific "name brands" that fall into this category.

2. List the four methods of assessment for myofascial tissue.

3. Explain what makes a myofascial technique direct or indirect.

4. List five regional contraindications to myofascial techniques.

5. What criteria must be met for deep transverse friction to be effective?

MULTIPLE CHOICE

6. What is the common intention of all myofascial techniques?
   a. Realignment of collagen fibers
   b. Improve range of motion
   c. Stretch, broaden, or loosen connective tissue
   d. Increase circulation

7. Which is the best site-specific technique to facilitate proper fiber alignment of a specific myofascial lesion during healing?
   a. Muscle rolling
   b. Deep transverse friction
   c. Pin-and-stretch
   d. Reverse-J

8. A myofascial technique that applies tissue stretch in the same direction as the restriction barrier is categorized as a(n)_____ technique.
   a. direct
   b. indirect
   c. linear
   d. site-specific

9. Two of the best assessment techniques for finding myofascial restrictions in the lumbosacral aponeurosis are skin rolling and _____.
   a. the athlete's pain rating
   b. general back massage
   c. review of the medical history
   d. tissue excursion

10. Deep transverse friction should first be introduced during which stage of the healing cycle?
    a. Acute
    b. Subacute
    c. Maturation flexibility
    d. Maturation strength

11. For deep transverse friction to be effective when applied over a sheathed tendon, the tendon should be placed in a _____ position.
    a. short
    b. relaxed
    c. semi-stretched
    d. stretched

12. Which of these steps in the DTF application formula immediately follows the friction strokes?
    a. A short heat application over the site of friction
    b. Isometric contractions while the muscle is in a shortened position
    c. General massage to the full muscle group
    d. A brief cold application followed by mild stretch

13. In which of these lesions would deep transverse friction be applied in a direction that parallels the humerus?

a. Origin of the extensor carpi radialis brevis
b. Insertion of the supraspinatus
c. Insertion of the subscapularis
d. Bicepital tendonitis

14. What are the three anatomic areas in which broad plane pin-and-stretch releases should regularly be applied?
a. Lumbosacral aponeurosis, patellar retinaculi, and the popliteal space
b. Anterior neck, shoulders, and hips
c. Iliotibial band, abdomen, and pectoral region
d. Anterior thigh, knee, and ankle

15. All broad plane myofascial techniques must be held for approximately how long for all movement barriers to be release?
a. 1 minute
b. 1 hour
c. 6 to 10 minutes
d. 3 to 5 minutes

16. What is the correct direction of application for deep transverse friction to the supraspinatus insertion?
a. Across the anterior edge of the acromion process
b. In line with the humerus
c. Across the posterior edge of the acromion process
d. Circular, around the lesser tubercle

17. The hamstring tendons should be in a(n) _____ position for effective deep transverse friction.
a. anatomic
b. stretched
c. short
d. contracted

18. The muscle rolling myofascial technique is best suited for muscles such as the sternocleidomastoid, upper trapezius, and _____.
a. erector spinae and latissimus dorsi
b. wrist flexors and extensors
c. hamstrings and adductor group
d. gastrocnemius and rectus abdominis

19. The correct hand position for the pelvic floor release is _____.
a. one hand vertical under the sacrum and the other across the lower abdominal cavity just superior to the pubic bone
b. both hands in parallel vertical alignment in the lower abdominal cavity just superior to the pubic bone
c. one hand horizontal under the lumbar spine and the other horizontal directly opposite it in the abdominal cavity
d. both hands in parallel vertical alignment over the sacrum

20. What two points of application are changed to make pin-and-stretch an effective broad plane fascial release?
a. The pressure is increased, and the movement is sped up.
b. The direction of tissue pinning is reversed, and the movement is created by the athlete.
c. A broader area of tissue is engaged, and the stretching movement is slower.
d. A smaller area of tissue is engaged, and the stretch is accomplished through tissue excursion.

REFERENCES

1. Denegar CR. Persistent pain and kinetic chain dysfunction: Making the link. Proceedings of NATA Annual Meeting and Clinical Symposium Los Angeles, CA, 2000.
2. Greenman PE. Principles of Manual Medicine, 3rd ed. Philadelphia: Lippincott Williams & Wilkins, 2003.
3. Barnes JF. Myofascial Release I. Paoli, PA: self published MFR Seminars, 1989.
4. Barnes JF. Myofascia Release: The Missing Link in Traditional Treatment. In: Davis CM, ed. Complementary Therapies in Rehabilitation. Thorofare, NJ: Slack, 1997.
5. Manheim CJ. The Myofascial Release Manual, 3rd ed. Thorofare, NJ: Slack, 2001.
6. Roth GB. New dimensions in the treatment of fascial tissue: Matrix re-patterning™. www.wellnesssystems.com.
7. Murphy J. Myofascial treatment proves beneficial in acute and sports medicine settings. Advance for Physical Therapists 1996, September 2.
8. Keirns M. Myofascial Release in Sports Medicine. Champaign, IL: Human Kinetics, 2000.
9. Scheumann DW. The Balanced Body: A Guide to Deep Tissue and Neuromuscular Therapy, 2nd ed. Philadelphia: Lippincott Williams & Wilkins, 2002.
10. Chaitow L, DeLany JW. Clinical Application of Neuromuscular Techniques, vol. 1: The Upper Body. Edinburgh: Churchill Livingstone, 2000.
11. Chaitow L. Soft-Tissue Manipulation: A Practitioner's Guide to the Diagnosis and Treatment of Soft Tissue Dysfunction and Reflex Activity. Rochester, VT: Healing Arts Press, 1988.
12. Cyriax J. Textbook of Orthopaedic Medicine: vol. 1: Diagnosis of Soft Tissue Lesions, 8th ed. London: Bailliere Tindall, 1982.
13. Benjamin BE. Frustrating neck injuries part 2. Massage Therapy Journal 1988, 27:3.
14. Hammer WI. Functional Soft Tissue Examination and Treatment by Manual Methods: The Extremities. Gaithersburg, MD: Aspen Publishers, 1991.
15. Juhan D. Job's Body: A Handbook for Bodywork, expanded edition. Barrytown, NY: Station Hill, 1998.
16. Meyers TW. Anatomy Trains: Myofascial Meridians for Manual and Movement Therapists. Edinburgh: Churchill Livingstone, 2001.
17. Sahrmann S. Movement and muscle impairments of the lower extremity. Advanced Track Seminar; 2000 NATA National Convention and Clinical Symposium Nashville, TN.
18. Sahrmann SA. Diagnosis and Treatment of Movement Impairment Syndromes. St. Louis: Mosby, 2002.
19. Roth GB. Scoliosis—new hope: A preliminary report on the use of Matrix Repatterning™. June 2004, www.rothinstitute.com.
20. Roth GB. A new approach to frozen shoulder: A pilot study using matrix re-patterning™. June 2004, www.wellnesssystems.com.
21. Hammer WI. Matrix Repatterning™. Dynamic Chiropractic 2001, March 12.

Protocols for Massage Used in Athletics

Chapter

10

Massage for Sports Events

After completing this chapter, the reader will be able to:

- List the goals for pre-, inter-, and post-event massage
- Explain the benefits and physiologic changes created by event sports massage.
- List the general stroke sequence for each category of event sports massage with and without the use of an emollient.
- Describe the most appropriate time frame for giving pre- and post-event massage in relation to the start/ finish of the activity.
- Estimate the appropriate duration of massage for each category of event massage.
- Conduct an appropriate pre-massage interview for pre-, inter-, and post-event massage.
- List and demonstrate the proper sequence of action steps for cramp management.
- List the common signs and symptoms of heat exhaustion, heat stroke, hypothermia, and frostbite.
- List and demonstrate the proper sequence of action steps for first aid with each of these conditions.
- Demonstrate an appropriate event massage sequence both with and without an emollient for upper and lower body sports.
- List and demonstrate an appropriate event massage sequence with an emollient for both upper and lower body.

E vent massage is designed to help athletes prepare for and recover from athletic endeavors. Therefore, it is delivered at the site of the activity and is generally fast paced. The three categories of event massage—pre-event, inter-event, and post-event—all combine the basic sports massage strokes to create the intended effects and benefits for the athlete as he/she participates. This chapter compares and contrasts the goals, strokes, pace, and duration of each category of event massage and also gives some examples of appropriate stroke combinations for lower and upper body either with or without an emollient.

Goals of Event Massage

Event sports massage must be designed to support the athlete in creating optimal internal conditions for the preparation and recovery from physical exertion. All three categories of event sports massage assist the normal physiologic processes inherent in each stage of the athlete's physical performance. For example, pre-event massage is designed to enhance the warm-up process by loosening myofascial structures, whereas the inter-event and post-event massages assist in recovery from exercise by addressing general tension and specific problem areas that are common to the athlete's activity. Because the physiologic status of the athlete differs in each category, the therapeutic goals for each of these are also different.

PRE-EVENT MASSAGE GOALS

It is a well-accepted concept that athletes should warm up before vigorous activity to decrease their risk of injury and enhance their perform potential. The general warm-up routine is intended to increase circulation and core temperature, facilitate the necessary neuromuscular pathways for the upcoming activity, and stretch muscles and connective tissue to ensure full range of motion and proper biomechanics during activity.[1] The overall intention of this is twofold: to reduce the risk of injury and to improve the athlete's *performance potential,* a term first coined by Benny Vaughn, LMT, ATC, CSCS. Ultimately, the athlete's performance is the result of a multitude of variables with the massage being only one of these factors. All that the pre-event massage can do is improve the athlete's potential for a winning performance. A pre-event massage has the same overall intention as the warm-up, and it makes some unique contributions to the process. However, because no amount of soft tissue manipulation can create the circulatory and core temperature increases needed for most athletic endeavors, pre-event massage is designed to complement the athlete's regular warm-up routine, not replace it. The goals of pre-event massage include[2–8]:

1. Soften and loosen the fascia and other connective tissue structures.
2. Decrease excess muscle tension.
3. Enhance the hyperemia response in the muscles to be used in the activity.
4. Provide *kinesthetic* feedback that helps create a positive state of mind; that is, athletes *feel* muscles relax and a greater sense of ease with movement.

The cardiovascular changes that can be attributed to pre-event massage are indirect or secondary responses to the loosening and decreased muscle tension created by the massage. When these mechanical changes are made in the tissue, there is a reduced resistance to blood flow, and the capillary beds can carry larger volumes. In addition, the manual pressure of a vigorous pre-event massage has been shown to cause a slight increase in local arterial pressure and emptying of veins, which creates a momentary negative pressure that tends to draw blood into the capillaries.[9] Although several authors list increased circulation as a goal of pre-event massage,[2–7,10] only active movement

can create sufficient increases in cardiac rate and output to actually increase circulation.[11] Creating a deep hyperemia is a better way to describe the "circulatory" improvements of the pre-event massage.

If one were to ask an athlete "why do you warm-up," a common response would be simply to "loosen up." This *feeling* of loose muscles has documented psychological benefit that is generally presumed to positively influence the athlete's performance.[2–5,10,12] However, the athlete's warm-up and stretch routine is often too general to address specific tender points or fascial restrictions. Although the general warm-up routine may serve to identify these tight and restricted areas, only direct soft tissue manipulation can address tension and restriction at specific anatomic sites such as musculotendinous junctions and bony attachments of muscles. Site-specific frictions directed to the tendons and musculotendinous junctions of the large muscle groups can accomplish two goals: (1) mechanical loosening of connective tissue and (2) stimulation of the proprioceptors (Golgi tendon organs) to inhibit muscle tension. In addition, all forms of massage do what stretching cannot—broaden the muscle to help balance the length–strength ratio. Because an athlete's sense of tension or ease during movement can be related to restrictions in either the lengthening or broadening capacity of a muscle, the broadening strokes used in pre-event massage are important contributions. Therefore, the structural effects of massage, that is, reduced muscle tension and loosening of tendons and fascia, contribute to enhanced performance potential in two ways: measurable improvements in range of motion and power[2–5,11,12] and the enhanced psychological benefit of feeling loose.

INTER-EVENT MASSAGE GOALS

An inter-event massage is given between bouts of exercise occurring on the same day and within a specific time frame, that is, between heats or events at a track meet, swim meet, tennis tournament, or even at half-time of a basketball game. Just as pre-event massage cannot take the place of the warm-up, the inter-event massage is merely an adjunct to the athlete's normal inter-event routine.

The primary goal of inter-event massage is to identify and address any areas of excess tension that have developed during exercise. Athletes may be able to direct the therapist to a specific tight spot, or the therapist can quickly assess the major muscle groups with effleurage and/or pétrissage. If two or three events are scheduled in the same session, the goals also include improving lymphatic uptake,[1,13] which may improve the athlete's rate of recovery. As in pre-event massage, the therapist must avoid sedating the athlete.

■ POST-EVENT MASSAGE GOALS

Athletes cool down after activity with light exercise and stretches. Stretching helps return tight and tense muscles to their normal resting tone and length, and light exercise maintains the low-grade increase in metabolism that helps repay oxygen debt and continues the body's natural recycling of metabolic by-products. Post-event massage assists the body with these processes by reducing any general muscle tension that develops during exercise, facilitating edema uptake and lymph movement, and helping return muscles and fascia to full length and flexibility.[1-7,9-16] The goals of post-event massage include:

1. Return muscles to resting tone and length.
2. Assist venous return to support metabolic recovery.
3. Deactivate trigger/tender points that may have developed during activity.
4. Reduce risk of delayed-onset muscle soreness.

For athletes, the rate of recovery varies greatly owing to the complex physiologic processes related to muscle fatigue and recovery. These variables can include the athlete's fitness level and basal metabolic rate, aerobic versus anaerobic demands, nutrition, hydration, and many others. Even environmental factors can influence fatigue and recovery. To date, the limited amount of research that has studied the effect of post-event massage on the rate of recovery has shown equivocal evidence. For example, Smith et al.[15] studied the effect of massage rendered 2 hours after eccentric exercise and its effect on delayed-onset muscle soreness and serum creatine kinase, "an indirect marker of muscle tissue damage." This study had a well-defined 30-minute massage protocol with specific time controls for each element of the massage. Results demonstrated a significant reduction in the intensity of delayed-onset muscle soreness and serum creatine kinase for the 14 subjects involved. In contrast, Weber et al.[16] studied the impact of massage on muscle soreness and force deficits after high-intensity eccentric exercise. Results of this study showed no statistical difference among massage, microcurrent electrical stimulation, and simple rest on either muscle soreness or force generation. However, the massage plan in this study was not well defined and was only 8 minutes in duration. The massage was also applied immediately after exercise and again at 24 hours after exercise. In effect, reliable studies on the effects of massage specific to athletic performance and recovery are scarce. In addition, the variance in research methodologies, measurement and analysis tools, and the wide variety of massage techniques used in these studies explain the variable results in the few studies that do exist.

From the Field

Drs. William Donnelly and Allan March, physicians working with the University of Florida athletes, agree that even though many of the benefits of massage to athletes are based largely on subjective observations, both are firm in their support for its use.

Donnelly: "Massage makes a big difference to performing athletes. Whatever edge they can get is worth it."

March: "I'm convinced of its beneficial aspects. We use it as a restorative measure in athletes with sports injuries."

From: "Does Sports Massage Have a Role in Sports Medicine." Samples, Pat.[13]

Stroke Combinations and Massage Focus

In addition to deciding which areas to begin with and focus time on, therapists must decide which combinations of the basic massage strokes best address the massage goals and priorities. The first consideration is whether any emollient will be used. In cases in which the athletes wear full-coverage uniforms or workout gear, or at events in which residual lubrication on the skin might cause slipping or heat retention, it is recommended that the dry massage combination of strokes be used. As with all massage, the general guidelines of working from general to specific and superficial to deep are used to formulate good event massage sequences. It is particularly important for therapists to gradually increase their pressure during inter-event and post-event massage because of the increased sensitivity and tenderness in muscles from exertion. Refer to Table 2-2 to review the specific effects attributed to each basic sports massage stroke. Regardless of whether or not an emollient is used, muscle and limb jostling is used to transition and connect the individual strokes and to move between body areas. When no emollient is used, the suggested strokes and sequence are very simple:

- Rhythmic compression
- Dry pétrissage

- General and specific friction
- Finish with tapotement in pre-event massage

When using an emollient, the suggested combination of strokes is:

- Effleurage
- Pétrissage
- Active-assistive releases
- Finish with tapotement in pre-event and effleurage in post-event massage

For each category of event massage, the same stroke combinations and general sequences are used to give brief, but focused attention to all the major muscle groups, tendons, and fascial zones in the body region. However, in inter-event massage, the athlete may need only one tight or restricted area addressed, and the therapist may perform only a single neuromuscular or myofascial release rather than a full massage routine. In post-event massage, the only significant change in stroke selection or sequence is that effleurage takes the place of tapotement at the end of the massage. Also, recognize that the "frog-leg" position used to address the iliotibial band and other lateral structures in the leg may be too uncomfortable for an athlete in a post-event massage because of tense and fatigued muscles. Another option for inter-event and post-event massage is to use the lymphatic sequences for recovery from exercise outlined in Chapter 7. These lymphatic sequences can either replace or be added to the end of a standard post-event sequence for athletes involved in multi-day competitions or tournament situations.

Stretches should be added toward the end of an event massage sequence after all the major muscle groups have been thoroughly massaged. Because most athletes do their own preferred stretches in the warm-up and cool-down processes and because stretches should be chosen specific to the individual athlete, no stretches are included in the sequence examples that follow. It is recommended that all therapists develop a thorough knowledge of stretching methods and techniques and include them during their event massage work as is appropriate. One general guideline for stretching is to remember that the contract–relax stretching method may stimulate muscle cramps if used during post-event massage. Therefore, it may be best to use only static stretching during inter-event and post-event massages.

Timing, Pace, and Duration for Event Massage

The key distinctions among pre-event, inter-event, and post-event massage are the differences in timing, pace, and duration. Pre-event sports massage is most beneficial when performed 1 to 2 hours before the start of activity and must be timed to coincide with the regular warm-up routine. Generally, the massage should be performed toward the end of the warm-up. However, in some cases, it may be important to briefly address a specific tight muscle before an athlete begins the warm-up and do the full pre-event massage after the warm-up is finished. To avoid disrupting the athlete's normal "ritual" of preparation, the massage should finish at least 10 minutes before the start of activity and average between 10 and 15 minutes in duration, never exceeding 20 minutes. As with all event massages, the pace of the work is faster than that of traditional Swedish or the other two categories of sports massage. This brisk pace is necessary both to complete the work in the available time and to avoid sedation of the athlete immediately before activity. However, if an athlete is overanxious before activity, therapists must moderate the pace enough to calm the athlete but maintain their "competitive edge." To get an idea about the proper pace for pre-event massage, approximate the beat of your favorite "rock and roll" tune.

The timing of an inter-event massage is obvious, and, again, the massage complements the regular routine of the athlete between events. Because the focus of the inter-event massage is one or two specific muscles or small tissue zones, the pace can be slower than the pre-event, but it is still faster than traditional massage. There is no single correct pace for inter-event as long as the pace is upbeat enough to avoid sedation. The more important guideline to follow is to keep it brief. The duration of an inter-event massage ranges from 5 to 10 minutes, rarely extending to 15 minutes.

Because the activity is over, the post-event massage does not have as rigid a time frame in which it must be administered. Generally, the post-event massage is administered within 1 to 2 hours after the end of the activity because most of the athletes are still at the event site during this time frame. Just as in pre-event, the post-event massage should be considered an adjunct to the athlete's regular cool-down and must be administered after that routine is finished. Because therapists may need to do post-event massage on several athletes, each massage is still only 15 to 20 minutes in duration and focused only on the large muscle groups. The pace of post-event massage is slower than either the pre- or inter-event massage—more like a reggae beat—and therapists must use care not to increase the depth of their strokes too quickly. If the pace is too rapid or if tissue is handled too abruptly, it may stimulate a muscle cramp.

If the activity is early in the season and/or involves a lot of eccentric muscle work, the risk of delayed-onset muscle soreness is much higher for athletes.[14–16] In these cases, the post-event massage should be administered *no less than 2 hours after* the end of activity because research has established this as the optimal time frame for preventing or reducing delayed-onset muscle soreness.[14–16] It appears that massage administered 2 hours after activity disrupts a pivotal first step in the inflammatory process—neutrophil accumulation—which helps prevent the soreness. If the massage is given before the 2-hour mark, this benefit has not been measured, perhaps because neutrophil accumulation has not yet been established.[15]

Massage Interviews

Although event massage is brief and not intended to *treat* any injuries or specific problems, it is still important for therapists to identify the particular needs of each athlete with a brief interview. An interview before a pre-event massage helps therapists determine contraindications, where to begin their work, which muscle groups require extra focus, and the best time line for their work. A pre-event massage interview should include questions such as the following:

- How much time before the start of your event?
- Where are you in your warm-up routine?
- What previous injuries might still be affecting your workouts and/or performance?
- What general muscle groups or body areas would you like me to focus on?
- Do you have any specific points of tension or tenderness that you want addressed?
- Are there any muscles you have trouble stretching on your own?

An inter-event interview is even briefer than the pre-event interview. One simple question usually suffices: "What muscle or area do you need me to focus on?" It may also be helpful for the therapist to ask if an area feels tight or heavy. If the athlete reports that the area feels tight, the inter-event massage can focus on reducing muscle and fascial tension with the basic sports massage strokes and/or neuromuscular techniques. However, if the athlete responds that the area feels heavy or full, therapists should include lymphatic techniques to facilitate edema uptake and diminish this heavy sensation. When lymphatic techniques are included in post-event massage, they should be the last step in the massage sequence.

The post-event massage interview is the most important one to conduct because this is when therapists can be faced with several different first aid situations. The massage therapist must know the signs and symptoms and be alert for indications that the athlete has suffered a musculoskeletal trauma that requires a specific evaluation or that he or she may be at risk for muscle cramps, hypothermia, or hyperthermia. Although not a requirement, it may be a good idea to begin all post-event massages with the athlete sitting on the edge of the table for the interview so the therapist can observe facial expressions and determine whether the athlete is focused and able to maintain eye contact. In most cases, the post-event massage should avoid work on the athlete's feet because of the possibility of blisters and the extreme tenderness that commonly occurs here. A post-event massage interview should include questions such as the following:

- Have you completed your cool-down and stretches?
- Have you had enough water since the end of the event?
- Are you wearing dry clothing?
- How are you feeling? Hot, warm, cold?
- Did you have any problems during the activity?

- Do you have any old injuries or surgeries I need to be aware of?
- Have you had any problems with training for this event?
- In what areas do you want me to focus my work?
- What are you feeling in these areas? Tight? Heavy? Pain?

In general, an athlete must answer "yes" to the first three questions before the post-event massage can be given.

Post-Event First Aid

As indicated by the post-event interview, muscle cramps, hyperthermia, and hypothermia are common post-event situations. Therapists must be able to quickly identify these conditions and take the appropriate first aid measures to manage the problem until full medical attention is available. In most event situations, there are plenty of emergency medical people available to administer the appropriate treatment if a life-threatening condition should occur. However, it is not uncommon for an athlete to get a muscle cramp during a massage or to develop signs and symptoms of heat exhaustion or hypothermia shortly after the massage begins. In these cases, it is essential that the correct first steps be taken to ensure the athlete's complete and rapid recovery. It is also very important for massage therapists to recognize the limits of their first aid training and make getting the athlete to the appropriate emergency medical personal a high priority.

From the Field

"Having worked with all levels of athletes, from the weekend warrior to the elite, one thing rings true: their soft tissue gets abused. Ignoring this fact will slow their return to the playing field. I have found over the past 16 years that pre-competition/work-out soft tissue work improves my athletes' efficiency and effectiveness and post work-out/competition massage decreases their DOMS [delayed-onset muscle soreness]."

Thomas Burton, PT, EMT

Supervisor of Outpatient Services
Providence–Holy Cross Medical Center
Mission Hills, CA

■ MUSCLE CRAMPS

One of the primary reasons for slowing down the pace and using only static stretches in a post-event massage is to reduce the risk of stimulating muscle cramps. Muscle cramps are caused by a combination of factors that are common in post-event situations including fatigue, dehydration, and electrolyte imbalances. If the post-event interview indicates that the athlete has had a cramp before or during the event, the post-event massage may be modified to focus mostly on neuromuscular inhibition and stretching techniques rather than the basic sports massage strokes (Fig. 10-1).

One of the quickest and most effective methods of cramp relief is a simultaneous application of direct pressure and reciprocal inhibition. The direct pressure provides a mechanical resistance to the shortening, and the reciprocal inhibition provides reflex inhibition. Reversing the physiologic process of muscle shortening before full stretching can help the athlete avoid microtearing of the muscle and residual soreness. A good illustration of how to use this method of cramp management is with a calf cramp, one of the most common muscle cramps that athletes experience. The cramp involves the plantar flexors of the ankle, so the therapist must engage the ankle dorsiflexors in an isometric contraction with one hand offering resistance at the foot while the other hand presses firmly over the area of the cramp.

The isometric contraction should be held for approximately 10 seconds, and then the therapist can apply a gentle stretch to the muscle, still maintaining direct pressure. The reciprocal inhibition may need to be repeated a few times before complete resolution of the cramp is achieved and full stretch is possible. It is also important to remember that when a muscle is cramping, the athlete is not likely to understand complex verbal instructions about reciprocal inhibition. Therefore, the therapist must give firm and simple verbal instructions and clear kinesthetic information to the body. The instructions should be something like "pull this foot into my hand" while tapping the dorsum of the foot. It is also a good idea to ask for some deep breaths and coordinate the gentle stretch with the athlete's exhalations. With a little practice, the therapist can learn to use this combination of direct pressure and reciprocal inhibition for the most common muscle cramps such as the gastrocnemius, hamstrings, quadriceps, anterior tibialis, and peroneals because these muscles are in simple flexor–extensor relationship. However, in situations in which no single antagonist group can be identified, such as cramps that occur in the foot, reciprocal inhibition may not be effective. In such cases, the direct compression and mild stretch are used without reciprocal inhibition.

Another method of cramp management that stimulates an inhibition of the contraction is approximation. As depicted in Figure 10-2, this technique inhibits the cramp by firmly pushing the muscle fibers together on either side of the cramp creating increased tension in the tendons that stimulates the Golgi tendon organs to inhibit the contraction. However, this technique's effectiveness is limited to superficial and fusiform muscles such as the wrist flexors and extensors, gastrocnemius, hamstrings, biceps and triceps brachii. Another disadvantage to approximation as a method of cramp relief is that both hands are occupied in the approximation, which eliminates the easy use of direct pressure in most cases. When muscle cramps occur during a post-event massage, immediate action is necessary to relieve the cramp before the massage can continue. The following action list is suggested. It is most effective for muscles that have clear flexor–extensor relationships.

Action list for cramp relief:

1. Direct compression over the site of the muscle cramp.
2. Simultaneous application of reciprocal inhibition (engage antagonist of cramping muscle in isometric

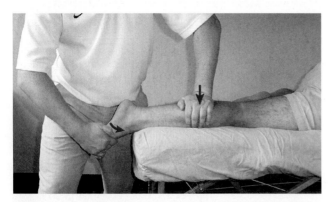

FIGURE 10-1 Reciprocal inhibition for cramp relief in the gastrocnemius. Therapist applies direct compression over the area of the cramp while simultaneously signaling an isometric contraction of the dorsiflexors.

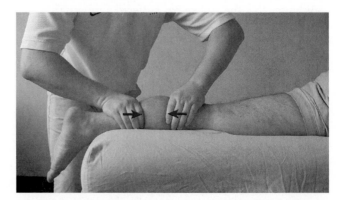

FIGURE 10-2 Approximation method of cramp relief for the gastrocnemius. Therapist grasps the muscle on either side of the cramp, and pushes the hands together, bunching the muscle fibers in the middle and stretching the Golgi tendon organs.

contraction) when possible. Maintain the compression and inhibition for 10 to 15 seconds.

3. When the athlete indicates that the cramp is subsiding, ask the athlete to take a deep breath and slowly stop the isometric contraction on the exhale. Therapists should slowly stretch the muscle at the end of the athlete's exhale.

4. Hold the stretch for 10 to 15 seconds and slowly return the muscle to its resting length. If the cramp returns during this process, repeat steps 1 to 3 as many as three times and try adding muscle approximation if the cramp is in a fusiform muscle.

5. Apply an ice pack to the muscle for 10 to 15 minutes after the cramp has been relieved, and encourage the athlete to drink more water and/or electrolyte drinks for the next 24 hours. Athletes should be instructed to continue stretching the affected muscle after the icing.

Therapists are encouraged to practice applying simultaneous compression and reciprocal inhibition to the gastrocnemius, hamstrings, and quadriceps because these muscles commonly sustain cramps. By practicing beforehand, therapists can respond quickly and confidently during this common post-event first aid situation.

■ HEAT STRESS SYNDROMES

Heat stress syndromes, or overheating conditions, require critical first aid decision making for therapists. Most commonly, heat stress syndromes are described as two separate conditions: heat exhaustion and heat stroke. Heat stroke is considered life-threatening, whereas heat exhaustion is not. However, if heat exhaustion is not recognized and treated properly, it may advance to heat stroke. Therapists must be alert for both conditions when events are held in hot and/or humid environments.

Heat exhaustion is a shocklike condition that occurs in athletes when the body has any combination of dehydrated, excess loss of electrolytes (sodium in particular) and depletion of energy. It is a type of peripheral vascular collapse that develops and progresses slowly and may occur in even the fittest of athletes. Heat exhaustion must be suspected when an athlete who has not suffered an injury begins to display signs and symptoms such as headache, light-headedness or dizziness, nausea, persistent muscle cramping, profuse sweating and chills, decreased urine output, pallor, and a sudden cessation of activity or fainting.[17,18] See Table 10-1 for the distinguishing signs and symptoms of both heat exhaustion and heat stroke. An athlete with heat exhaustion must be removed from activity and must rest in a cool environment while fluids and electrolytes are being replaced.

Heat exhaustion action steps:

1. Help the athlete to sit or lie on the table, and notify any surrounding therapists that you are treating a suspected case of heat exhaustion so they can remain available for assistance. It is preferable to keep the athlete sitting if he or she is stable enough to do so. This prevents a rapid decrease in blood pressure.

2. Cool down the athlete by removing heavy clothing or equipment (especially any form of head covering), fanning, draping wet towels over head, neck, and shoulders, and/or pouring cool water over him or her.

3. Replace fluids with water or an electrolyte drink. Do not allow the athlete to drink juice, soda, or caffeinated beverages and encourage small sips of fluid rather than gulping down large volumes. Too-rapid fluid replacement may cause vomiting and further dehydrate the system.

4. Engage the athlete in conversation, watch the eyes, and monitor vital signs closely. *Never leave an athlete with heat exhaustion alone during recovery.*

It is not uncommon for an athlete suffering from heat exhaustion to get goose bumps and begin shivering while cooling down. This is simply a superficial phenomenon that can be addressed by drying off the skin by lightly rubbing with a towel and having the athlete sit up if he or she has been lying down. *Do not* wrap or cover up the athlete. If the athlete does not stop sweating, and signs and symptoms continue after 15 minutes of treatment, he or she may require intravenous fluid replacement and must be referred for a full medical assessment. After signs and symptoms return to normal, athletes must be evaluated and cleared by a physician before being allowed to return to activity. Also, be aware that once athletes have suffered a bout of heat exhaustion, they are susceptible to repeated bouts of heat stress syndromes.

TABLE 10-1	Comparison of Signs and Symptoms in Heat Stress Conditions	
Signs	**Heat Exhaustion**	**Heat Stroke**
Skin	Pale or splotchy, and may be cool to touch	Red or flushed, and hot to touch
Sweat	Profuse	May or may not be sweating in initial stages; sudden cessation of sweating in advanced
Pulse	Weak and rapid	Strong and rapid
Respiration	Shallow and rapid (panting)	Deep and irregular; hyperventilation

Heat stroke occurs when all of the body's cooling mechanisms have failed and core temperature increases to a life-threatening level, for example, higher than 104° F. This heat buildup is due to some combination of dehydration, prolonged physical exertion, and environmental conditions of high heat and/or high humidity. Heat stroke can develop rapidly when all three of these elements coincide, and therapists must quickly recognize the following signs and symptoms to prevent severe or fatal damage to the athlete's nervous system. Disorientation or mental confusion; **tachycardia**; vomiting; hyperventilation; seizures; and a strong, rapid pulse all are clear indicators of heat stroke.[17-20] When an athlete is treated for heat exhaustion, therapists must be alert to a sudden shift to heat stroke. This is marked by a shift from profuse sweating to a cessation of sweating, indicating that the tissue has been dehydrated and the sweating mechanism has been shut down. The athlete may still feel damp, but the skin becomes flushed and hot to touch. The distinguishing signs and symptoms between these two heat stress conditions are summarized for easy reference in Table 10-1.

An athlete who displays any signs of heat stroke requires immediate cooling and should be transferred to an emergency room as soon as practical. Careful attention must be given to monitoring and maintaining the athlete's airway during all of the following action steps.

Heat stroke action list:

1. Immediately call for emergency medical attention, and remove any heavy clothing and equipment, especially from the head and torso.
2. Begin cooling down the athlete by any means available: full-body immersion in ice water is the best way to rapidly cool the athlete and should always be the first choice if available.[19,20] However, if this is not possible, pouring water over the athlete's head, draping the head and shoulders with wet towels, or applying ice bags to armpits, groin, forehead, back of neck, and wrists are alternate methods of cooling.
3. Monitor the vital signs and maintain an open airway. *Do not* concern yourself with fluid replacement because only intravenous fluids can reverse the level of dehydration associated with heat stroke.

■ HYPOTHERMIA AND FROSTBITE

Hypothermia is another shocklike condition brought on by an excess loss of heat. This condition is most likely to occur when there is a combination of cool temperature, wind, and wet clothing. For example, those playing autumn soccer or field hockey game in the rain or the last finishers of a marathon (wet from sweat but slow moving and not generating heat) are particularly susceptible to hypothermia. In each of these cases, the wet clothing acts like evaporating sweat on the skin and dissipates body heat. Those who exercise or work in cold conditions need to be made aware of the importance of proper layering of clothes to wick moisture away from their body and to create air pockets of insulation. Hypothermia is suspected when a previously uninjured athlete begins to act disoriented, irritable, and/or confused; loses coordination; appears pale and is cool to touch; has a slowed pulse and respiratory rates; and is shivering uncontrollably. Uncontrolled shivering is an indicator of advanced hypothermia, and immediate warming is necessary to avoid further progression of the condition.[17,21] Hypothermia can progress to death within 2 hours of the onset of symptoms,[21] making it a top priority medical emergency that therapists must recognize early and treat quickly with the appropriate first aid measures. The number one priority is to safely and quickly re-warm the athlete by following the recommended action list.

Hypothermia action list:

1. Help athlete sit or lie on the table, and notify any surrounding therapists that you are treating a suspected case of hypothermia and may need assistance. It is preferable to keep the athlete sitting if stable enough to do so. This prevents a rapid decrease in blood pressure.
2. Remove wet clothing (replace with dry if available), wrap the athlete in blankets, towels, or whatever is available. The important area to cover is the head and neck because a large percentage of body heat is dissipated from this region.
3. Warm the athlete with an *external* heat source such as hot water bottles, electric blankets, space heater, or body heat from the therapist.
4. If the athlete is conscious, warm liquids may be administered after steps 1 to 3 are accomplished.
5. When the athlete is coherent and focused with pulse and respiration returned to normal ranges, and he or she is able to stand, therapists may support the athlete and start some slow walking to encourage complete recovery.

Note: It is dangerous to use vigorous jostling or friction rubs to re-warm a hypothermic athlete because cold blood is more acidic than normal and the rapid vasodilation of the superficial blood vessels shifts the blood volume to a degree that mimics a shock response.[17,20]

Frostbite happens when prolonged exposure to extreme cold has caused tissue to freeze. In frostbite, the core temperature may be maintained, but skin temperature is dramatically decreased, resulting in localized freezing. It is unlikely that an athlete would suffer severe frostbite when participating in supervised athletic events. However, first-degree or superficial frostbite, sometimes called **frostnip**,[17,21] is a common cold injury that all therapists should be able to recognize and manage. The ears, nose, cheeks, chin, fingertips, and toes are the most susceptible body parts because these areas are far from the heart and often hot water (100° to 105° F) until the normal color returns to the tissue is preferred and may be necessary with second-degree frostbite. When using immersion, the container must be large enough to allow movement of the part being treated without touching the sides. It is expected that the athlete will experience an increase in tingling and aching of the area during the re-warming process. *Do not* rub, massage, or apply a dry external heat source such as a heating pad to frostbitten tissue. To do so, risks extensive tissue damage because the frozen superficial tissue is literally ripped apart by the rubbing, and dry heat may cause superficial burns before the underlying tissue can be warmed back up.[17,21]

Examples of Event Massage Sequences

Because the focus of event massage is the large muscle groups and fascial structures stressed by the activity, the sequence of strokes and the positioning of the athlete's body are generally the same for all categories. The example sequences in this section are well suited for both pre- and post-event massage, and therapists may choose only a few of the steps when doing inter-event work.

■ LOWER BODY FOCUS

Appendix B classifies each sport as being upper body or lower body dominant activities and outlines the muscle groups that should be included in the event massage for both areas of focus. In lower body massage there is one unique positioning method used while the athlete is in the prone position. The *prone figure-4 legs* or *frog-leg* position (Fig. 10-3) offers several advantages to the therapist during event massage. First, the position allows complete access to the iliotibial band without the therapist going into a deep squat at the side of the table or the athlete turning two more times for side lying. Second, the athlete's thigh is fully supported by the table, allowing the therapist to use both hands in the tissue and correct body mechanics (using body weight rather than hand/arm strength) for deep work. Third, both the quadriceps and hamstrings can receive three-dimensional treatment from this position. Finally, the position is anatomically advantageous because the external rotation and flexion of the hip shorten and soften the gluteal and the tensor fasciae latae muscles. Be sure to rotate the hip slightly by lifting with the upper hand before moving the thigh into abduction and external rotation (Fig. 10-3A and B), and you *must avoid* lifting the knee off the table during any portion of the movement. When the athlete is in the frog-leg position, the therapist should unwind the quadriceps, which tend to roll medially during the abduction and rotation process, and apply light traction to

exposed to the external environment. In first-degree frostbite, the tissue appears white or gray, and the athlete describes the area as numb, tingling, itchy, and/or painful. If the frostbite has advanced to second degree, the affected tissue takes on a white, waxy appearance that is extremely cold and firm to the touch. In both cases, the tissue must be carefully re-warmed to avoid extensive tissue damage.

Treatment of frostbite is to warm the tissue without damaging the tissue. Simple warming methods such as blowing through cupped hands onto the area and holding the frostbitten body part in a warmer body region such as the armpit, groin, or abdomen works for most cases. When available and practical, immersing the body part in

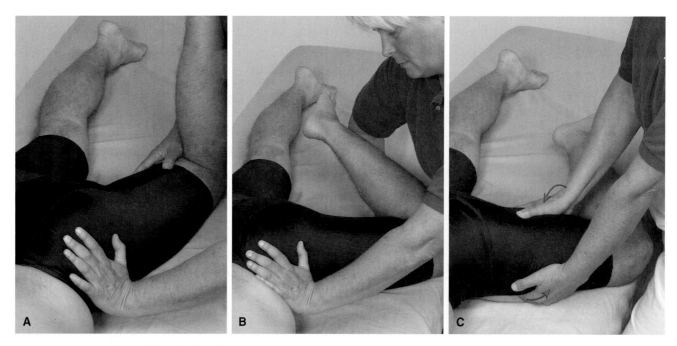

FIGURE 10-3 Frog-leg position for iliotibial band focus. (A) Starting position. **(B)** Therapist rotates the hip up slightly with a slight lift of the outside hand, and simultaneously supinates and slides the inside hand out and up the side of the table to achieve the finished frog-leg position. **(C)** To ensure the athlete's comfort, the therapist must "unwind" the quadriceps and apply light traction to the sacroiliac joint.

the hip joint (Fig. 10-3C). As a final precaution, visually and verbally check with the athlete for any strain in the hip or back in this position before proceeding with the massage. If the athlete's pelvic girdle is rotated high off the table in this position or if the leg does not rest flat on the table, it indicates a lack of hip and/or low back flexibility, which suggests that this position should not be used. In addition, if the athlete is taller than average, he or she should be moved to the opposite side of the table before positioning to ensure that the edge of the table will not press into the medial thigh during this portion of the massage.

In the examples of lower and upper body event massages that follow, one sequence is for event massage *without* an emollient, and another example is for massage *with* an emollient. If therapists choose to use an emollient with pre-event massage, a towel should be used after the massage to remove as much lubricant from the skin as possible before the start of the event. Both samples can be completed within the 10- to 15-minute time frame of a pre-event massage or the 15 to 20 minutes of a post-event massage by changing the overall pace of the massage and the amount of time spent in each major muscle group. In the following examples, the athlete begins in prone position, with the therapist standing at the side of the table facing the athlete's head. However, therapists may choose to begin with the athlete in supine position, especially in post-event massage.

No Emollient—Lower Body

Athlete prone (7 to 10 minutes)

HIP AND THIGH

1. Rhythmic *compressions* to gluteal (Fig. 10-4) and hamstring groups (see Fig. 2-13A).
2. *Pétrissage* and circular *friction* to gluteal (Fig. 10-5) and hamstring groups. *Jostle* full hamstring group.
3. Frog-leg position: Rhythmic *compressions* (Fig. 10-6A), *pétrissage* (Fig. 10-6B), and general to specific *frictions* (Fig. 10-6C)

LEG/ANKLE/FOOT

4. *Rhythmic compressions* (Fig. 10-7A), *pétrissage,* and general *friction* to calf (Fig. 10-7B).
5. Pincer *friction* (Fig. 10-8A) and *pincer pin-and-stretch* to Achilles tendon (Fig. 10-8B).
6. General *friction* around malleoli (Fig. 10-9A) plus *calcaneal lift* (Fig. 10-9B).
7. *Compression and circular friction* to plantar fascia (Fig. 10-10A and B).
8. *Footwave: pin-and-stretch* of plantar fascia (Fig. 10-11A–C).

Note: Steps 7 and 8 are optional and performed only when athletes request specific work on their feet.

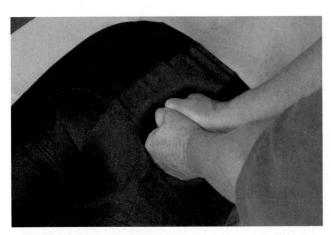

FIGURE 10-4 Rhythmic compressions in the gluteal muscles.
Compressions are applied with two thirds of the pressure directed
straight down to the table and one third of the pressure on a diag-
onal line to accommodate the oblique surface of the posterior ilium.

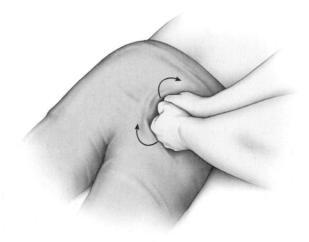

**FIGURE 10-5 Circular frictions engage the gluteal muscle
mass with moderate pressure and stretch the entire mass with
an up-and-out motion.** Fists do not slide over the surface of the
skin/shorts.

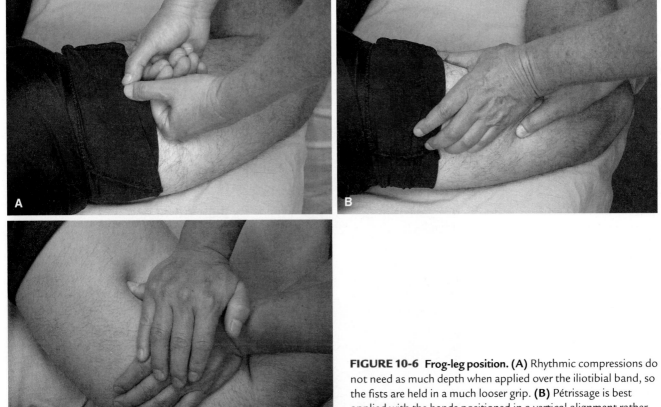

FIGURE 10-6 Frog-leg position. (A) Rhythmic compressions do
not need as much depth when applied over the iliotibial band, so
the fists are held in a much looser grip. **(B)** Pétrissage is best
applied with the hands positioned in a vertical alignment rather
than the standard side-by-side. **(C)** Site-specific friction with a
braced thumb over the posterior edge of the iliotibial band.

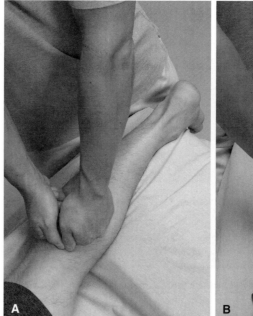
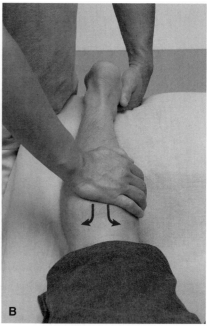

FIGURE 10-7 Calf. (A) Rhythmic compressions of the calf muscles. **(B)** Circular friction stretched the tissue toward the knee, then out to medial and lateral sides.

ANTERIOR COMPARTMENT OF LEG

9. *Rhythmic compression* (Fig. 2-13A or 10-12A) and *knuckle circular friction* (Fig. 10-12B).
10. Repeat sequence on opposite leg.
11. *Tapotement* to both legs (if this is a pre-event massage).

SUPINE LOWER BODY (5–8 MINUTES)

The other half of the lower body sequence is with the athlete in supine position and the therapist standing at the side of the table facing the athlete's head. This part of the massage should take 5 to 8 minutes to complete.

HIP, THIGH, AND KNEE

1. *Jostle* quadriceps and full limb.
2. *Rhythmic compressions* over hip flexors and upper *ad*ductors (Fig. 10-13A), then over quadriceps (Fig. 10-13B).
3. *Pétrissage* quadriceps and adductors followed by *friction with passive motion* across hip flexors (Fig. 10-14).

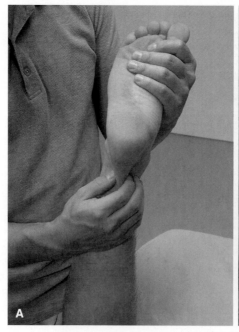
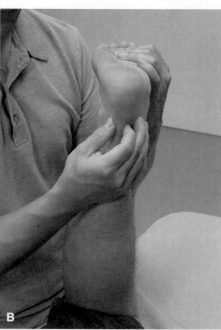

FIGURE 10-8 Friction to Achilles tendon. (A) Pincer pin-and-stretch of the Achilles. Gently squeeze the tendon and pull the tendon away from the ankle (drop the heel of your hand to the calf creating a fulcrum) while simultaneously dorsiflexing the ankle. **(B)** Finish position.

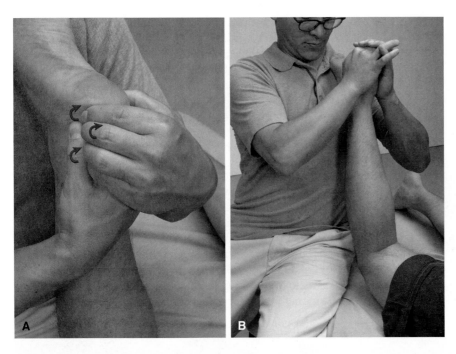

FIGURE 10-9 Ankle and foot. (A) Pincer friction to the retinaculi of ankle. Gently squeeze the tissue between the thumbs and first three fingers of both hands, and pull the tissue through a circular motion. Move the fingers and tissue as one unit. **(B)** Calcaneal lift: Decompress the subtalar joint by squeezing the calcaneous and lifting while resting the forefoot against your shoulder to maintain plantarflexion.

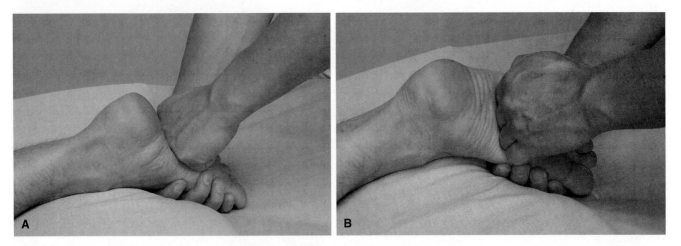

FIGURE 10-10 Compression and friction of the plantar fascia. (A) Support the dorsum of the foot with one hand while applying rhythmic compression with other fist. **(B)** Use the knuckles of the proximal interphalangeal joint to engage the plantar fascia in circular friction. Use the underneath hand to add inversion/eversion for modulation of the friction.

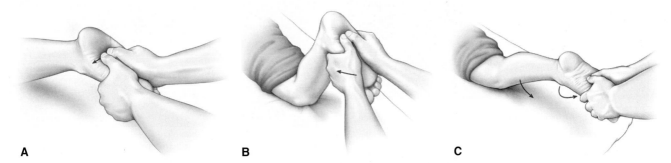

FIGURE 10-11 Foot-wave pin-and-stretch. (A) Begin by pressing both thumbs into the middle of the sole while the foot is in a relaxed (plantar-flexed) position. **(B)** Maintaining thumb pressure, press the foot into full dorsiflexion with the weight of your full hand by leaning forward. Knee flexion is maintained at 45 degrees or less during this push, and lean to achieve maximal stretch of the plantar fascia. **(C)** After the stretch, allow the ankle to gently roll into plantar flexion, and repeat the stretch with the thumbs in a new point in the fascia.

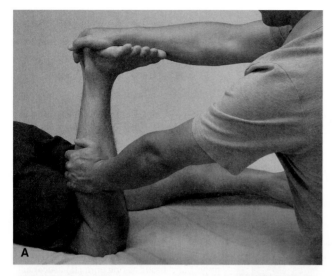

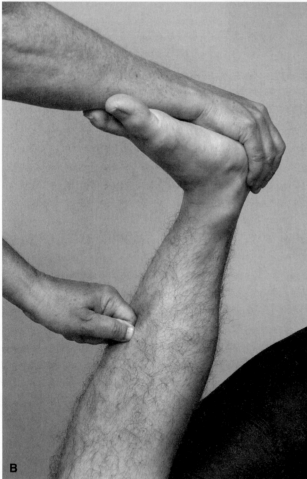

4. *Patellar frictions:* Scooping lateral edges, S-friction, and *myofascial lift* (Fig. 10-15 A-C).
5. Adductors: Rhythmic *compressions* (Fig. 10-16A), *pétrissage* (Fig. 10-16B), and *circular friction* (Fig. 10-16C).
6. *General fascial release* of anterior thigh (Fig. 10-17A and B).
7. *Jostle* ankle and foot (foot boogie) (Fig. 10-18).
8. Repeat sequence on opposite leg.
9. *Tapotement* both legs (if this is a pre-event massage).

If the anterior compartment of the leg was not addressed while the athlete was prone, it can be inserted as step 8 in this supine sequence of strokes. Even when an emollient is used, following the same general order of addressing muscle groups and beginning with rhythmic compression is still a good strategy. Therefore, an event massage using an emollient that is focused on the lower body also begins with the athlete in a prone position and the therapist standing at the side of the table facing the athlete's head. The example below

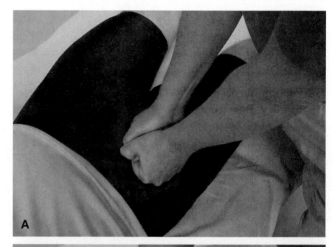

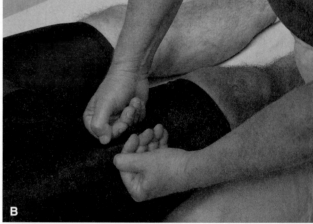

FIGURE 10-12 Anterior compartment of the leg. (A) The heel of the hand can be used for compressions in this small muscle group **(B)** Circular frictions. Use the pad of the thumb braced into the proximal interphalangeal knuckle of the index finger to create a point-specific stretch.

FIGURE 10-13 Hip and quadriceps. (A) Rhythmic compressions over the hip flexors and upper *add*uctors moves along the line of the inguinal ligament. **(B)** A very loose fist is used for compressions over the quadriceps to accommodate the anterior curve of the femur and firm muscle septum through the middle of the muscle group.

is written as a basic event massage and uses only the basic sports massage strokes. If time allows and it is deemed necessary, therapists may include active-assistive releases for a few more or all major muscle groups.

Emollient—Lower Body

Athlete prone (8 to 12 minutes)

HIP/THIGH

Step 1 is without an emollient.

1. Rhythmic *compressions, pétrissage,* and general *friction* to gluteals and hamstrings.
2. Apply emollient with brisk *effleurage:* Two to three full-extremity strokes, then three to four strokes specific to the hamstrings.
3. *Pétrissage* full hamstrings and *add*uctors.
4. *Active-assistive release* for hamstrings: Minimum of three strokes broadening and two to three lengthening (Fig. 10-19A-C).
5. *Frog-leg position* (steps 5 to 7): Effleurage, pétrissage, and circular fist friction over the iliotibial band.

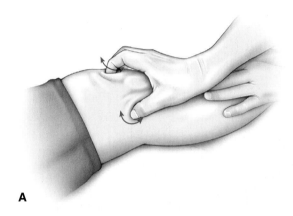

A

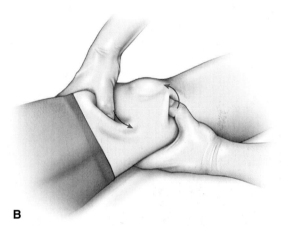

B

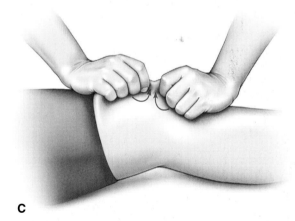

C

FIGURE 10-15 Friction around the patella. (A) Scoop the tissue on both sides of the patella with the thumb and fingers for a general friction. **(B)** Place the thumbs above and below the patella on opposite sides of the patellar tendon and ligament. Push thumbs together three times for "S friction," then trade thumb positions and repeat three more strokes. **(C)** Roll the tissue directly over the patella into one large fold, and firmly lift it upward to decompress the patellofemoral joint.

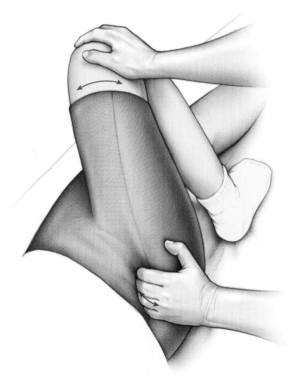

FIGURE 10-14 Site-specific friction over the hip flexor tendons. The fingers of the therapist's uppermost hand apply pressure and movement over the tendons while the other hand rotates the hip in opposition to the tissue movement. Positioning the hip into full flexion creates deeper tissue engagement without the need for extreme pressure from the therapist.

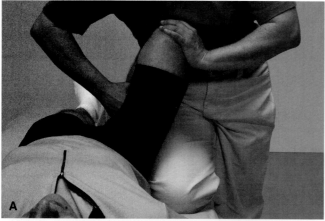

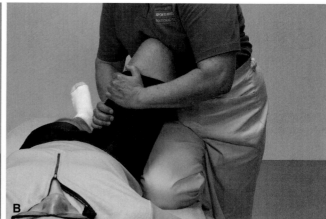

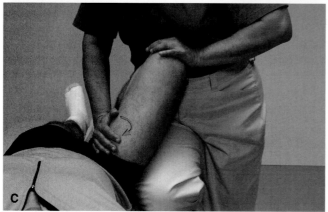

FIGURE 10-16 **Adductors.** The knee of the therapist's inside leg is placed on the table next to the athlete's flexed (90 degrees) and slightly abducted (less than 45 degrees) hip for support while holding the athlete's knee in the outside hand. The therapist's inside hand is used for this series of strokes. **(A)** Rhythmic compressions. **(B)** Pétrissage. **(C)** Circular friction.

6. *Braced-thumb friction* gliding along the posterior edge of the band as in Figure 10-6D.

LEG/ANKLE/FOOT

7. *Effleurage* and *twisting fist friction* over the anterior compartment (Fig. 10-20).

8. Return leg to normal position: *Effleurage and pétrissage* of calf.
9. *Pincer grip friction* to the Achilles and retinaculi followed by *pincer pin-and-stretch.*
10. *Bilateral fascial pull* through the gastrocnemius (Fig. 10-21).
11. Circular fist and linear friction to plantar fascia.

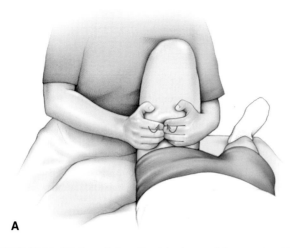

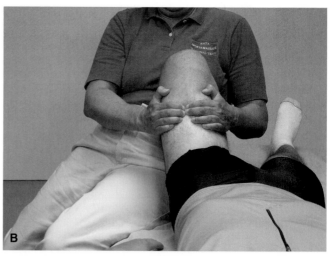

FIGURE 10-17 **Broad plane fascial release of the anterior thigh. (A)** Bring the hip and knee into full flexion and sit in front of the athlete's leg. Wrap both hands around the thigh and curl the fingers into the tissue on the anterior thigh—slide all of the tissue upwards to the knee. **(B)** Lean back while maintaining this fascial stretch to maximize the release.

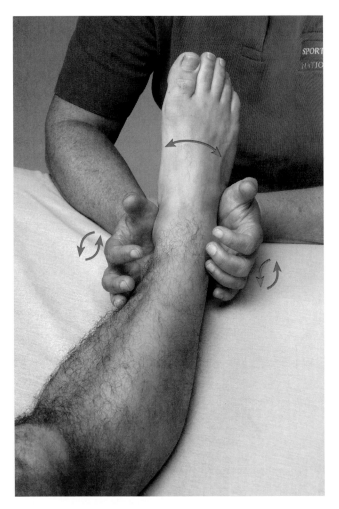

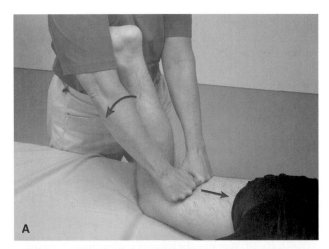

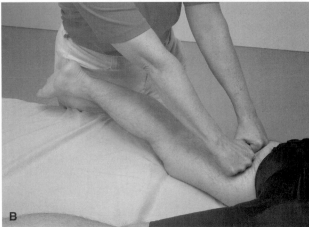

FIGURE 10-18 Foot-boogie mobilization. Cup the calcaneous between the heels of your hands and jiggle the foot back and forth by rolling your hands in a small circle.

12. Repeat sequence on opposite leg, and finish with tapotement (pre-event) or effleurage (post-event) to both legs.

　Note: Therapists may choose to address the anterior compartment in the frog-leg position or wait for the supine part of the massage. Step 11 is optional and performed only when athletes request specific work on their feet.

　To finish the lower body sequence with emollient, the athlete is in supine position with the therapist standing at the side of the table facing the athlete's head.

Emollient—Lower Body

SUPINE (5 to 8 minutes)

HIP/THIGH/KNEE (TABLE 10-2)

1. No emollient for steps 1 to 3: Jostle quadriceps and full limb.

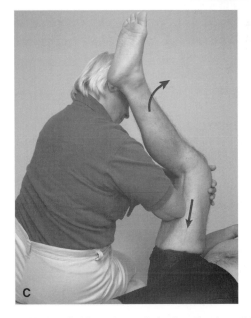

FIGURE 10-19 Active-assistive lengthening of the hamstrings. **(A)** Start with the athlete's leg in flexion. **(B)** Slide both fists toward the muscle origins as the athlete slowly extends the knee. **(C)** Therapists may choose to do this release when the athlete is supine.

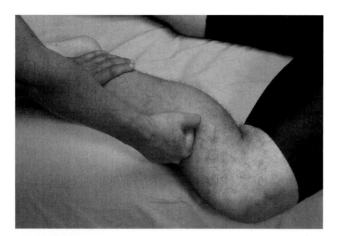

FIGURE 10-20 Working the anterior compartment from the frog-leg position. This position is used primarily for work in the iliotibial band, but also allows good access to the anterior and lateral compartments of the leg.

2. *Rhythmic compressions* hip flexors and upper *adductors.* (see Fig. 10-13).
3. *Friction with passive motion* across hip flexors (see Fig. 10-14).
4. Add emollient: *Effleurage:* Three full-length strokes, then two to three focused on anterior thigh.
5. *Pétrissage* full quadriceps, iliotibial band, and *adductors.*
6. Double-fist *fanning friction* through middle of quadriceps (Fig. 10-22).
7. Lift athlete's knee to 90 degrees hip and knee flexion to address the *adductors: Kneading* (Fig. 10-23A) and *circular fist friction* (Fig. 10-23B).
8. Put leg back down on table for *friction* and *myofascial lift* around patella (see Fig. 10-15).

LEG/ANKLE/FOOT

9. *Twisting fist friction* through anterior compartment— one up and one down (Fig. 10-24A and B).
10. Repeat on opposite leg and finish with tapotement (pre-event) or effleurage (post-event) to both legs.

▊ UPPER BODY FOCUS

As with the lower body sequences, refer to Appendix B for sports/athletes classified as upper body–dominant and the list of muscles that should be included in the event work. One special technique is used in the upper body massage sequences—hip lift–compress—which can also be used in the lower body sequences. This technique is designed to give a slight torsion stretch to the lumbar muscles and lumbosacral fascia (Fig. 10-25 A–C). The hip lift–compress

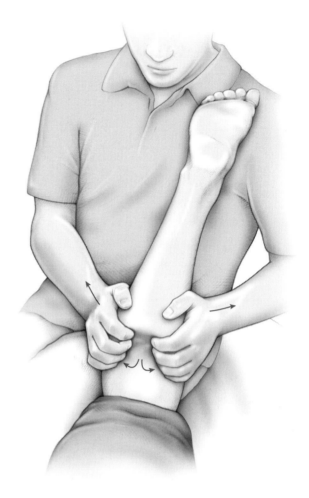

FIGURE 10-21 Pulling friction through the septum between the two heads of the gastrocnemius.

is included in the upper body sequences because so many of the upper body–focused sports require torso rotation. However, therapists may choose to include this technique in the lower body sequences as well, especially when athletes request or require focus in the low back and hips. Again, two examples of upper body sequences are given: one without and one with an emollient. See Table 10-3 for a synopsis of upper body sequences. Begin the sequence with the athlete in prone position with the therapist standing at the side of the table facing across the athlete's body.

No Emollient—Upper Body

PRONE (8 to 10 minutes)

HIPS AND BACK

1. *Rhythmic compressions* to lumbar paraspinal muscles (see Fig. 2-13A).

TABLE 10-2	Abbreviated Lower Body Sequences	
Body Region	**No Emollient**	**Emollient**
Prone: Hip and thigh	1. Gluteals and hamstrings: Compressions 2. Gluteals and hamstrings: Pétrissage and friction 3. Frog-leg/iliotibal band (ITB): Compressions, pétrissage and friction	1. Same steps 1–2 no emollient sequence, then apply emollient to full limb 2. Hamstrings and adductors: Effleurage and pétrissage 3. Hamstrings: Active-assistive broaden and lengthen 4. Frog-leg/ITB: Effleurage, pétrissage, and circular fist friction 5. Frog-leg/ITB: Braced-thumb friction posterior edge
Leg/ankle/foot	4. Calf: Compressions, pétrissage, and friction 5. Achilles: Pincer friction and pin-and-stretch 6. Ankle: General friction around malleoli + calcaneal lift 7. Plantar fascia: Compressions and knuckle friction 8. Footwave: Pin-and-stretch of plantar fascia 9. Anterior compartment: Compression and knuckle friction (if not included here, can be inserted after step 17)	6. Frog-leg/anterior compartment: Effleurage and twisting fist friction 7. Return leg to original prone to massage calf: Effleurage and pétrissage 8. Achilles: Pincer friction and pin and stretch 9. Gastrocnemius: Bilateral fascial pull 10. Return leg to table for foot massage. Plantar fascia: circular fist and linear frictions
Completion/transition	10. Repeat steps 1–9 opposite leg 11. Full-leg tapotement/jostle	11. Repeat steps 1–10 opposite leg 12. Full leg tapotement and/or effleurage
Supine: Hip, thigh, and knee	12. Quadriceps: Jostle 13. Hip flexors: Compressions 14. Quadriceps and adductors: Pétrissage and friction with passive motion 15. Patella: Friction lateral edge, S-friction to tendons, and myofascial lift 16. Adductors: Compression, pétrissage and circular friction 17. Anterior thigh: General fascial release	13. Hip flexors: Compressions and friction with passive motion, then apply emollient to full limb 14. Full thigh: Effleurage and pétrissage 15. Quadriceps: Fist fanning friction 16. Reposition leg to 90 degrees hip and knee flexion to address adductors: Wringing and circular fist friction 17. Return leg to table to address patella: Friction and myofascial lift
Leg/ankle/foot	18. Jostling (foot-boogie)	18. Anterior compartment: Twisting fist friction
Completion/transition	19. Repeat sequence opposite leg 20. Full-leg tapotement/jostle	19. Repeat sequence opposite leg Full-leg tapotement and/or effleurage

2. Low back mobilization with *hip lift–compress* (see Fig. 10-25A–C).

3. *Rhythmic compressions* through thoracic paraspinal muscles and upper trapezius. *Note:* Therapists must move to the head of the table and face toward the feet to apply compressions to the upper trapezius (see Fig. 1-6C).

4. *Dry pétrissage* to full back: Begin posterior neck and upper trapezius, progress out to deltoids, down lateral torso from axilla through latissimus dorsi to crest of the ilium (Fig. 10-26A). Continue with bilateral pétris-

sage of the paraspinal muscles from ilium back up to the posterior neck (Fig. 10-26B).

5. *Circular friction* through posterior neck, upper trapezius, infraspinous fossa (Fig. 10-27A), and full paraspinal muscles (Fig. 10-27B).

6. *Friction and point releases* in the interscapular muscles (see Figs. 8-15 and 10-38). *Note:* Therapists may choose to take more time and do specific neuromuscular release in this step if necessary. However, because of the time and patience it takes to properly apply these techniques, extensive point deactivation should not be

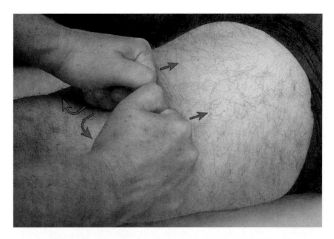

FIGURE 10-22 Fanning friction over the anterior thighs. Both fists are used to engage the tissue in a linear stretch toward the hip. Fanning the fists open several times during the linear stroke also helps to broaden the muscle slightly.

considered a standard part of an event massage sequence.

SHOULDERS/ARMS/HANDS

7. The therapist changes position to sit on the side of the table facing the head of the athlete, with the athlete's arm *ab*ducted off the side of the table (Fig. 10-28A) for *rhythmic compressions and muscle rolling* (Fig. 10-28 B) from deltoids through triceps.
8. *Site-specific friction* at the long head of triceps tendon (see Fig. 2-7B) followed by pin-and-stretch through the middle of the full muscle group (see Fig. 2-8).
9. The therapist now stands at the side of the table and places the athlete's arm back up on the table with palm up. *Rhythmic compressions, dry pétrissage, muscle rolling, and circular fist friction* to the anterior forearm muscles.

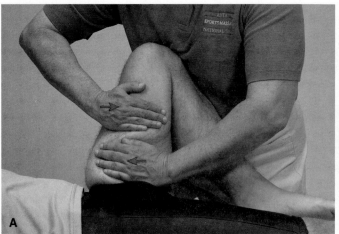
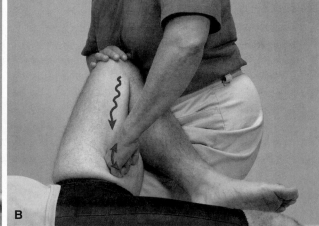

FIGURE 10-23 *Adductors.* (A) Kneading or wringing. **(B)** Twisting fist friction.

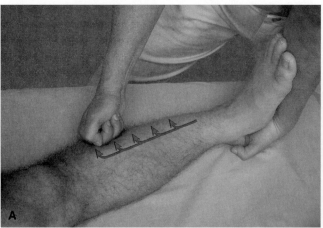
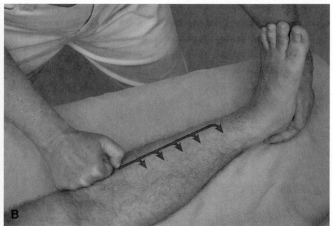

FIGURE 10-24 Twisting friction through the anterior compartment is most effective when two passes are used. (A) Twisting up and away from the crest of the tibia. **(B)** Twisting down and toward the tibia.

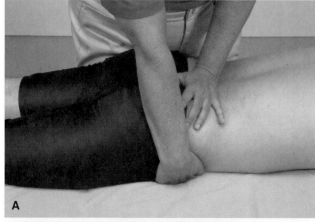

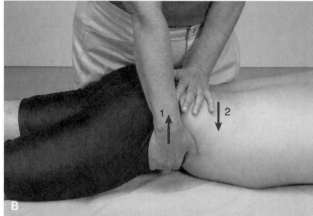

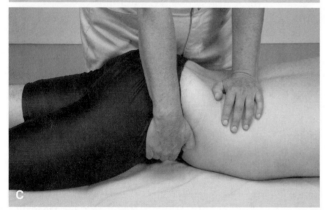

FIGURE 10-25 Hip lift–compress. **(A)** Starting hand position with therapist cupping the athlete's anterior superior iliac spine in the palm of the lower hand and the heel of the upper hand over the sacrum. **(B)** First, lift the ilium straight up, then push with the upper hand back to the table. The lift–compress is repeated several times; each time the therapist moves the upper hand superiorly through the paraspinal muscles to the bottom of the rib cage **(C),** then back down to the sacrum. **Caution:** Be sure the top hand is pressed straight down into the erector spinae as it travels through the lumbar zone. If the top hand is pressed down lateral to the erector, floating ribs may endanger abdominal organs.

10. *Rhythmic compressions* to palm of the hand and fingers, plus knuckle friction to the heel of the hand (Fig. 10-29A–C).
11. Tapotement (pre-event) or effleurage (post-event) over mid and upper back.

To finish the dry massage for the upper body, the athlete is in a supine position with the therapist standing at the head of the table facing the athlete's feet.

No Emollient—Upper Body

SUPINE (5 to 8 minutes)

CHEST AND NECK

1. *Rhythmic compressions* (Fig. 10-30), *pétrissage,* and general *pin-and-stretch* of the pectoralis major (Fig. 10-31).
2. Pétrissage and friction to posterior neck muscles: *Head bob* (Fig. 10-32).
3. Therapist moves to the side of the table and faces the athlete's head for application of *general neuromuscular and myofascial release* to the sternal-costal junctions (Fig. 10-33). REPEAT to opposite side.

SHOULDERS AND ARMS

4. *Rhythmic compressions, pétrissage, and pin-and-stretch* over the biceps brachii (Fig. 10-34). Finish with *site-specific friction* to the deltopectoral junction (Fig. 10-35).
5. *Rhythmic compressions, dry pétrissage, muscle rolling and circular fist friction* over the posterior forearm.
6. *Combination stretch* for wrist flexors, triceps, and latissimus (Fig. 10-36A). Site-specific friction to the teres-subscapularis junction of the posterior axilla (Fig. 10-36B).
7. Repeat steps 5 to 7 on the opposite arm, and finish with tapotement (pre-event) to both arms; no tapotement over the chest.

Emollient—Upper Body

Athlete **PRONE** (8 to 12 minutes)

When event massage is done with an emollient, the suggested sequence begins with the athlete in prone position and the therapist standing at the side of the table.

HIPS AND BACK

1. Rhythmic compressions to lumbar muscles (see Fig. 2-12B) and hip lift–compress (see Fig. 10-25).
2. Apply emollient: *Effleurage and pétrissage* to full back.
3. *Tracing of the ilium* in two zones: Figure 10-37A over the crest of the ilium; Figure 10-37B traces through the muscles and fascia between the greater trochanter and crest.

TABLE 10-3	Abbreviated Upper Body Sequences	
Body Region	**No Emollient**	**Emollient**
Prone: Hips and back	1. Lumbar erectors: Compressions and hip lift–compress 2. Mid and upper back: Compressions and pétrissage all major muscles 3. Full paraspinals: Circular fist friction 4. Interscapular: Site-specific friction and point releases	1. Same step 1 no-emollient sequence, then apply emollient to full back and arms 2. Full back: Effleurage and pétrissage 3. Hip and lumbar: Tracing ilium (2 zones if available) and pétrissage up paraspinals to transition to head of table 4. Paraspinals: Circular fist friction full length 5. Interscapular: General friction and neuromuscular with scapula retracted
Shoulders/arms/hands	5. Abduct athlete's arm off side of table for work in posterior brachium. Deltoid and triceps: Compressions, dry pétrissage, and site-specific friction to origin of long head of triceps 6. Triceps: Pin-and-stretch, then reposition arm back on table 7. Anterior forearm: Compressions, pétrissage, muscle rolling, and circular fist friction 8. Palm and fingers: Compressions and frictions	6. Abduct athlete's arm off side of table for work in posterior brachium. Deltoid and triceps: Effleurage, pétrissage, and site-specific friction to origin of long head of triceps 7. Reposition arm back on table. Anterior forearm: Effleurage, pétrissage, circular fist and reverse-J frictions 8. Anterior forearm: Active-assistive broadening and lengthening (include when wrist/hand flexors are focal group of sport, eg, tennis) 9. Palm and fingers: Compressions and frictions
Completion/transition	9. Repeat steps 5–8 opposite arm 10. Full back and both arms: Tapotement/jostle	10. Repeat steps 6–9 opposite arm 11. Full back and both arms: Tapotement and/or effleurage
Supine: Chest/neck	11. Pectoralis major: Compressions, pétrissage, and pin-and-stretch 12. Head/neck: Pétrissage and friction (head bob) 13. Therapist moves to side of table for sternocostal work: General neuromuscular and circular friction. Repeat to other side of sternum	12. Pectoralis major: Compressions and pin-and-stretch 13. Chest, shoulders, and neck: Apply emollient with effleurage, then pétrissage full area 14. Sternocostal junction: General neuromuscular release and circular friction. Repeat to other side
Shoulders/arms	14. Biceps: Compressions, pétrissage, and pin-and-stretch 15. Deltopectoral junction: Site-specific friction 16. Posterior forearm: Compressions, pétrissage, muscle rolling and circular friction 17. Combination stretch for wrist flexors, triceps and latissimus dorsi, then site-specific friction posterior axilla	15. Apply emollient to full arms. Biceps: Effleurage, pétrissage, and linear fist friction 16. Deltopectoral junction: Site-specific friction 17. Biceps and deltoid: Active-assistive broadening to both 18. Posterior forearm: Effleurage, pétrissage, and active-assistive broadening and lengthening (include active-assistive when wrist/hand extensors are focal group of sport, eg crew) 19. Combination stretch and site-specific friction as in step 17 of no emollient sequence
Completion/transition	18. Repeat steps 14–17 opposite arm 19. Full arm tapotement/jostle	20. Repeat steps 15–19 opposite arm 21. Full arm tapotement and/or effleurage

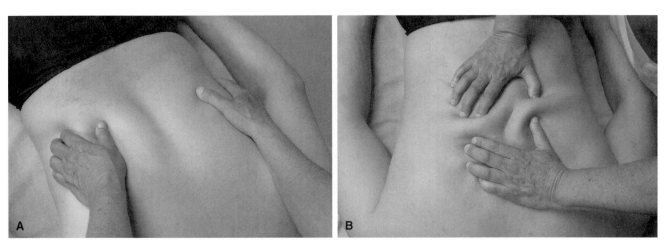

FIGURE 10-26 Dry pétrissage. (A) Latissimus dorsi down to ilium. **(B)** From ilium up the paraspinals to the neck.

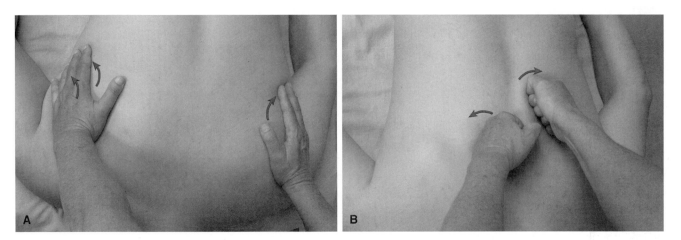

FIGURE 10-27 Infraspinous fossa and paraspinals. (A) Circular friction over the infraspinous fossa. **(B)** Alternating circular fist friction over the paraspinals.

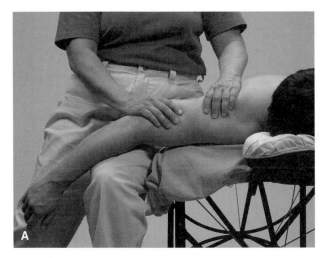 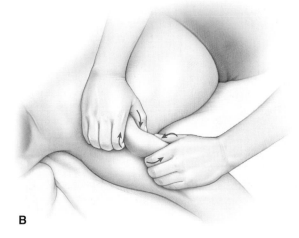

FIGURE 10-28 Posterior brachium and triceps. (A) Position the athlete's arm over the edge of the table for deep work in the posterior brachium. **(B)** Muscle rolling of the triceps.

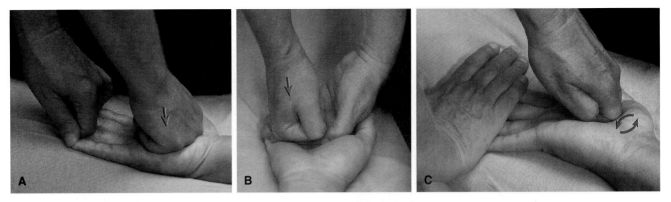

FIGURE 10-29   Hand. (A) Compressions of the palm of the hand. **(B)** By placing your own fingers across the athlete's and for compression, the pressure is evenly applied to all fingers at the same time. **(C)** Engage the tissue mass over the heel of the hand with the distal interphalangeal knuckles for effective circular friction.

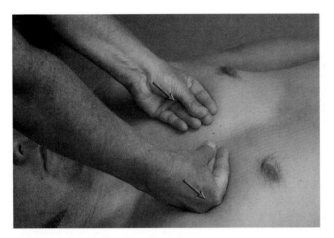

FIGURE 10-30   Rib cage. For moderate pressure over the ribcage, therapists must use flat fingers or palms of the hands for rhythmic compression of the pectoralis major. Loose fists may be used only in heavily muscled athletes.

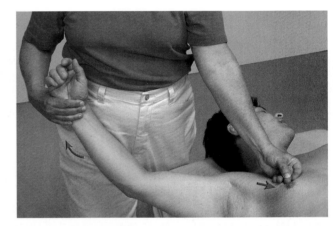

FIGURE 10-31   Pin-and-stretch for the pectoralis major.
Engage the tissue in light compression and stretch toward the feet while bringing the athlete's arm into hyperflexion and *ab*duction.

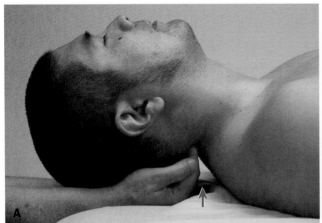
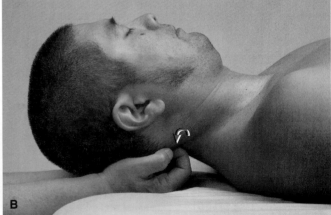

FIGURE 10-32   Head-bobbing friction up the cervical paraspinals. (A) With the athlete's head cradled on the heels of your hands, press fingers straight up into the paraspinal muscles causing the chin to point up to the ceiling. **(B)** Now curl the pads of the fingers into the tissue and pull it toward the occiput, which should cause the chin to roll back to level, and repeat the full length of the neck.

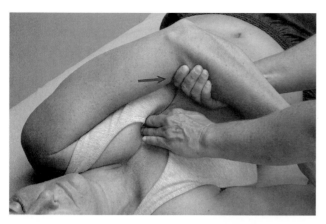

FIGURE 10-33 General tender point and friction through the sternocostal borders.

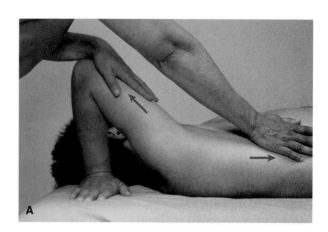

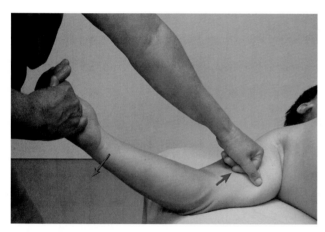

FIGURE 10-34 Pin-and-stretch for biceps brachii. Remember to moderate the amount of pressure applied directly down into the muscle mass.

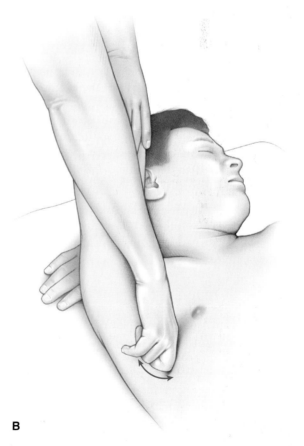

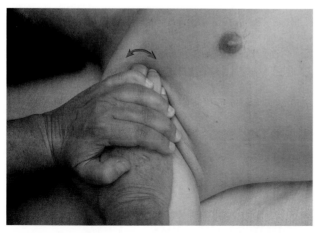

FIGURE 10-35 Site-specific friction over the deltopectoral junction is applied with braced fingers. The athlete's arm is supported in slight flexion.

FIGURE 10-36 Combination stretch for wrist flexors, triceps, and latissimus and site-specific friction to the teres–subscapularis junction of the posterior axilla. (A) Combination stretch for the wrist flexors, triceps, and latissimus dorsi. Slide the tissue apart between the hands to create an oppositional stretch. If the athlete's palm cannot rest flat on the table in this position, modify by having him or her make a fist to rest on the table. **(B)** Site-specific friction to the subscapularis–teres junction. Use the outside hand to scoop and stretch the tissue of the posterior axilla.

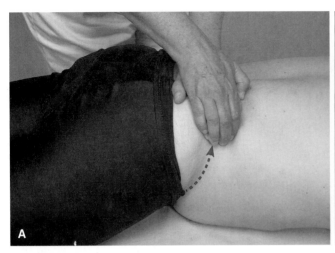
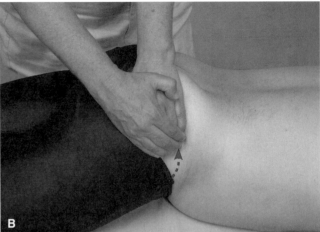

FIGURE 10-37 Tracing the ilium. (A) Use a cupped hand to pull tissue up over the full iliac crest from the anterior superior iliac spine to sacrum. **(B)** A second pass from the superior edge of the greater trochanter up through the middle of the gluteal fossa. Use your body weight to create depth with this stroke.

4. *Pétrissage* up the erector spinae as a transition stroke to the head of the table. Pétrissage from neck out to the upper trapezius to deltoids and transition to pétrissage in the axilla and down the lateral torso to the ilium.

5. *Circular fist friction,* starting at the posterior neck and progressing through the upper trapezius, infraspinous fossa, and down the erector spinae to the iliac crest.

6. *General friction and tender point release* in interscapular muscles (Fig. 10-38).

Note: Again, therapists may choose to spend more time in the interscapular area for more specific neuromuscular or fascial work. However, it is not considered a standard part of event massage.

SHOULDERS/ARMS/HANDS

7. Position arm *ab*ducted over side of table (see Fig. 10-28A) for *effleurage and pétrissage* through the triceps followed by *site-specific friction* to the long head of the triceps tendon. *Note:* There should be no need to apply emollient to the triceps for these strokes. The amount of emollient on the therapist's hands from the back massage should be sufficient.

8. The therapist now stands at the side of the table and places the athlete's arm back up on the table with the palm up, applies emollient to full arm with *effleurage,* and follows with *pétrissage and circular fist friction* to the anterior forearm muscles.

9. *Active-assistive* broadening and lengthening of anterior forearm (active-assistive releases are optional in all major muscle groups for event massage with emollient).

10. *Rhythmic compressions* to palm of the hand and fingers plus *knuckle friction* to heel of the hand (see Fig. 10-29A–C).

11. Tapotement (pre-event) or effleurage (post-event) over mid and upper back.

Emollient—Upper Body

Athlete **SUPINE** (8 to 12 minutes)

Therapist begins standing at the head of the table facing the athlete's feet.

CHEST AND NECK

1. *Rhythmic compressions* (see Fig. 10-30) and general *pin-and-stretch* of the pectoralis major (see Fig. 10-31).

2. *Apply emollient with effleurage* from sternum out over pectoralis to deltoids, then under upper trapezius and posterior neck.

3. *Pétrissage* the pectoralis major, deltoids, upper trapezius, and posterior neck.

4. Therapist moves to the side of the table and face the athlete's head to apply *general neuromuscular and circular friction* through the sternocostal junctions (see Fig. 10-33).

5. Apply emollient to the full arm with effleurage and pétrissage over the biceps, triceps, and deltoids.

6. *Site-specific friction* over the deltopectoral junction (see Fig. 10-35).

SHOULDERS AND ARMS

7. Active-assistive broadening with the thumbs to the biceps (Fig. 10-39A) and deltoid (Fig. 10-39B).

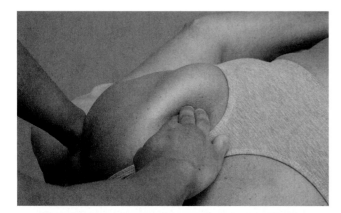

FIGURE 10-38 **Friction and trigger/tender point work in the interscapular zone is facilitated with passive retraction of the scapula.**

8. Pétrissage to the forearm, followed by active-assistive release of the posterior forearm muscles.
9. Combination stretch and posterior axilla friction (see Fig. 10-36A and B).

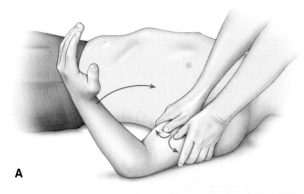

A

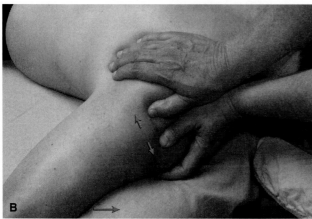

B

FIGURE 10-39 **Active-assistive broadening. (A)** For the biceps brachii, therapist strokes across the muscle fibers as the athlete slowly flexes the elbow. Two to three hand positions are required to fully cover the muscle. **(B)** For the deltoids, therapist may use the thumbs to stroke across the muscle during abduction.

10. Repeat steps 4 to 8 to other arm, and finish with tapotement (pre-event) or effleurage (post-event).

To develop their ability to smoothly and efficiently apply a *comprehensive* event massage, therapists are encouraged to practice each example sequence as written several times before eliminating steps. Because these example sequences are designed so that *all* the major muscle groups in the upper or lower body are thoroughly addressed, it is unlikely that a therapist will be able to complete them in the standard event massage time frame during the first few attempts. However, it is generally not necessary to work this thoroughly in all the major muscle groups for all athletes. For example, both tennis players and swimmers are considered upper body athletes, but tennis players require more time focused in their forearms and palms than a swimmer does. In fact, pre-event massage for a particular swimmer may include the upper back, chest, neck, and shoulders and none of the hips, back, forearms, or hand massage that a tennis player might need. When therapists have sufficient practice with the full sequences, the confidence in their strokes, positioning, and transition maneuvers makes the event massage time frame more realistic. Eventually, the massage is easily completed in the standard time frame, and selecting and combining the specific techniques to fit the needs of individual athletes becomes second nature.

SUMMARY

- Event massage is designed to help athletes prepare for and recover from physical activity, and uses several Swedish/classic massage plus all basic sports massage strokes.
- Each event massage is brief and delivered at the site of the activity. Standard time frames are 10 to 15 minutes for pre-event, 5 to 10 minutes for inter-event, and 15 to 20 minutes for post-event.
- Event massage is focused on the large muscle groups that are stressed during the individual activity. Therefore, event massage generally addresses only the upper or lower body region for any one athlete.
- Event massage is ancillary to the athlete's primary warm-up and cool-down routines and not a replacement for either.
- Event massage may be administered with or without an emollient.
- The general sequence of basic sports massage strokes is rhythmic compressions, pétrissage, and frictions.
- Therapists must conduct a brief interview before each event massage to ascertain areas of focus, contraindications, or the need for first aid.
- Therapists must be able to recognize and apply appropriate first aid measures for these common situations: muscle cramps, heat exhaustion, heat stroke, hypothermia, and frostbite.

Review Questions

SHORT ANSWERS

1. List the goals of pre-event sports massage.

2. List the goals of post-event sports massage.

3. What are the most distinguishing features between pre-event and post-event massage routines?

4. Describe the steps involved in placing the athlete in the frog-leg position for iliotibial band focus and the indicators that this position should not be used.

5. What is the general sequence of basic sports massage strokes when no emollient is being used?

MULTIPLE CHOICE

6. Which of these basic sports massage strokes would be most appropriate to eliminate from a post-event massage?
   a. Effleurage
   b. Broad friction
   c. Jostling
   d. Tapotement

7. What is the standard duration of a pre-event massage?
   a. 10 to 15 minutes
   b. 15 to 30 minutes
   c. 5 to 10 minutes
   d. 20 to 40 minutes

8. What is the general sequence of basic sports massage strokes when an emollient *is* being used?
   a. Effleurage, pétrissage, effleurage
   b. Compressions, pétrissage, friction
   c. Effleurage, pétrissage, friction
   d. Pétrissage, friction, tapotement

9. In which of the following pre-event situations would dry massage be preferred to massage using an emollient?
   a. Basketball
   b. Gymnastics
   c. Rowing
   d. Cross-country running

10. Pre-event massage should be given within what time frame before the beginning of activity?
   a. No more than 30 minutes before the event
   b. 24 hours before the activity
   c. 4 hours to 30 minutes before activity
   d. No more than 1 hour before activity

11. What is the best time after the end of activity to give post-event massage to decrease the likelihood of delayed-onset muscle soreness?
   a. 1 hour
   b. 30 minutes
   c. 3 hours
   d. 2 hours

12. The first aid actions steps for heat exhaustion are to first stabilize the athlete (sit or lie) on the table and call for assistance; the second step is _____.
   a. cooling the athlete by any means available
   b. giving the athlete cold water to drink
   c. covering the athlete's head and neck
   d. giving the athlete an electrolyte drink

13. Contract–relax stretching is best used in which event massage situation?
   a. Pre-event
   b. Inter-event
   c. Post-event
   d. Within 30 minutes of the end of activity

14. Which of these signs is the best indicator that an athlete has heat stroke?
   a. Sweating profusely with disorientation
   b. Disorientation and fainting
   c. Skin is very red and hot to touch
   d. Skin is cool, damp, and pale

15. Proper first aid for hypothermia says that the most important body region to cover in the warming process is the _____.
   a. torso
   b. head and neck
   c. legs and feet
   d. arms and shoulders

16. Which of these action steps is contraindicated for treatment of hypothermia?
   a. Vigorous rubbing and shaking of the extremities
   b. Removal of athlete's wet clothing
   c. Giving the athlete warm broth to sip
   d. Having the athlete walk with assistance and support after initial warming

17. What is the best first action step for cramp management?
   a. Athlete does active stretch
   b. Approximation + reciprocal inhibition
   c. Contract–relax
   d. Direct compression + reciprocal inhibition

18. Which of these actions is contraindicated for treatment of frostbite?
    a. Re-warm first-degree frostbite with body heat and warm breath
    b. Immerse the body part in warm water
    c. Rub the area to increase circulation
    d. Remove wet gloves and/or sox and replace with dry

19. Inter-event massage is most common in which of these sports?
    a. Swimming and track
    b. Golf and tennis
    c. Gymnastics and rowing
    d. Volleyball and basketball

20. Athletes should not receive post-event massage until they can answer yes to these three questions: "Have you completed your cool-down?" "Have you replaced your fluids?" _____
    a. "Have you had any problems training for this event?"
    b. "Are you wearing dry clothing?"
    c. "What body areas do you want me to focus on?"
    d. "Do you have any old injuries?"

REFERENCES

1. Archer PA. Massage for Sports Health Care. Champaign, IL: Human Kinetics, June 1999.
2. King RK. Performance Massage: Muscle Care for Physically Active People. Champaign IL: Human Kinetics, 1993.
3. Benjamin PJ, Lamp SP. Understanding Sports Massage. Champaign IL: Human Kinetics, 1996.
4. Meagher J, Boughton P. Sports Massage. Barrytown, NY: Station Hill Press, 1990.
5. Phaigh R, Perry P. Athletic Massage. New York: Simon & Schuster, 1984.
6. Boone T, Cooper R, Thompson WR. A physiologic evaluation of the sports massage. Athletic Training 1991;25:51–54.
7. Cafarelli E, Flint F. The role of massage in preparation for and recovery from exercise. Sports Med 1992;14(1):1–9.
8. Rodenburg JB et. al. Warm-up, stretching and massage diminish harmful effects of eccentric exercise. Int J Sports Med 1994;15:414–419.
9. Yates J. A Physician's Guide to Therapeutic Massage: Its Physiologic Effects and Their Application to Treatment. Vancouver B.C.: Massage Therapists' Association of British Columbia, 1990.
10. Weerapong P, Hume PA, Kolt GS. The mechanisms of massage and effects on performance, muscle recovery and injury prevention. Sports Med 2005;35(3):235–256.
11. Braverman DL, Schulman RA. Massage techniques in rehabilitation medicine. Comp Ther Phys Med Rehab 1999;10:3:631–649.
12. Prentice WE, Lehn C. Therapeutic massage. In: Therapeutic Modalities, 2nd ed. New York: McGraw-Hill, 2002.
13. Samples P. Does sports massage have a role in sports medicine? The Physician and Sports Medicine 1987;5(3):177–183.
14. Tiidus PM. Manual massage and recovery of muscle function following exercise: A literature review. JOSPT 1997;25(2):107–112.
15. Smith LL et al. The effects of athletic massage on delayed onset muscle soreness, creatine kinase, and neutrophil count: A preliminary report. JOSPT 1994;19(2).
16. Weber MD, Servedio FJ, Woodall WR. The effects of three modalities on delayed onset muscle soreness. JOSPT 1994;20(5):236–242.
17. Flegel MJ. Sports First Aid. Champaign, IL: Human Kinetics, 1992.
18. Binkley HM, Beckett J, Casa DJ et al. National Athletic Trainer's Association Position Statement: Exertional Heat Illnesses. Journal of Athletic Training 2002;37(3):329–343.
19. Eichner ER. Heat stroke in sports: Causes, prevention, and treatment. Sports Science Exchange 2002;15(3).
20. Clements JM, Casa DJ, Knight C et al. Ice-water immersion and cold-water immersion provide similar cooling in runners with exercise-induced hyperthermia. Journal of Athletic Training 2002;37(2):146–150.
21. Safran MR, McKeag DB, VanCamp SP. Manual of Sports Medicine. Philadelphia: Lippincott-Raven, 1998.

11 Maintenance Massage

After completing this chapter, the reader will be able to:

- Explain the major differences between event massage and maintenance massage, and list the goals of maintenance massage.
- List eight common injury prevention measures other than massage taken by sports health care therapists.
- Explain some common methods for prioritizing the sports and athletes who will receive regular maintenance massage.
- Describe how maintenance massage contributes to injury prevention efforts.
- Describe appropriate maintenance massage schedules for competitive and recreational athletes as well as the weekend warrior.
- Explain general guidelines used to determine the areas of focus and sequence of maintenance massage.
- List several techniques that should be included in a maintenance massage for an upper body athlete.
- List several techniques that should be included in a maintenance massage for a lower body athlete.
- Demonstrate an appropriate maintenance massage for both upper and lower body athletes.

*A*ll athletes experience some level of muscle tension and soreness that may interfere with their regular training and competitive routines. Maintenance massage is intended to minimize the negative effects of repetitive movement by identifying and treating areas of tenderness and restriction. This keeps the athlete participating at the highest level and decreases the risk of injury. Compared with event massage, maintenance massage is a more anatomically directed style of work, which is directed toward the origins, insertions, tendons, ligaments, musculotendinous junctions, and myofascial structures of the body. Maintenance massage combines the basic sports massage strokes with general myofascial and neuromuscular techniques to create sport-specific and effective massage sequences that can be administered on a regular basis.

The duration of maintenance massage sessions range from 30 to 90 minutes, and each session can be focused on specific body regions or may be a full-body massage. Because the soft tissue specialist on the sports health care team may be responsible for many athletes, it may not be practical to provide preventive massage to everyone on the team. For this reason, it is helpful to establish some method of prioritizing the sports and the athletes to be treated. Chronic repetitive stress syndromes are common in sports such as swimming, track and field, crew, tennis, and cross-country running and skiing. Therefore, athletes on these teams might be scheduled for maintenance massage on a more regular basis than members of the football or basketball team. Other methods for prioritizing athletes include treating only the top point getters, the first-string team members, or those with chronic injury histories. These priorities must shift as seasons change and injuries occur or progress through the healing cycle. Regardless of how priorities are established, athletes are best served when the sports health care team includes a qualified and experienced sports massage specialist.

Goals and Benefits of Maintenance Massage

It is impossible to say with any certainty that the regular use of massage in athletics will prevent injury. Acute injury in particular will happen even when all possible preventive measures are used because the causes of acute injury are variable, unpredictable, and ultimately unpreventable. However, we still apply as many preventive measures as possible, being certain that the risk of acute injury is diminished and that a few chronic injuries may be prevented. The acknowledged tools for injury prevention include[1-3]:

- Training and conditioning
- Pre-season physicals
- Teaching proper skills and mechanics
- Proper equipment
- Bracing and taping
- Proper nutrition and diet
- Warm-up and cool-down procedures
- Flexibility and strength training

Regular therapeutic massage would also have a positive impact on injury prevention in several ways. Pre-season physicals could be expanded to include soft tissue assessment to identify restricted fascial planes and stress points in muscles. These soft tissue dysfunctions could lead to injury or lost time in training if they go untreated. The warm-up/cool-down processes could be enhanced with event/performance massage (Chapter 10). Regular myofascial and neuromuscular massage added to standard stretching routines enhances general flexibility and therefore indirectly enhances muscle power. In addition, regular massage provides regular and thorough assessment of the muscles and fascia, allowing therapists to identify and address problem areas before incapacitating injuries occur.

Although the positive effects of maintenance massage are difficult to measure with standard research protocols, they are overwhelmingly supported by anecdotal evidence and athlete testimonials. This may be because massage has its greatest impact through gradual and cumulative changes created in the tissues rather than immediate or daily changes.[4] The physiologic effects of massage outlined in Chapters 1 and 2 provide support for the following goals of maintenance massage:

1. Reduce general muscle hypertonicity/spasm—both the general and localized points that often occur with physical training.
2. Stretch, broaden, and loosen connective tissue in the areas of common stress for that sport.
3. Enhance general flexibility and range of motion (via the points mentioned above).
4. Decrease the likelihood and impact of delayed-onset muscle soreness and the low-grade strains associated with intensive training schedules.

As mentioned in previous chapters, the psychological benefit of helping the athlete "feel good" should not be underestimated, suggesting that maintenance massage may enhance the effectiveness of the other injury prevention measures previously listed.

Guidelines for Maintenance Massage

A solid understanding of the common training methods, techniques, schedules, and biomechanics for a wide variety of sports is essential for the soft tissue specialist providing maintenance massage. As with all massage, maintenance massage follows the guidelines for combining and organizing strokes, that is, working from general to specific, superficial to deep, and according to the needs of the athlete. The needs of the athlete in maintenance massage are generally those body areas that are placed under the greatest demand during their sport/activity. Appendix B provides a general outline of the large muscle groups to be included in event massage and also identifies areas of focus to be added for maintenance massage in various athletes.

■ SUGGESTED SCHEDULING

Commonly, training schedules have intense and light workout days. It is most appropriate for the maintenance massage sessions to be scheduled on the light days. These light days are generally scheduled by coaches to allow recovery time for the athletes. Because maintenance massage is intended to facilitate this recovery process, it makes sense to schedule this work on these light days. However, athletes reap the greatest benefits when maintenance massage is scheduled on a regular basis.

A competitive athlete who trains in a specific sport at least 5 days per week year-round and who competes regularly should receive a minimum of one full-body preventive massage per week. When this regular schedule of massage has been established and sustained for several weeks—that is, enough massage for the cumulative effects to occur—the frequency of massage might be decreased to once every 2 or 3 weeks for some athletes and benefits can still be maintained. During periods of intense training, it is better to schedule two or three short sessions (approximately 30 minutes) each week rather than the one full-body session. An individual who regularly exercises three or four times per week will benefit from at least one massage per month. For those training for a particular event like a 10K race or a triathlon, the schedule should increase to two to three times per month. The weekend warrior, an individual who exercises once a week or only on occasion really needs maintenance massage only once a month as related to their activity level.[5] Again, maintenance massage is for athletes who are training regularly and are injury free.

■ AREAS OF FOCUS

Because the biomechanics of each sport create several areas of stress in the muscles, tendons, fascia, and joints, these areas must be addressed on a regular basis to prevent overt injury and/or diminished capacity for training. Therefore, maintenance massage must be designed to systematically address the common stress areas in a thorough and efficient manner. As established in the event massage chapter, the first consideration is to determine whether the athlete's activity is upper body dominant or lower body dominant. The focus of the maintenance massage is to address all the key myofascial elements of that region first, then move into the other major muscle groups that are also commonly under stress. For example, cyclists are categorized as lower body dominant athletes, so a 1-hour maintenance massage should begin at the lower body, and a minimum of 30 minutes should be spent working in the key anatomic areas of the lower extremity. The additional 30 minutes of maintenance massage then includes deep Swedish, myofascial, and neuromuscular massage in the back, neck, and chest because these areas are also considered as stress points for a cyclist.

It is generally easy for therapists to categorize athletes/sports as upper body dominant or lower body dominant, and with knowledge of the specific demands of that sport, to identify the additional areas of focus. In maintenance massage, therapists must always remember to assess and address the musculotendinous junctions, bony stations of the myofascial chains (Chapter 9), and major fascial bands, planes, and septa in all the major muscle groups of the massage (Figs. 11-1 and 11-2).

Maintenance Massage for the Lower Body

In maintenance massage, therapists use more active-assistive and neuromuscular releases and both the general and site-specific myofascial techniques to expand the basic sports massage routines. The specific muscle releases listed in Tables 11-1 and later in Table 11-2 are suggested for inclusion in the maintenance massage routines because they address key anatomic areas. The phrase **specific muscle release** is used to describe any method that reduces muscle tension and/or fibrous adhesion in muscle(s). These *releases* generally use a combination of site-specific myofascial and neuromuscular release techniques. The tables provide several examples of techniques that can be added to the event massage sequence to create a more thorough and specific massage for athletes as part of their regular training routine. However, the tables are not designed as comprehensive lists of every possible release or specialty option that might be effectively used. As therapists gain experience and training in new techniques, they naturally expand their therapeutic repertoire and modify their maintenance massage as needed.

Even though a maintenance massage routine is based on the same general sequence of strokes as in an event massage, the maintenance routine is more detailed and comprehensive and applied at a much slower pace. Moreover, during maintenance massage the athlete is disrobed and draped as in classic Swedish massage. However, it is a good general rule to have both male and female athletes leave their underpants on to make it easier to perform any broad fascial releases and/or stretches included in the massage. The maintenance routine adds thorough broad plane myofascial work and active-assistive releases and takes the time to search for and address specific tender/trigger points as well as contract–relax techniques in several major muscle groups. The example sequences given here takes approximately 75 minutes to complete and should be adjusted and abbreviated according to information from the athlete regarding specific areas of tension and soreness. Only the techniques that have not been shown in previous chapters are called out and pictured in the following maintenance sequences.

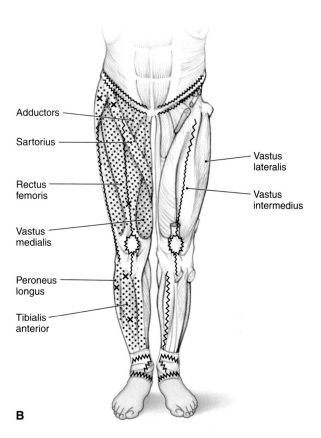

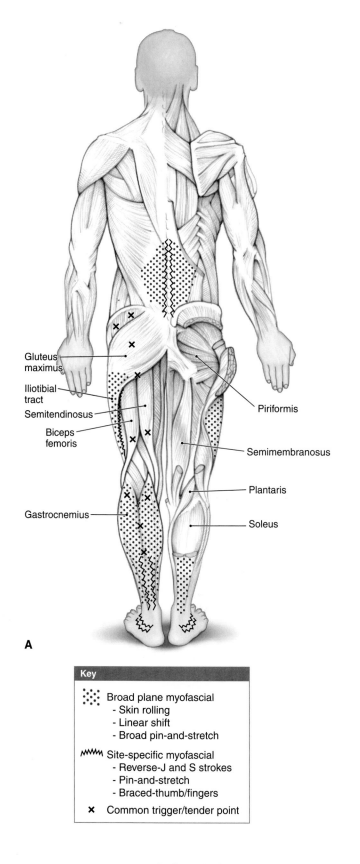

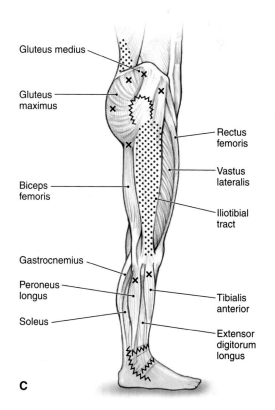

Key

Broad plane myofascial
- Skin rolling
- Linear shift
- Broad pin-and-stretch

Site-specific myofascial
- Reverse-J and S strokes
- Pin-and-stretch
- Braced-thumb/fingers

✕ Common trigger/tender point

FIGURE 11-1 Focus areas for lower body preventive massage.
(A) Posterior view. **(B)** Anterior view. **(C)** Lateral view.

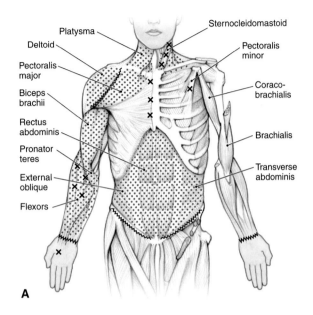

A

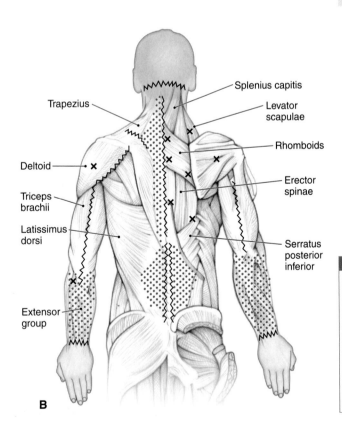

B

Key

⠿ Broad plane myofascial
- Skin rolling
- Linear shift
- Broad pin-and-stretch

〰 Site-specific myofascial
- Reverse-J and S strokes
- Pin-and-stretch
- Braced-thumb/fingers

✕ Common trigger/tender point

FIGURE 11-2 Focus areas for upper body preventive massage. (A) Posterior view. (B) Anterior view.

TABLE 11-1	Specific Techniques for Maintenance Massage: Lower Body Focus		
Category	**Technique**	**Region/Site**	**Figure #**
Neuromuscular	Contract–relax	**Hip:**	
		Internal/external rotators	11-9 A, B
		Flexors/extensors	11-10 A, B
		Abductors/adductors	11-12
		Quadratus lumborum	13
	Trigger/tender point	Gluteus medius and minimus	13
		Piriformis	8-16
		Tensor fasciae latae	8-12 A, B
		Adductors	Ch.13
		Anterior tibialis	Ch.13
		Plantar fascia	Case study 8-2
Myofascial	Site-specific friction	**Hip/thigh:**	
		Origin hamstrings	2-7 A
		Greater trochanter	11-5 B
		Insertion of iliotibial band	11-5 C
		Distal tendons of hamstrings	11-4
		Posterior and anterior edge of iliotibial band	10-6C
		Hip flexor tendons	10-14
		Knee/leg:	
		Patellar tendon	10-15 B
		Edges of patella (as needed)	10-15 A
		Posterior medial tibia (tibialis post)	11-7 A, B
		Retinacula of ankle	10-9 A
		Plantar fascia	10-10 B
	Broad plane	**Back/hip/thigh:**	
		Lumbosacral aponeurosis	9-1
		Iliotibial band	11-5 A
		Anterior hip pin-and-stretch	9-20 A, B
		Pelvic floor (if needed)	9-24 A, B
		Knee/leg/foot:	
		Posterior/anterior compartment	As in 9-1
		Patellar lift	10-15 C
	Muscle and skin rolling	Lumbosacral aponeurosis	9-2
		Iliotibial band	As in 9-2
		Anterior/posterior/lateral compartments	11-6
		Achilles and gastrocnemius	As in 9-2

■ SAMPLE MAINTENANCE MASSAGE FOR A DISTANCE RUNNER

Posterior Legs

Athlete **PRONE**. Steps 1 to 9 are carried out *without* an emollient.

1. Lumbar: *Rhythmic compressions* and *hip lift–compress*.
2. Gluteal: *Rhythmic compression, circular friction,* and *pin-and-stretch* (Fig. 11-3A). Finish with *tender/trigger points* as needed (Fig. 11-3B).
3. Hamstrings: *Rhythmic compressions, pétrissage, general and site-specific friction* to origin and distal tendons (Fig. 11-4).
4. Frog-leg/iliotibial band: *Compressions, pétrissage,* and *broad plane shift* both linear and across (Fig. 11-5A). *Site-specific friction* at greater trochanter (Fig. 11-5B) and insertion (Fig. 11-5C). Return leg to table.
5. Lateral compartment: *Skin rolling* (Fig. 11-6) across lateral and posterior compartments, and *tender points* as necessary.
6. Posterior leg: *Compressions, pétrissage, general friction,* and *muscle rolling* through the Achilles tendon.

TABLE 11-2	Specific Techniques for Maintenance Massage: Upper Body Focus		
Category	**Technique**	**Region/Site**	**Figure #**
Neuromuscular	Contract–relax	**Back/neck:**	
		Quadratus lumborum	Ch.13
		All neck motions	Ø
		Shoulder/arm:	
		Internal/external rotators of shoulder	Ch.13
		Flexion/extension of wrist	Ch.13
	Trigger/tender point	**Back/neck:**	
		Quadratus lumborum	8-7 A, B
		Upper and mid-thoracic paraspinals	8-13 A, B
		Scalenes and sternocleidomastoid	Ch.13
		Suboccipitals	8-5 B, C
		Shoulder/scapula:	
		Levator/upper trapezius	8-6 B
		Rhomboids/mid trapezius	8-15 A, B
		Latissimus/teres major	Ø
		Subscapularis	8-9
		Pectoralis major and minor	11-17
		Arm/hand:	
		Wrist flexors and extensors	8-8 B, C
Myofascial	Site-specific friction	**Back/neck/head:**	
		Mastoid process	Ø
		Temporomandibular joint	Ø
		Shoulder/scapula/arm:	
		Vertebral border of scapula	10-38
		Deltopectoral junction	10-35
		Origin of long head of triceps	2-7 B
		Subscapularis (posterior axilla)	10-36 B
		Superior angle of scapula	11-14 A
	Broad plane	**Chest/neck/back:**	
		Full back	9-1
		Full chest	10-31
			11-18 A-C
		Anterior neck pin-and-stretch	9-18 A, B
		Anterior shoulder pin-and-stretch	9-19 A, B
		Horizontal planes (2)	9-22 A–C, 9-23 A, B
	Muscle rolling	**Chest/neck/back:**	
		Pectoralis major and minor	11-16
		Sternocleidomastoid	9-16 A
		Upper trapezius/levator	9-14 A
		Shoulder/arm:	
		Latissimus/teres major junction	9-15
		Biceps and triceps	10-28 B
		Wrist flexors and extensors	9-16 B
	Skin rolling	Full back with sacral lumbosacral aponeurosis	9-1
		Anterior and posterior forearms	As in 9-1
		Abdominal aponeurosis	Ch.13

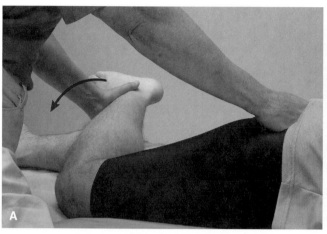 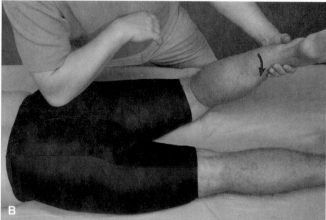

FIGURE 11-3 Pin-and-stretch and positional release for gluteals. (A) Pin-and-stretch for gluteals. Engage the tissue with a loose fist while the hip is externally rotated and maintain the tension as internal rotation is applied. **(B)** Positional release through the gluteal–sacral junction. Position the hip in external rotation to decrease the tension in the gluteus maximus and deep external rotators. Press the elbow into a tight/tender point at the gluteal-sacral junction and wait until the tension and tenderness diminish (90 seconds). Make small adjustments to the pressure and hip rotation while holding the point to make sure you are holding the softest position for the muscle. Repeat as needed through the full sacrum.

7. Achilles tendon: *Pin-and-stretch* of tendon progressing to *friction* of retinaculi and *calcaneal lift.*
8. Plantar fascia: *Rhythmic compressions, knuckle friction,* and *tender point* as necessary.
9. Medial tibia: *General friction* and *trigger/tender points* as needed (Fig. 11-7).

Repeat steps 1 to 9 on opposite leg. **Apply emollient.**

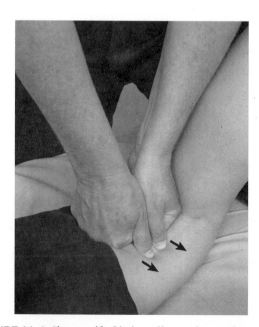

FIGURE 11-4 Site-specific friction of hamstring tendons. Press firmly into the muscle mass to tighten the tissue and stabilize the distal tendons. Press the tendon until it feels taut; then sweep across it to increase its pliability.

10. Full leg: *Effleurage.* Minimum of three strokes from foot to iliac crest followed by two to three strokes focused over thigh.
11. Hamstrings: *Pétrissage* (start in gluteals if exposed), plus *active-assistive* broadening and lengthening.
12. Frog-leg for iliotibial band: *Pétrissage,* then *braced-finger friction* through posterior edge (return leg to normal prone position).
13. Gastrocnemius/soleus: *Pétrissage* fully through the Achilles tendon, then *active assistive* broadening and lengthening (Fig. 11-8).
14. Anterior compartment: *Linear and twisting friction* (fist) and *tender point* as necessary.

Repeat steps 10 to 14 on the opposite leg.

Back Massage

1. Apply emollient to the full back with three to four *effleurage* strokes.
2. Hip (opposite side): *Pétrissage* from greater trochanter to bottom of the rib cage. *Trace the ilium* in two zones.
3. Full back: Continue *pétrissage* to cover full back, and *repeat the tracing of ilium* on opposite hip. Use pétrissage up the paraspinals to transition to the head of the table.
4. Paraspinals: *Reverse-J and linear friction* with fists.
5. Interscapula: Trigger/tender points as needed, and finish with linear friction strokes.
6. Full back: Deep effleurage full paraspinals, and stop to release trigger/tender points as needed.

Turn athlete to supine.

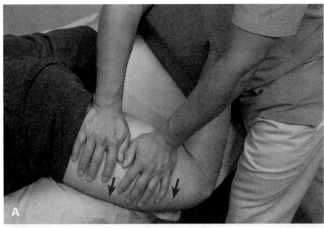

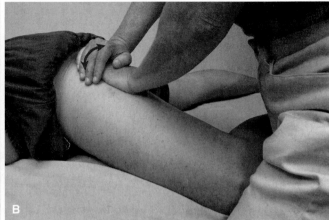

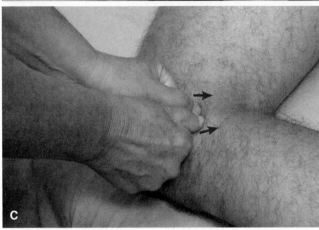

FIGURE 11-5 Fascial releases for the iliotibial band progress from general to specific. (A) Apply linear shift both in-line and across the iliotibial band. **(B)** Braced-finger friction over the greater trochanter to loosen the fascial connections of tensor fasciae latae, gluteals, and external rotators of the hip. **(C)** Site-specific friction at the insertion of the band completes the series of specific strokes over the iliotibial band.

Front of Legs

Steps 1 to 4 are carried out without emollient.

1. Anterior thigh: Rhythmic *compressions, site-specific friction* with movement (flexor tendons), and *broad plane pin-and-stretch* across anterior hip if needed.

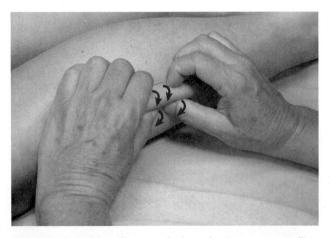

FIGURE 11-6 Skin rolling over the lateral compartment. Rolling should be continued throughout the calf, covering the area from fibula to tibia.

2. Adductors: *Rhythmic compressions, pétrissage,* and general *friction.*
3. Quadriceps/knee: Rhythmic *compressions,* dry *pétrissage,* and patellar *frictions* plus *fascial lift.* Include specific friction to any tender points/zones along the edges of the patella.
4. Hip/thigh muscles: *Assess and balance muscle tension in all major muscle groups of the hip/thigh. Assess with passive range of motion, and use contract-relax techniques to balance this range of motion between legs as depicted in Figures 11-9 through 11-12.*

Note: These neuromuscular release techniques may be performed at this point during the massage, or therapists may prefer to do them before or after the massage.

Repeat steps 1 to 4 on the opposite leg before application of emollient to full leg.

5. Quadriceps: Full *effleurage, pétrissage, and active assistive broadening* (Fig. 11-13).
6. The anterior compartment and posterior medial crest of the tibia can be addressed in the supine position if preferred (see Fig. 11-7B).
7. Repeat steps 5 and 6 on opposite leg.

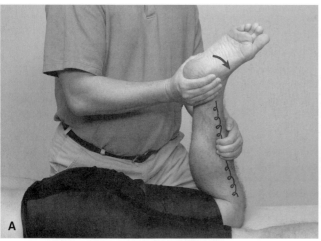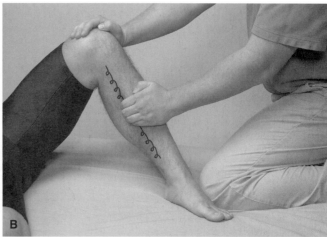

FIGURE 11-7 Site-specific friction to the edge of the posterior tibialis muscle. (A) In a prone position the knee is flexed to 90 degrees or more to make the muscle mass of the posterior compartment fall away from the tibia. Note that the thumb of the therapist is held in a relaxed position on the same side of the leg as the fingers to avoid squeezing the tissue too firmly between thumb and fingers, and to avoid excess stress on the therapist's hand/wrist. **(B)** Friction same area with the athlete in supine.

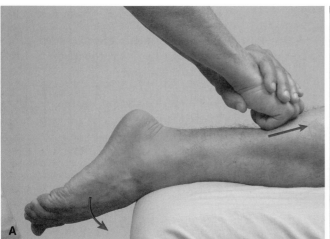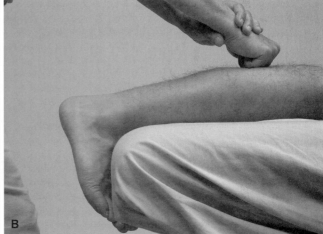

FIGURE 11-8 Active-assistive lengthening of gastrocnemius soleus. (A) Start. **(B)** Finish.

Chest/Neck/Arm Massage

General Swedish massage to chest, neck, and arms unless otherwise directed by the athlete.

Maintenance Massage for the Upper Body

Maintenance massage for an athlete in upper body dominant sports, such as tennis, swimming, and baseball, can be more challenging for therapists because the athletes are still standing, running, or using their legs. Because of this, maintenance massage for these athletes often requires that the routine/sequence include some focus on specific lower extremity areas. For example, it is not uncommon for tennis

players to develop patellar or Achilles **tendinopathies,** or for baseball players to have recurrent hamstring strains or plantar fasciitis. Therefore, therapists must remember to investigate these areas on a regular basis and occasionally include some detailed work in these structures. Familiarity with the athlete's past injuries, training/workout routines as well as a thorough pre-massage interview will help therapists adjust their maintenance massage according to an athlete's needs on a daily basis. Table 11-2 lists several of the myofascial, neuromuscular, and active-assistive techniques that most likely need to be included in a generic maintenance massage for athletes in upper body dominant sports. Following is a sample massage sequence for a tennis player. Although the upper body is the general focus of the routine, it includes more detail in the forearms, hands, and knees than would be necessary for a swimmer or baseball outfielder (review Appendix A for more detail).

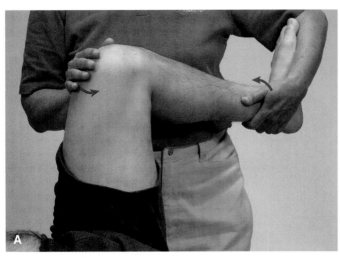
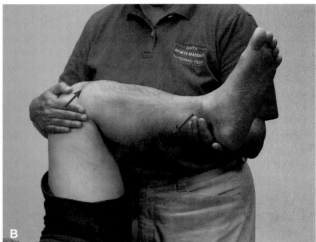

FIGURE 11-9 Contract–relax for internal and external rotators of the hip. Therapist holds both hip and knee in 90 degrees flexion for the contract-relax method of neuromuscular release. Arrows indicate the direction of resistance from therapist. **(A)** Limited internal rotation is related to tension in the external rotators. To reduce this tension the therapist applies resistance at the knee and lower leg as the athlete gently contracts the external rotators as if to cross the leg over the other. **(B)** The opposite hand position and resistance is used for the contract–relax technique used to reduce tension in the internal rotators.

■ SAMPLE MAINTENANCE MASSAGE FOR A TENNIS PLAYER

Back

The athlete is prone. Steps 1 to 4 are carried out *without* an emollient.

1. Lumbar: Rhythmic *compressions, circular friction, hip lift–compress* and *skin rolling* in lumbosacral aponeurosis.
2. Full back: *Compressions, circular friction,* broad plane *fascial shift,* and *skin rolling.*

3. Interscapular: *Trigger points* and/or *tender points* throughout, plus *site-specific friction and pin-and-stretch* for levator scapulae (Fig. 11-14).
4. Posterior brachium: Rhythmic *compression, pétrissage, and pin-and-stretch* over the triceps. *Site-specific friction* over the long head of triceps tendon.

Back Massage

Apply emollient.

5. Full back: *Effleurage, pétrissage, and frictions;* include *tracing of ilium.*

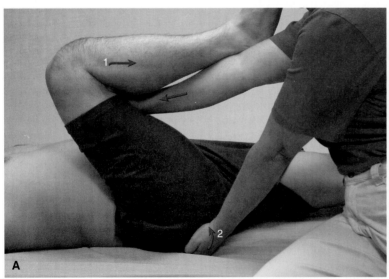
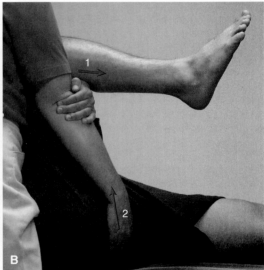

FIGURE 11-10 Contract–relax for the gluteals and upper hamstrings. Photos **(A)** and **(B)** depict two different options for the technique.

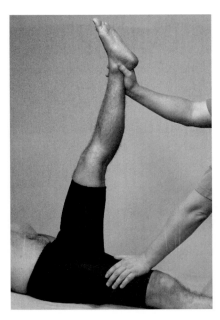

FIGURE 11-11 Contract–relax for hamstring group. Focus on engaging the full muscle group by asking the athlete to begin with slight flexion of the knee before attempting to push the full leg down to the table.

Trigger and/or tender points as needed in all major muscles.

6. Brachium and forearm: *Active-assistive broadening* for deltoids, triceps, and flexor group.

   Active-assistive lengthening for triceps and wrist/finger flexor group.

Back of Legs

Steps 7 to 11 are carried out *with* emollient.

7. Full leg: *Effleurage.* Minimum of three strokes from foot to iliac crest followed by two to three strokes focused over thigh.
8. Hamstrings: *Pétrissage* (start in gluteals if exposed), plus *active-assistive* broadening and lengthening.
9. Frog-leg for iliotibial band: *Pétrissage, linear and twisting, fist friction* through full iliotibial band and posterior edge (return leg to normal prone position).
10. Gastrocnemius/soleus: *Pétrissage* fully through the Achilles tendon, then *active-assistive* broadening and lengthening (see Fig. 11-8).
11. Anterior compartment: *Linear and twisting friction* (fist) and *tender points* as necessary.

Repeat steps 7 to 11 on the opposite leg. **Turn athlete to supine.**

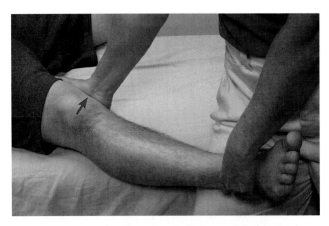

FIGURE 11-12 Contract–relax for the *ad*ductors. Position the athlete in supine with one leg off the opposite side of the table to provide stability during the contract–relax. Therapist holds the athlete's leg in *ab*duction and approximately 30 degrees external rotation to better isolate the *ad*ductor group.

Chest/Neck/Arms

Steps 12 to 15 are carried out *without* emollient.

12. Pectoralis major: Rhythmic *compressions, pin-and-stretch, lift and unwind* (Fig. 11-15). If necessary, *broad plane pin-and-stretch* across the anterior shoulder.

> ### From the Field
>
> "Most complaints I see clinically revolve around soft tissue, that is, muscle, fascia, ligaments, and tendons. When these four components are not functioning optimally and in kinetic sync, they result in movement dysfunction. The majority of athletes' complaints are not those that prevent participation, but those that hinder performance. Therefore, the sports health care of athletes is incomplete without soft tissue therapy."
>
> Benny Vaughn, LMT, ATC, NCTMB, CSCS
>
> Sports Massage Specialist, Fort Worth, TX

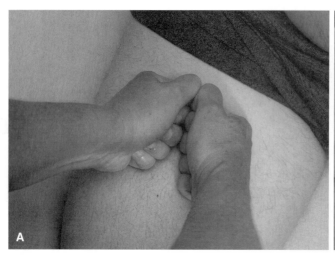

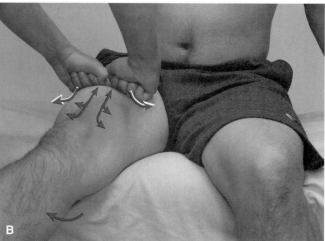

FIGURE 11-13 Active-assistive broadening of the quadriceps. (A) Have the athlete sit at the edge of the table with the knee hanging in flexion over the side. The therapist fans their fists open across the oblique fiber run of the muscles while the athlete slowly extends their knee. Several repetitions are necessary to cover the full length of the muscle group. **(B)** Finish position of the second or third repetition.

13. Sternum/pectorals: *General friction and tender point Release* through sternocostal borders. *Specific trigger/tender points* as needed in pectoral muscle (Fig. 11-16).

    Muscle rolling and/or pincer grip *trigger point* pectoralis minor (Fig. 11-17).

14. Neck: *Broad plane pin-and-stretch* for anterior neck if needed.

    Head-bob friction to posterior neck.

    Muscle rolling for the sternocleidomastoid and *linear friction or pin-and-stretch* to scalenes.

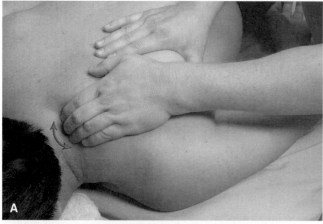

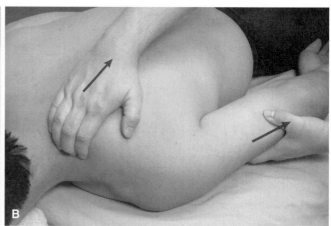

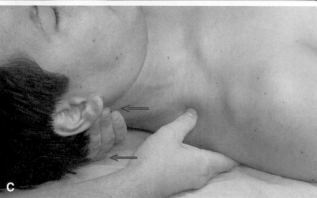

FIGURE 11-14 Site-specific friction and pin-and-stretch for the levator scapulae (A) Site-specific friction at the insertion of the levator scapulae. Elevate the scapula slightly with one hand at the inferior angle, then hook the fingers of the other hand around the superior angle (first scoop under the edge of the upper trapezius) and friction across the muscle mass. **(B)** Pin-and-stretch of the levator. Engage the tissue at the superior angle and pull downward with both hands to apply a stretch to the levator scapulae. **(C)** Supine pin-and-stretch for the levator scapulae. First, elevate the scapula slightly to soften and fully engage the tissue, then depress the scapula for the stretch.

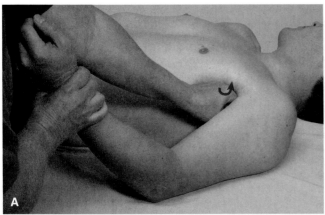

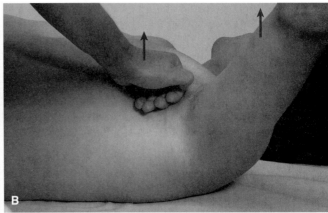

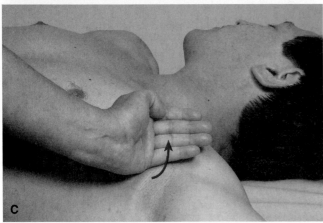

FIGURE 11-15 **Pectoralis lift and unwind. (A)** Therapist positions the knuckles of the inside hand under the lateral edge of the pectoralis major and holds the athlete's wrist in the outside hand. Lift both hands simultaneously so the muscle mass of the pectoralis is lifted away from the thorax. **(B)** Continue to lift under the muscle mass as the arm is moved through flexion and external rotation. **(C)** When the shoulder reaches full flexion, rotate the loose fist under the edge of the muscle to create a full unwinding effect.

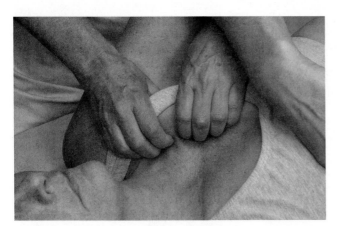

FIGURE 11-16 **Muscle rolling of the pectoralis muscles.** This technique is performed by laying the athlete's flexed and adducted arm over your own and engaging the muscle mass in a light pincer grip between the thumbs and fingers of one or both hands. The hand underneath the scapula is used to apply more protraction, elevation, or depression as needed during the muscle rolling.

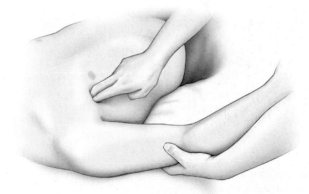

FIGURE 11-17 **Trigger point deactivation for the pectoralis minor.** This technique is done with the arm held in slight *ab*duction. The therapist must scoop under the axillary edge of the pectoralis major to locate the trigger point.

15. Biceps brachii: *Compressions, pétrissage, and pin-and-stretch.*

    Site-specific friction to deltopectoral junction.

16. Full arm: *Combination stretch* for wrist flexors, triceps, and latissimus dorsi.

    Site-specific friction in latissimus/teres–subscapularis junction, and *specific trigger/tender points* as needed.

Apply emollient.

17. Chest/neck/abdomen: *Effleurage and pétrissage* full chest and neck. Add appropriate neck stretches.

    Active-assistive broadening and lengthening for pectoralis major (Fig. 11-18).

18. Abdomen: *Effleurage, pétrissage* full abdomen, and *tracing friction* of diaphragm (Fig. 11-19).

Arms

19. Full arm: *Effleurage, pétrissage,* and *active-assistive release* for all major muscle groups (deltoid, biceps, wrist extensors).

SUMMARY

- Maintenance massage combines all the basic sports massage, myofascial, and neuromuscular techniques into a thorough and muscle specific therapeutic massage.
- It is best delivered in a clinical environment and is most often a full-body massage.
- Because of the duration of a maintenance massage session, it may not be practical to offer this regular body work to all teams and/or athletes, and therapists must prioritize the maintenance massage schedule accordingly.
- The maintenance massage sequences are based on those used for event massage, but the pace is much slower and the work in each muscle group is more specific and thorough.
- Maintenance massage routines focus more time in the muscle groups stressed by the athlete's activity and are further directed by the requests and needs of the athlete on that day.
- Maintenance massage should include some massage with and some without emollient.
- Maintenance massage includes more of the time-consuming and specific strokes such as active-assistive releases, broad plane and site-specific myofascial techniques, trigger point deactivation, and/or tender point release.

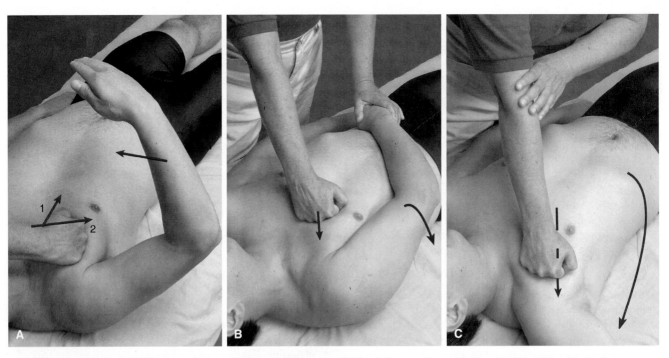

FIGURE 11-18 Active-assistive broadening of the pectoralis major. (A) Begin by standing at the head of the table with single or double fists positioned just under the clavicle. As the athlete engages in active horizontal adduction, gently press the fists across the full muscle mass. **(B)** Active-assistive lengthening begins with the athlete's hand on the opposite hip so the arm is fully adducted. The therapist stands on the opposite side of the table and positions fist(s) at the sternum. **(C)** As the athlete engages in active horizontal *ab*duction and external rotation, therapists slide their fist(s) from the sternum to the coracoid process.

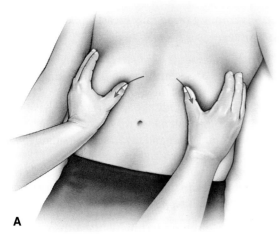

A

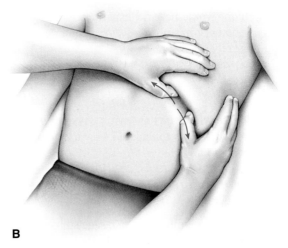

B

FIGURE 11-19 Tracing the diaphragm. (A) Bilateral stretch is applied to the diaphragm by curling the thumbs centrally under the rib cage and sliding out as the athlete exhales a deep breath. **(B)** Unilateral tracing of the diaphragm is done with the therapist standing on the opposite side of the table.

Review Questions

SHORT ANSWERS

1. Explain four ways in which regular maintenance massage may have a positive impact on injury prevention.

2. Define "specific muscle release."

3. List three goals of maintenance massage.

4. List five sports that are categorized as *upper body–dominant* in Appendix B.

5. List five sports that are categorized as *lower body–dominant* in Appendix B.

MULTIPLE CHOICE

6. Which of these settings is most appropriate for maintenance massage?
   a. Site of competition
   b. Locker room
   c. Clinic treatment room
   d. Weight room

7. The major differences between maintenance massage and event massage include the longer duration and slower pace of maintenance and _____.
   a. maintenance is more anatomically specific
   b. event is more anatomically specific
   c. no myofascial work can be done in event
   d. maintenance uses a completely different set of strokes than event

8. Generally, the minimum duration of a preventive massage is
   a. 30 minutes
   b. 15 minutes
   c. 45 minutes
   d. 60 minutes

9. What type of massage techniques/strokes are added to the basic sports massage strokes to make it a maintenance massage?
   a. More effleurage and pétrissage
   b. Lymphatic facilitation
   c. More jostling and tapotement
   d. Neuromuscular and myofascial

10. An individual who exercises three to four times a week should have a maintenance massage schedule a minimum of _____.
    a. one massage a month
    b. one massage per week
    c. two massages per month
    d. three massages per month

11. Athletes training five or more times per week on a year-round basis should have a preventive massage schedule of _____.
    a. one per month
    b. one per week
    c. two per month
    d. three per week

12. From the lower body sports listed in Appendix B, which one would have the expanded focus of abdominals and neck in a preventive massage?
    a. Basketball
    b. Lacrosse
    c. Soccer
    d. Field hockey

13. An athlete who trains at least 5 days per week on a year-round basis is considered what a kind of athlete?
    a. Recreational
    b. Part-time
    c. Weekend warrior
    d. Competitive

14. How often is maintenance massage suggested for an individual who exercises three to four times a week?
    a. 1 per week
    b. 1 per month
    c. 3 to 4 per month
    d. 2 to 3 per week

15. In addition to maintenance massage, several acknowledged tools for injury prevention include year-long training and conditioning, pre-season physicals, using proper equipment, and _____.
    a. keeping athletes out of activity until injuries are completely healed
    b. including plyometrics in pre-season training for all sports
    c. teaching proper biomechanics for all sport-specific skills
    d. emphasis on daily high weight–low rep strength training

16. Athletes who should receive regular maintenance massage include top point getters or the first string members of a team and _____.
    a. those with a history of chronic injury
    b. the team captains
    c. the star point guard on the basketball team
    d. any athlete who requests regular full body massage

17. Of the upper body sports listed in Appendix B, which sport would have the expanded focus of gluteals, thighs, and knees in a preventive massage?

    a. Rowing
    b. Lacrosse
    c. Swimming (especially breast stroke)
    d. Golf

18. Which statements best describe why maintenance massage is best scheduled on light training days?
    a. Coaches prefer those days.
    b. These are the only days when athletes have enough time for maintenance massage.
    c. Neuromuscular and myofascial techniques cannot be used on heavy training days.
    d. Light training days allow the athlete's body time to recover from stress and maintenance massage facilitates this process.

19. The muscle-rolling technique used in maintenance massage for a lower body–dominant athlete should be applied to what muscle groups or areas?
    a. Lumbar paraspinals and tensor fasciae latae
    b. Pes anserine group and the Achilles tendon
    c. Biceps femoris and patellar tendon
    d. Flexor and extensor retinaculi of the ankle

20. Therapists should always consider using the frog-leg position in maintenance massage when athletes need specific work in the _____,
    a. Hamstrings and quadriceps
    b. Gastrocnemius and peroneals
    c. Adductors and iliotibial band
    d. Serratus posterior inferior and quadratus lumborum

REFERENCES

1. Prentice WE. Rehabilitation Techniques in Sports Medicine, 2nd ed. St. Louis: Mosby, 1994.
2. Arnheim DD, Prentice WE. Principles of Athletic Training, 8th ed. St. Louis: Mosby, 1993.
3. Benjamin PJ, Lamp SP. Understanding Sports Massage. Champaign, IL: Human Kinetics, 1996.
4. Archer PA. Massage for Sports Health Care. Champaign, IL: Human Kinetics, June 1999.
5. Meagher J, Boughton P. Sports Massage. Garden City, NY: Doubleday & Company, 1980.
6. Kuprian W. Physical Therapy for Sports. Philadelphia: WB Saunders, 1982.

Evaluation: Identifying Problems and Assessing Needs

OBJECTIVES

After completing this chapter, the reader will be able to:

- List the three key pieces of information that evaluation must identify and explain how this information helps to guide therapists through the treatment decision-making process.
- Define and make clear distinctions between acute injuries and chronic injuries and the severity of injury and stage of healing.
- Name the five steps of a thorough injury evaluation, and list the standard sequence for this process.
- Name the five key pieces of subjective information, and give examples of information from each of these areas.
- Name the four components of objective information gathering.
- Name and explain the two parts of functional assessment.
- Name and describe the three normal end-feels of passive range of motion.
- Explain how strength is assessed, and name the three general levels of strength.
- Name several common neurologic tests, and identify each as a true or peripheral neurologic test.
- Carry out a thorough evaluation and identify the key problems for most athletic injuries and complaints

To be therapeutic, a massage must be designed to address the unique needs of each athlete within the context of his or her training and competitive requirements. When an athlete suffers an injury or has a specific complaint, the therapist must gather and note the signs and symptoms and carefully consider the data to create a current picture of an athlete's condition. From this information, it is possible to establish appropriate treatment goals and priorities and to choose the most effective techniques to meet these goals. For example, if an athlete demonstrates a limited and painful range of motion, a therapist must choose the appropriate neuromuscular and/or myofascial techniques to help improve pain-free range of motion. However, if the athlete's condition includes signs of acute inflammation, the therapist would choose lymphatic techniques to support the stabilization and reduction of swelling. This chapter outlines the key elements of the evaluation process and discusses the purpose of each step. The process is designed to help therapists identify the problems and limitations of an athlete's condition rather than give a specific name to any injury or condition. This is an important distinction because it helps soft tissue specialists remain clear about their role within the sports health care team and focus on thinking critically and choosing appropriate tools rather than following rote procedures or protocols for specific injuries.

The Purpose of Evaluation

The overall purpose of any injury evaluation process is to identify the anatomic or physiologic problems that are limiting an athlete's ability to train or perform at his or her

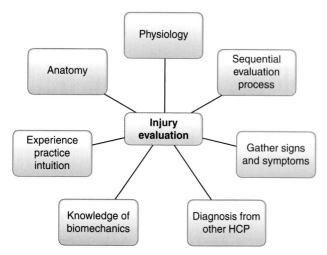

FIGURE 12-1 **Elements of good injury evaluation.** A good evaluation is based on a combination of all of these factors. HCP, health care provider.

highest level (Fig. 12-1). Naming the condition is secondary to identifying the problems because treatment is dictated by signs and symptoms rather than by specific protocols or recipes attached to any named condition. Specifically, the evaluation process should identify three key pieces of information:

1. The *structure(s)* involved in the problem. The most basic foundation for all evaluation of injuries/complaints is a thorough knowledge of anatomy and physiology. This is a simple and unarguable concept: If you do not know the normal structure and function of a system or body region, you cannot recognize that things are out of place or working incorrectly. Because of this, it is vital that all evaluations are based on *bilateral comparisons* and begin with assessment of the unaffected side to establish what is *normal* for that athlete. By comparing the status of the region or system at the time of evaluation with the normal model, therapists can identify problems in structure and/or function and make appropriate treatment decisions. Specific soft tissue techniques and strokes can then be applied to the affected structures.

2. The *stage of healing*. All musculoskeletal traumas heal through the same general physiologic processes. As described in Chapter 6, there are external indicators for each stage in the healing process that correlate with the ongoing physiologic processes in that tissue, and the evaluation process is designed to identify these external signs of the internal physiology. By determining the stage of healing, therapists can choose treatment and rehabilitation modalities and techniques that support the normal physiologic processes for that stage to theoretically improve the rate of healing. Knowing the stage of tissue healing is arguably the

single most important piece of information for therapists because all therapeutic interventions can be harmful if used at the wrong time in the cycle. It is not therapeutic if the treatment is creating physiologic changes that the body is working against.

3. The *severity* of the trauma. Severity refers to the amount of tissue damage. The most basic descriptors for injury severity are mild, moderate, and severe. These are the terms most universally used and understood across the many branches of sports health care. The severity rating of an **acute injury** (sudden onset) is based on the degree of **s**welling, **h**eat, **a** loss of function and/or asymmetry, **r**edness, and **p**ain (S.H.A.R.P.). Of these signs and symptoms, the loss of function, that is, limited/painful movement and loss of strength, is the most reliable indicator of the severity in acute injuries. Because **chronic injuries** (gradual onset) rarely have much swelling, heat, and redness, for example, severity is rated by when the pain occurs and whether disability is associated with the pain (Table 12-1). The most important reason for determining the severity of injury is to decide whether the athlete must be referred to another health care professional for specific diagnosis and/or treatment with modalities that are outside the scope of practice for that sports health care therapist. For example, an athlete who is suspected of having a torn meniscus must be fully tested and diagnosed by a physician because resolution of the injury may require surgical intervention. Once diagnosed and treated, massage therapists can use appropriate pain and edema management techniques in the pre- and

TABLE 12-1	Indicators of Injury Severity	
Acute Injury	**Severity**	**Chronic Injury**
Little or no S.H.A.R.P.	Mild	Pain after activity and activity is still normal
Moderate S.H.A.R.P.	Moderate	Pain during and after activity with or without disability
Severe S.H.A.R.P.	Severe	Pain all the time + disability

S.H.A.R.P., **s**welling, **h**eat, **a** loss of function and/or asymmetry, **r**edness, and **p**ain.

postsurgical treatments. Identifying the severity of an injury also helps a therapist establish reasonable treatment schedules with specific goals that help athletes focus on recovery rather than being injured.

When the initial evaluation process has identified the problems and treatment begins, therapists must periodically reevaluate to determine how the condition is progressing through the stages of healing. Quick post-massage assessments of how well the treatment has addressed specific problems, that is, range of motion and postural changes or tissue excursion, are important to determine the effectiveness of the session and ensure that progress is being made. This does not mean that every massage completely resolves a problem, but there should be positive changes that keep the athlete motivated.[1-6]

The Evaluation Process

The evaluation must be an organized process that ties together all the pieces of information to create a full picture so that therapists can make the best choices for care. Think of putting a jigsaw puzzle together. Each piece of the puzzle must be put into perspective by looking at the whole picture. Without this view of the big picture, each puzzle piece is a disconnected piece of information that is confusing rather than clarifying. Therefore, it is important to follow a step-by-step procedure to gather all the signs and symptoms necessary—all the puzzle pieces—to determine stage, structure, and severity. The most basic organizational concept for evaluation is to divide the information-gathering process into two large categories: the *subjective* information or **symptoms**, which is what the athlete tells you about the problem, and the *objective* information or **signs**, which is all of the measurable and quantifiable information.

It is recommended that therapists follow a set procedure of evaluation until the numbers and variety of conditions seen allow a few short-cuts. A good analogy for this is to imagine that you have been given driving directions to a new destination. The first few times you go to this new place, you must follow the directions very carefully and may

get confused or lost if a construction detour takes you only a few blocks off-course. However, when you have traveled in that area enough, a few mental connections between roads can be made and shortcuts become more apparent. You may then begin to travel to your intended destination a little faster.

Even though the process of evaluation is generally a linear and logical process, a few intangibles enter into the step-by-step procedure. How well the therapist knows the athlete, the biomechanical demands of the athlete's sport, and even intuition can play important roles in the evaluation process. In other words, practice and experience are vital to fully develop evaluation skills and to gain confidence in your conclusions.

Throughout the evaluation process, therapists identify specific problems related to the stage of healing, the structures involved, and the severity of injury. This information is used to establish treatment goals and plans and to help therapists track progress. Reevaluations must be made at regular intervals to make appropriate adjustments to the plan as improvements are made.[1-6]

■ SUBJECTIVE INFORMATION

Step 1 in the evaluation process is to gather the subjective information beginning with the athlete's medical history, the current pre-participation physical examination, and the athlete's description of the current complaint. The medical history and pre-participation exam may link the current complaint to previous injuries or conditions that can clarify or complicate this problem. When the athlete's complaint is chronic injury or pain, the history is of particular importance because it helps establish links along the myofascial chain that may be affecting the current problem and may indicate the need for a more comprehensive rehabilitation plan that addresses some of these old injuries along with the current complaint.

One of the most important pieces of subjective information for sports health care therapists is the **mechanism of injury**, or the description of how the injury happened. A key element of the mechanism is the athlete's description of a sudden or gradual onset of injury. When the athlete describes a specific movement or incident when he or she got hurt, it is an *acute* injury. When the athlete cannot describe an acute episode, but describes a gradual onset of signs and symptoms, it indicates a *chronic* injury. The description of an acute injury mechanism includes what position the athlete was in and the direction and amount of force applied. This gives therapists important clues about what structures have been placed under stress and the possible severity of injury to those structures. Additional information about the mechanism should include whether the athlete heard anything like a pop or crunch or felt anything unusual like a ripping sensation or a joint displacement at the time of injury.

The terms "acute" and "chronic" refer only to the onset and duration of an injury, not to the severity or the stage of healing. Although the first stage in the healing cycle is also called the acute stage, without the specific reference to healing cycle, the phrase "acute injury" means an injury with a sudden onset and a short duration, which can be mild, moderate, or severe, and in any stage of healing (Table 12-2). Chronic injuries may also be any level of severity and are generally in the subacute or maturation stage of healing before the athlete seeks help.

The rest of the subjective information includes having the athlete give a precise *location* of the problem/pain, the *intensity*, *frequency*, and *duration* of pain, and pain *descriptors* such as sharp, dull, throbbing, shooting, burning, stabbing, and so on. All this information can be summarized with the mnemonic: Locate F.I.D.D.O: location, frequency, intensity, description, duration, onset. It is not necessary to gather or write down this information in this exact order. However, all these pieces of information must be noted before proceeding to the objective information gathering.

■ OBJECTIVE INFORMATION

The measurable and quantifiable information that must be gathered includes simple visual and palpation assessments of the athlete's loss of function (Box 12-1). Traditional guidelines for objective assessments recommend that therapists make a bilateral comparison of all injuries and evaluate the unaffected side first to establish what is *normal* for that athlete. The following order of presentation and discussion of each step in the process is the suggested sequence for gathering this objective information: (1) pos-

tural assessment, (2) tissue inspection, (3) functional tests, and (4) special tests.

From the Field

"I had two bulging discs in my lumbar spine that were irritating nerves with every single stroke, and I really didn't like the thought of taking lots of pain medication. For me, massage was the alternative to pain killers. Why would I take medication with all the bad side effects when there is another way that has only good side effects? The massage I received from our team massage therapist was amazing. He was able to get me back into activity when nothing else I had tried, including the pain meds, had been able to. I credit my being able to get back in the boat and compete in Nationals to the regular massages I received in the weeks prior to competition."

Sanda Hangan

University of Washington Women's Crew 2002-2005

Postural Assessment and Tissue Inspection

The first part of the objective information gathering is a postural assessment and/or tissue inspection. Postural assessments are of greater importance when evaluating

TABLE 12-2	Comparison of Acute and Chronic Injuries	
	Acute	**Chronic**
Onset	Sudden	Gradual
Duration	Short/measurable gradual	Long/difficult to measure

BOX 12-1 STEP-BY-STEP PROCESS FOR GATHERING INFORMATION

OBJECTIVE INFORMATION

↓

Postural Assessment

↓

Tissue Inspection
Visual and Palpation

↓

Functional Tests
Active Range of Motion
Passive Range of Motion
Strength

↓

Special Tests

complaints of chronic conditions because they are often due to the combination of previous traumas or repetitive motions that manifest as postural adaptations. In acute injuries, there is no question about the cause of the pain, and the postural assessment is not vital to determining initial treatment. A good postural assessment helps therapists to identify and connect areas of muscle tension and fascial restriction that may be causing or responding to the chronic condition. By assessing the full myofascial chain, areas far removed from the area of pain can be identified as being related to that problem and treated accordingly. Therefore, a postural assessment should be a full-body visual inspection of the athlete while standing. Therapists must view the athlete from front, back, and both profiles and note any imbalances or differences in position between head and torso, shoulders, hips, soft tissue contours, and so on.

Tissue inspection is a more local examination of the area of the complaint, but is still not limited to only the exact area of pain. This inspection involves both visual observation and palpation of the area. Tissue inspection identifies such things as swelling, inflammation, discoloration, loss of contour, trigger points, tissue hydration, and point tenderness. All these signs are indicators that will help identify the structures involved and the stage of healing.

A thorough tissue palpation includes two anatomic components: bony landmarks and the soft tissues. Palpation of the bony landmarks is important for assessing mus-

cle attachments and joint structures such as menisci and bursae. It also helps a therapist gain proper anatomic orientation for other structures. It is recommended that the major bony landmarks in a region of pain be palpated in a sequential manner. For example, with a complaint of knee pain therapists can begin with the tibial tuberosity, palpate up and out to the medial and lateral tibial epicondyles, move from the lateral epicondyle to the head of the fibula, back to the epicondyles and joint line, from there to the femoral condyles and epicondyles, and finally around the edges of the patella. Each of these landmarks serves as an attachment for important soft tissue structures, and therapists can use the bony landmarks as a sort of home base for palpating the muscle, tendon, or fascia leading into or out of that point.

Palpation pressure is deeper for bony landmarks than for soft tissue. However, the goal is to find the landmark without creating too much discomfort for the athlete. Soft tissue palpation must begin with lighter pressure to assess skin and superficial fascia (fascial excursion as described in Chapter 9) and gradually increase in depth to assess the muscle mass and deeper fascial layers.

Functional Tests

It is not practical or necessary to measure all changes in neuromuscular, circulatory, and musculoskeletal functions related to a specific injury to formulate an appropriate treatment plan. For assessment purposes, an athlete's loss of function is measured by loss of range of motion and strength. These findings are the strongest indicators of the severity of an acute injury and can also clarify the structures involved in the injury.

During all functional assessments, two follow-up questions must be asked whenever an athlete indicates pain during the movement: "Where is the pain?" "Describe the pain." Answers to these questions help determine structure. For example, different structures are indicated as the source of the problem when shoulder flexion causes a stabbing pain on the anterior side, or a pulling/stretching sensation in the muscles over the rib cage. This information also directs the therapist to perform additional range of motion and resistive tests.

RANGE OF MOTION

Range-of-motion assessments are the first steps in functional testing because painful and/or limited movement is commonly the athlete's first indicator of a problem. This includes both active and passive range of motion assessments. During subjective information gathering, the athlete indicates the area of the problem and often describes a certain pain or limitation during a complex movement related to the sport, such as throwing. Therapists must evaluate the active range of motion for each movement of that complex motion to systematically engage specific muscle groups and joint structures(s) involved in that motion. For example, an athlete complaining of pain in the thigh or knee during squats should be asked to perform slow knee extension and flexion while non–weight bearing (sitting) in addition to standing in front of the therapist and doing a slow squat. If pain is associated with motion of a complex joint such as the hip or shoulder, evaluation of the individual movements may be of particular importance. However, rather than doing an individual assessment of all the motions, that is, flexion, extension, *ab*duction, *add*uction, medial and lateral rotation, and horizontal *ab*duction and *add*uction, therapists may be able to choose two or three of these movements for active range-of-motion assessment based on the athlete's subjective description of the pain and/or limitation. The active range-of-motion assessment also establishes the athlete's usable or **functional range of motion.** Knowing the functional range can help determine the severity of the trauma; it is also an important method of evaluating the progression of the injury through the healing cycle.

After the active range of motion, a passive range-of-motion assessment should be performed by the therapist, moving the body part through the movement without any muscular engagement on the athlete's part. The **available range of motion** is measured via the passive range of motion, and the limits of that motion are due to anatomic or physiologic restrictions. In other words, the structural elements of the joint are what stop and limit the movement. At this stopping point, therapists experience a distinct feeling at the end of the movement called **end-feel.** The end-feel of a passive range of motion helps to determine what structures might be limiting the movement, and therapists must become practiced at taking a joint to its limit and applying a slight overpressure at that point to sense the end-feel.

There are three normal end-feels: hard, soft, and firm. A **hard end-feel** indicates that bone has run into bone to stop the passive movement. The sensation is similar to pushing your hand into a table or wall. There is a sudden and hard stop to the pushing motion. Only two joints/motions in the body should have a hard end-feel: the elbow during extension and the temporal mandibular joint when closing the jaw. Actively hyperextend your own elbow, and close your mouth a few times to reinforce the sensation of a hard end-feel. If the hard end-feel occurs during passive range of motion of any other motion or in the mid-range of elbow extension and closing the jaw, it is considered an *abnormal hard* end-feel. This indication of an abnormal hard end-feel is that pain and limitation may be due to calcium deposits, bone spurs, or a dislocation in that joint.

The soft end-feel is at the opposite end of the spectrum. A **soft end-feel** occurs when a mass of soft tissue stops the movement, as occurs in elbow flexion when the forearm muscles press into the muscle mass of the biceps brachii and in knee flexion when the calf muscles press into the hamstrings. An abnormal soft end-feel generally occurs in cases of muscle hypertrophy or obesity.

The most common normal end-feel in the body is a **firm end-feel,** which indicates that tension in the soft tissue is stopping the movement. The sensation of a firm end-feel is like stretching an elastic cord to the limit. A few examples of normal firm end-feel are ankle dorsiflexion and plantar flexion, wrist flexion, extension, and *ab*duction and *add*uction. If a firm end-feel occurs before the normal end of a range of motion, it is termed an *abnormal firm* end-feel, and therapists must suspect abnormal muscle tension and/or fascial restrictions as causes of the movement limitation. Therefore, taking a joint through a passive range of motion and applying overpressure to sense the end-feel gives the therapist a strong indication of whether bone (hard), a soft tissue mass (soft), or tension (firm) is limiting the movement, and this helps to distinguish the exact structures involved and the severity of injury.[2–4]

Because the athlete is not using the muscles to create the movement, passive range of motion can help the therapist isolate and evaluate the inert tissues of the joint as possible sources of pain and limitation. The **inert tissues**— articular cartilage, menisci, ligaments, bursae, and joint capsules—are moved and stressed by both the active and passive movements of the joint. Theoretically, it is *only* the inert tissues that are moved and stressed during the passive range of motion. However, myofascial or neuromuscular restrictions cannot be eliminated from the passive range-of-motion assessment in all cases, making the questions of location and description of the pain by the athlete imperative follow-up questions. Generally, when pain and/or limitation occur with a passive range of motion, it is a strong indicator that one or several of the inert tissues has been damaged. The point in the range of motion at which pain occurs during passive range-of-motion assessment also helps to specify structures involved. For example, if there is pain with passive movement in all directions, the inert structures that surround the joint, that is, articular cartilage and joint capsules, are more likely to be involved. When pain occurs in only one direction, the inert structures in that location, such as a bursa or ligament, are more strongly indicated. Table 12-3 is an example of an assessment of a tennis player.[2]

STRENGTH ASSESSMENT

The other half of functional assessment is a strength assessment (Box 12-2). Information from the strength assessment clarifies the severity of the injury and confirms or denies muscles and tendons as primary sources of the athlete's pain. To isolate the contractile elements (muscle and tendon) during the assessment, an isometric manual-resistive exam applied in the mid-range of motion must be used. An isometric contraction does not create movement in the joint, and the mid-range of motion keeps inert structures in a somewhat neutral position. Therefore, even if there is no loss of strength (mild severity), pain during an isometric resistive test confirms muscle or tendon strain as part of the problem.

The information from the active range of motion can be combined with the results of the manual-resistive exam to rate the athlete's strength. Average strength is demonstrated by the ability to move through a full range of motion against gravity. Normal strength is demonstrated by the ability to resist, and good strength is shown by the ability to move through the full range of motion against resistance. Even though manual-resistives are not the most accurate measures of strength, this scale is sufficient for quantifying severity of injury and progression through the healing cycle.

TABLE 12-3	Tennis Player With Anterior Shoulder Pain: Part 1	
Evaluation	**The Narrative**	**Key Signs/Symptoms**
History and mechanism	Tennis player complains of sharp aching pain in the anterior shoulder of racket arm. Through questioning, athlete relates that the pain first occurred the day before during practice: A sudden sharp pulling sensation and stabbing pain in the anterior shoulder while serving. After a few more hits, he felt increased pain and weakness especially with the forehand stroke and could not serve again. Stopped activity and iced for 15 minutes.	1. Acute onset 2. Sharp pain/pulling 3. Anterior shoulder 4. Immediate weakness and pain
Postural assessment and tissue inspection	Postural assessment not relevant in acute trauma. Tissue inspection reveals mild swelling and heat over the anterior shoulder. Point tenderness over the medial bicipital groove and lesser tubercle.	Swelling and heat Point tender over lesser tubercle and bicipital groove.
Functional tests	Active range of motion shows mild pain over anterior aspect of the shoulder during all movements, but all are normal ranges. No painful arc. In passive range of motion, there is mild anterior shoulder pain (stretch/pull) at the end range of extension and external rotation. Resistive tests find moderate pain and weakness during internal rotation, and all other tests are normal. Negative Spee's and impingement special tests.	Active range of motion painful but full. Passive range of motion: Stretch pain at end of shoulder extension and external rotation. Resistives show painful and weak medial rotation. Negative Spee's (not biceps brachii). Negative impingement (not bursitis or supraspinatus).

Determination: Moderate subscapularis muscle strain in the acute stage of healing

BOX 12-2 GENERAL TERMINOLOGY FOR LEVELS OF STRENGTH

Average	Can perform active range of motion for the area against gravity
Normal	Can resist or hold against an isometric force
Good	Moves through full concentric range of motion against resistance

From the Field

"Having the team hire a sports massage specialist that was able to work with me on a regular basis was very beneficial. His work with me over the past 2 years has improved my flexibility, and the amount of general aches and pains that I get throughout the season has been reduced. I don't think I would have been able to play at my best in some of the games if I did not have [the therapist] to help relieve the stress and tension."

Betty Lenox #22

Guard for the Seattle Storm of the WNBA

Special Tests

The final step in objective information gathering and the full evaluation process is to carry out a few special tests. These are specialized functional tests that isolate and evaluate the function of specific structures. The evaluation findings up to this point should give therapists a pretty good idea of what structure(s) are suspected, and so performing a special test for that particular structure can confirm or eliminate it as a primary source of the problem. If the special test elicits a specific movement or pain, it is considered a *positive response* to the special test, and that structure has been confirmed as a part of the problem. However, a negative response does not necessarily rule out that structure. A negative result may mean that the therapist was not able to perform the test properly because of the athlete's apprehension, pain, or another injury or that the severity of injury is too mild to yield a positive result.

In general, therapists are cautioned not to overemphasize the results of special tests but to consider the results in context with the findings of the full evaluation.

STRUCTURAL STRESS TESTS

Most special tests fall into the category of structural stress tests, so named because therapists place the body in certain positions and apply a specific stress (movement and direction of force) to isolate a structure. Perhaps the most universal structural stress tests are the **ligament laxity tests.** They are used to evaluate the integrity of ligaments in synovial joints throughout the body. In these tests, moderate force is applied to a specific ligament by pushing or pulling the bones of attachment in the direction of the ligament. Because the ligament's job is to stabilize the bone, it is normal for this stress to result in only a fraction of movement and a firm end-feel, indicating that the ligament is intact and fully functional (Fig. 12-2). To get a feeling of this, perform a quick ligament laxity on the collateral ligaments of your index finger. Hold the finger out straight and place the thumb of your opposite hand on the side of the middle joint. Stabilize the distal end with your fingers as you apply lateral pressure to the hinge joint with the thumb to feel the slight shift of the bone and the firm end-feel that the intact ligament gives to the movement. In addition to the ligament laxity tests, other structural stress tests are used to evaluate specific cartilage (Fig. 12-3) myofascial chains (Figs. 12-4 and 12-5), tendons (Fig. 12-6), and bursae (Fig. 12-7). Some of the more common and useful tests are outlined in Appendix D.

NEUROLOGIC AND CIRCULATORY ASSESSMENTS

Any description of numbing and tingling sensations or shooting, burning pain may indicate neurologic or circulatory impairment. These sensations may be caused by compression or tension over a specific peripheral nerve, nerve root/spinal cord segment, a specific artery, or a combination of nerve and blood vessel (neurovascular bundle). The athlete's choice of pain descriptor can be the first clue to whether the problem is circulatory or neurologically based. Nerve pain is most often described as a shooting or

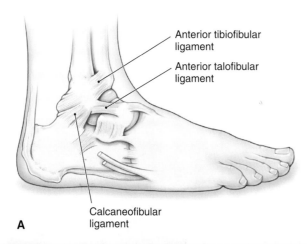

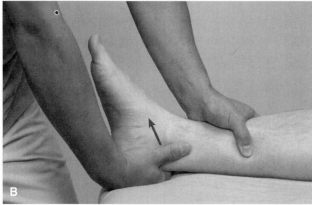

FIGURE 12-2 Ligament laxity test. (A) The anterior talofibular ligament prevents anterior displacement of the talus. **(B)** The anterior drawer sign for integrity of anterior talofibular ligament of the ankle. Stabilize the ankle in slight plantar flexion and lift the calcaneous toward the ceiling. Excess forward movement of the talus with less than a firm end-feel indicates the talofibular ligament is probably torn.

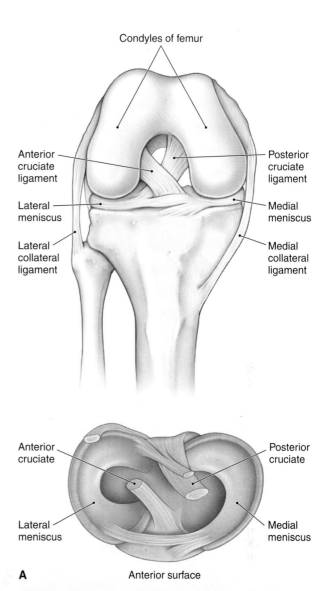

FIGURE 12-3 Apley's compression test for possible meniscal tear. (A) The menisci of the knee serve both as shock absorbers and as stabilizing structures by an edge or outer rim around the femoral condyles. **(B)** Evaluator firmly compresses the knee joint and rotates the tibia medially and laterally. Pain and/or a clicking–clunking sensation indicates a probable meniscal tear.

shocking pain that radiates down the spine or extremity, or as a complete loss of sensation or numbness. Circulatory impairments are more commonly described as a pins and needles tingle, technically called **paresthesia**, or as a burning and aching. Because pain descriptors are considered symptoms or subjective information, therapists must use more specific objective testing to first confirm that there truly is neurologic or circulatory impairment and then distinguish one from the other.

The most basic circulatory test is to check the pulse points in the area of the athlete's complaint. Circulatory impairments can be complications related to traumas such as fractures and dislocations, or it can be the primary pathology of such conditions as compartment syndromes. Therefore, it is vital to the check pulse points when athletes have a fracture or dislocation injury to avoid secondary damage to the major blood vessels and nerves. With compartment

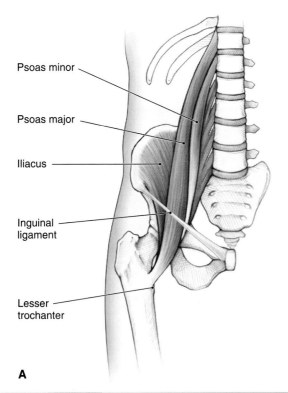

Psoas minor

Psoas major

Iliacus

Inguinal
ligament

Lesser
trochanter

A

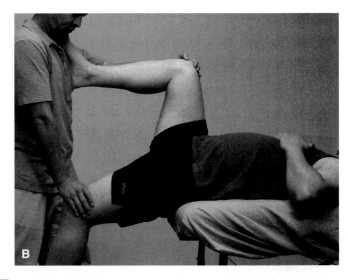

B

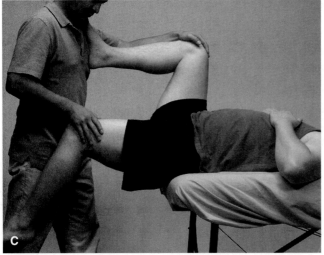

C

FIGURE 12-4 Muscle length test. (A) Tension in the iliopsoas can be related to increased lumbar lordosis, excess anterior pelvic tilt, and limited hip extensions. **(B)** Ask the athlete to sit on the edge of the table and then to roll back with buttocks at the edge of the table. Bring both knees to the athlete's chest, and slowly lower one knee while stabilizing the other in the flexed position. Normal flexibility in iliopsoas. **(C)** Excess tension in the iliopsoas is indicated when the thigh does not easily extend to a level position. *Note:* Tension and restriction in the quadriceps may cause the knee to hang at less than 90 degrees, and iliotibial band restrictions and/or abductor muscle tension may cause the thigh to "drift" laterally as it is lowered.

syndromes, a key indicator of the syndrome is a diminished pulse or absence of a pulse (Fig. 12-8). Therefore, checking the pulses are special tests that confirm or rule out the pathology.

When neurologic impairment is suspected, such as an athlete describing radiating pain during subjective information gathering, the therapist's first challenge is to determine whether the impairment is more likely due to a peripheral nerve compression–tension, or from a nerve root/spinal cord compression–tension (Table 12-5). Because nerve root and spinal segment functions can be measured via dermatomes, myotomes, deep tendon reflexes, and organ function (enterotome/visceratome), checking these functions is

extremely important.[2,5,6] The athlete can be asked about any loss of sensation, noticeable weakness, or change in organ function, that is, bowel and bladder changes for lumbar injuries and speech, hearing, and vision changes for cervical injuries. These answers will raise or lower a "red flag" for the evaluator, but special tests are necessary regardless. If the athlete reports any numbness, rudimentary dermatome tests for that body region can be done by pressing a finger and/or a fingernail into at least two points along each dermatome. The loss of sensation in a dermatome is a strong indicator of nerve root/spinal segment impairment.

Myotomes are tested by having the athlete resist a series of manual movements. The evaluator systematically tests

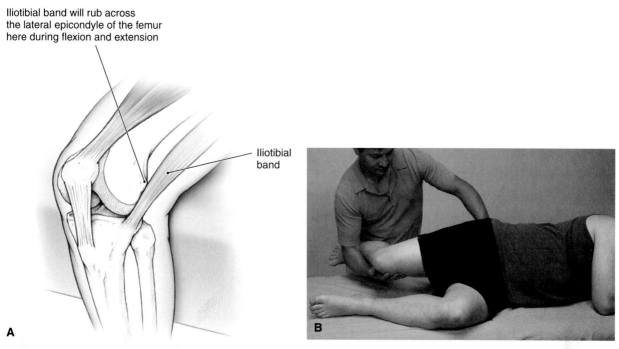

Iliotibial band will rub across the lateral epicondyle of the femur here during flexion and extension

Iliotibial band

A

B

FIGURE 12-5 Ober's test. (A) The iliotibial band inserts on the lateral tibial condyle. When the knee is extended, the iliotibial band rests over the lateral femoral epicondyle, slips over the epicondyle when the knee is flexed, and rests posterior to the epicondyle. **(B)** Ober's test helps identify excess tension in iliotibial band and hip abductors. Position the athlete in side-lying position and bring the top leg into slight extension, then passively lower it to the table. If the knee will not go down to the table, it indicates excess tension in the iliotibial band and/or abductor muscles.

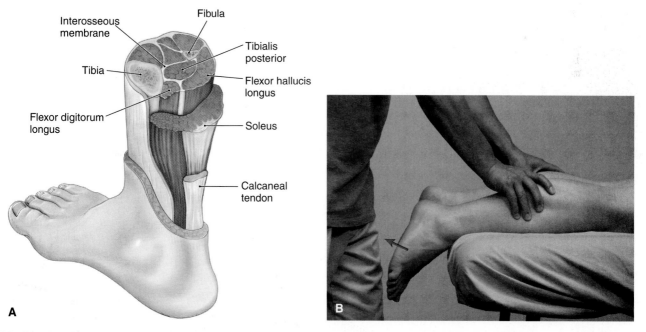

Interosseous membrane

Fibula

Tibialis posterior

Tibia

Flexor hallucis longus

Flexor digitorum longus

Soleus

Calcaneal tendon

A

B

FIGURE 12-6 Thompson's test. (A) Both gastrocnemius and soleus attach to the calcaneous via the Achilles tendon and are prime movers in plantar flexion. **(B)** Thompson's test for integrity of the Achilles tendon is performed by squeezing the muscle belly of the gastrocnemius and measuring the level of plantar flexion. The movement should be strong and equal if the Achilles is intact.

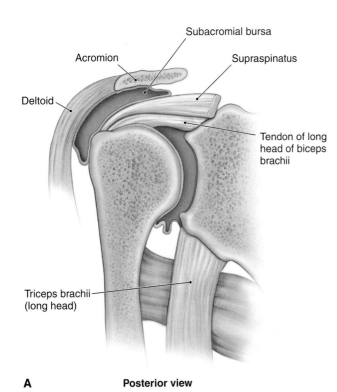

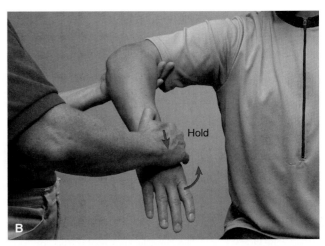

FIGURE 12-7 Impingement test. (A) The subacromial bursa and insertion of the supraspinatus muscle occupy the narrow space under the acromial arch, and inflammation of either can cause a sharp pinching/stabbing pain during this test. **(B)** The impingement test begins with the therapist passively positioning the athlete's shoulder in 90-degree flexion, approximately 45 degrees abduction, and full internal rotation. Ask the athlete to externally rotate as you gently resist that motion. The test is positive if it elicits pain and weakness.

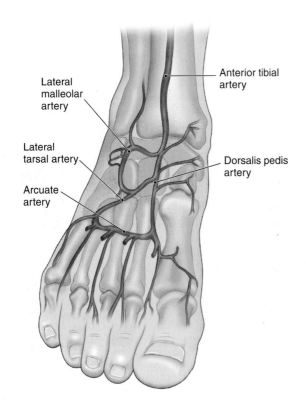

FIGURE 12-8 A diminished or absent pulse of the dorsal pedis artery is a strong indicator of anterior compartment syndrome.

the athlete's ability to resist each movement of the proximal joint first, then does the same for each joint moving distally down the extremity. For example, myotome testing for a suspected concussion or cervical nerve root compression would be to have the athlete resist the following:

1. Shoulder flexion, extension, and *ab*duction (the adductor muscles are the flexors/extensors)
2. Elbow flexion and extension
3. Wrist flexion and extension (ab/add movers are the same)
4. Finger and thumb flexion and extension

If the athlete has a loss of strength with any of these manual-resistive tests, it is a strong indicator of nerve root/spinal segment impairment. The deep tendon reflex tests are more complicated assessments and are not a recommended part of the special testing process for soft tissue specialists. Therapists can also perform special tests that stress either the nerve roots and spinal segment or a specific peripheral nerve to clarify the probable source of neurologic pain. Several of the common neurologic tests are depicted and described in the following section, including the straight-leg raise (Fig. 12-9), Kernig's sign (Fig. 12-10), cervical spine compression (Fig. 12-11), Tinel's sign (Fig. 12-12), Adson's maneuver (Fig. 12-13), and the hyperabduction

TABLE 12-4	Tennis Player With Anterior Shoulder Pain: Part 2	
Evaluation	**The Narrative**	**Key Signs/Symptoms**
History and mechanism	Tennis player complains of sharp aching pain in the anterior shoulder of racket arm. Athlete cannot remember a distinct time when sudden pain was felt: "It's just been bugging me and getting worse for about a week." The aching increases with activity, and it is felt during activity and for an hour or so after activity stops. Reports that the tennis player has been working on developing a top-spin backhand, and this stroke plus serving causes a sharp increase in the pain during activity. Because of this, the athlete had reduced overall practice time and specific work on these two strokes.	Chronic onset Anterior shoulder Aching pain felt during and after activity Pain related to the backhand and serving motions Intensity and duration of practice decreased because of pain
Postural assessment and tissue inspection	Postural assessment finds bilateral protraction and medial rotation of the shoulders plus mild kyphosis. Point tenderness over and around the bicipital groove. There is no swelling or heat, but the biceps tendon feels a little thicker than the unaffected side.	No swelling or heat Point tender over bicipital groove; thickening in the area of the tendon
Functional tests	Active range of motion shows mild pain over anterior aspect of the shoulder during all movements, but all are normal ranges. No painful arc. In passive range of motion, there is mild anterior shoulder pain (stretch/pull) at the end range of extension and horizontal *ab*duction. Resistives find moderate pain and weakness during shoulder flexion, and all others are normal. Positive Spee's and negative impingement special tests.	Active range of motion painful but full Passive range of motion: Stretch pain at end of extension and horizontal *ab*duction Resistives show painful and weak flexion Positive Spee's (biceps brachii is involved) Negative impingement (not bursitis or supraspinatus)

Determination: Biceps brachii strain or tendonitis; grade 3 (moderate); subacute stage

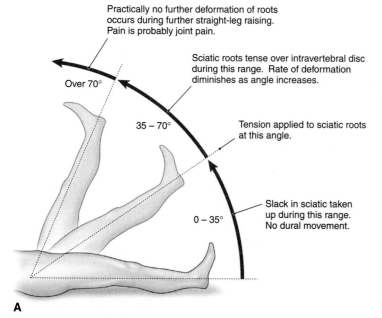

Practically no further deformation of roots occurs during further straight-leg raising. Pain is probably joint pain.

Sciatic roots tense over intravertebral disc during this range. Rate of deformation diminishes as angle increases.

Over 70°

35 – 70°

Tension applied to sciatic roots at this angle.

0 – 35°

Slack in sciatic taken up during this range. No dural movement.

A

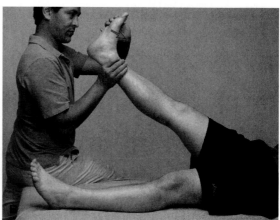

FIGURE 12-9 Straight-leg raise. (A) The lumbar spine and nerve roots are stretched/stressed most during the 35- to 70-degree range of motion of the straight-leg raise. **(B)** To perform the test, the athlete lies supine as the therapist passively raises the straight leg into hip flexion. If the athlete experiences radiating pain in the back or hip during this middle range, it indicates possible nerve root and/or spinal segment impairment.[2]

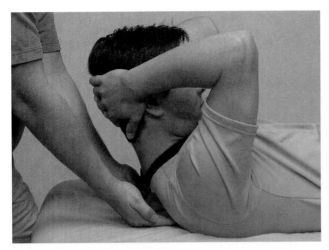

FIGURE 12-10 Kernig's sign is a test for true neurologic signs. The athlete lies supine and actively flexes the neck and head, then applies slight overpressure with hands behind the head. Radiating pain down the spine is a positive test and indicates possible nerve root and/or spinal segment impairment.

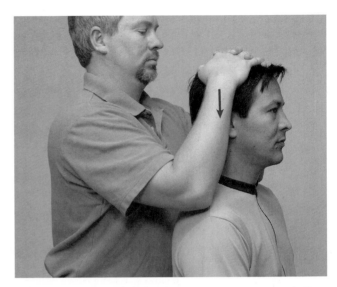

FIGURE 12-11 Cervical compression test for true neurologic signs. Stand behind the athlete to slowly and firmly press down over the crown of the head as he or she exhales a deep breath. Radiating pain down the spine is a positive response and indicates possible nerve root and/or spinal segment impairment.

test (Fig. 12-14) for the pectoralis minor tension. Several other neurologic special tests are depicted in Appendix D. Table 12-5 identifies each of these special tests as an indicator of either peripheral nerve or spinal cord/nerve root impairment. Therapists can apply safe and effective massage to help relieve signs and symptoms in both cases. However, when the evaluation indicates the possibility of spinal cord/nerve root involvement, the athlete must be referred to other health care professionals for definitive diagnosis and treatment plans.

The peripheral nerve impairment tests depicted in Figures 12-13 and 12-14 are special tests related to a condition called **thoracic outlet syndrome.** Thoracic outlet syndrome is a compression–tension syndrome of the neurovascular bundle that passes through the posterior triangle of the neck out to the upper extremity. The brachial plexus nerves plus the subclavian artery make up this bundle, which first passes between the middle and anterior scalene muscles, then over the first two pairs of ribs and under the clavicle,

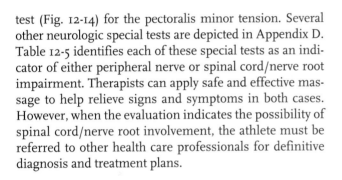

Flexor tendons

Posterior tibial nerve

Flexor retinaculum

A

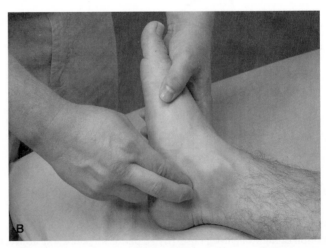

B

FIGURE 12-12 Tinel's test for neurologic compression–tension can be performed to evaluate any of the superficial nerves. (A) The common peroneal nerve is a fairly common site for this problem to occur, creating a condition called tarsal tunnel syndrome. **(B)** In this test, firm tapping over a superficial nerve elicits a shooting pain or tingling sensation to confirm peripheral nerve impairment.

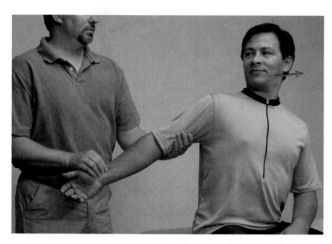

FIGURE 12-13 Adson's test confirms or rules out compression–tension between the scalene muscles. In this test, the athlete's arm is passively *ab*ducted and extended with palm up. The athlete then turns the head toward and/or away from that side, takes a deep breath, and holds it as the evaluator checks the radial pulse. Re-creation of the pain and/or a decreased radial pulse indicate compression–tension of the neurovascular bundle from the scalenes.

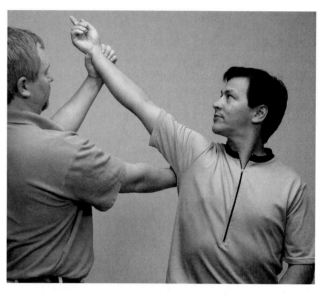

FIGURE 12-14 Hyperabduction + flexion (pectoralis minor) test for thoracic outlet syndrome. The athlete's arm is hyper*ab*ducted, flexed, and externally rotated as the therapist checks the radial pulse. Re-creation of the pain and/or a decreased radial pulse indicate compression–tension of the neurovascular bundle between the pectoralis minor and the first two pair of ribs.

TABLE 12-5	Neurologic Special Tests: Complaint of Radiating-Burning-Shooting Pain or Tingling and Numbness	
Special Test	**Positive Response = Radiating Pain (Indicates Spinal Cord and/ or Nerve Root Involvement)**	**Positive Response = Re-creating the Pain in the Complaint (Indicates Peripheral Nerve Involvement)**
Loss of a dermatome	√	
Loss of a myotome	√	
Change or decrease in organ function	√	
Decrease in deep tendon reflexes	√	
Straight-leg raising: ⊕ in the 30- to 75-degree range	√	
Kernig's	√	
Valsalva	√	
Cervical compression	√	
Tinel's		√
Phalen's		√
Straight-leg raising above 75 degrees		√
Adson's		√
Roos		√
Military/Wright's		√
Hyperflexion + abduction: Pectoralis minor test		√

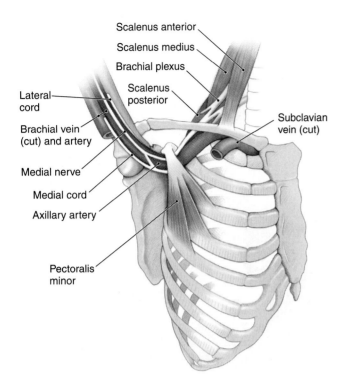

Scalenus anterior
Scalenus medius
Brachial plexus
Scalenus posterior
Lateral cord
Brachial vein (cut) and artery
Medial nerve
Medial cord
Axillary artery
Pectoralis minor
Subclavian vein (cut)

FIGURE 12-15 Thoracic outlet syndrome. Thoracic outlet syndrome is a condition in which the neurovascular bundle of brachial plexus and/or subclavian artery is directly compressed or given excess tension by a variety of structures.

and finally underneath the coracoid process and pectoralis minor tendon into the axilla (Fig. 12-15). Although the axillary artery does not pass between the scalene muscles, it can be part of the condition, especially when there is excessive tension in the pectoralis minor. Compression or tension can be applied to the neurovascular bundle at any or all of these sites, and this series of special tests is used to help determine the most likely site of the impairment. The Roos test (Appendix D) is a generic test for thoracic outlet syndrome, which confirms that there is a peripheral impairment of this neurovascular bundle, but does not specify the site of impairment. Table 12-6 associates the other thoracic outlet syndrome tests to the structures being evaluated. Therapists can better prioritize their order of treatment and

the amount of time devoted to each segment after the most likely site of compression–tension has been determined via these tests.

The special tests depicted in this chapter represent a small sample of tests that therapists should be able to perform. Appendix D depicts and explains several other helpful special tests and organizes the tests according to the complaint of the athlete.

SUMMARY

- Effective treatment goals and plans are based on determining the structures involved, the stage of healing, and the severity of the athlete's injury or complaint.
- Signs and symptoms must be gathered via a systematic process of injury evaluation and interpreted to create a complete and coherent picture of the athlete's problems.
- Each step of the evaluation process contributes unique pieces of information to the puzzle, and when assembled and considered together, provides therapists with a solid foundation for decision making throughout the treatment and rehabilitation process.
- The terms "acute" and "chronic" refer to the onset and duration of an injury, not the severity of tissue damage.
- Postural assessment is of greater importance in chronic injury syndromes than in acute injury.
- The best indicators of the *severity* of injury with acute trauma are the results of the range-of-motion and resistive tests. The amount of pain and swelling present with the trauma is a very poor indicator of severity.
- Information from the passive and active range of motion must be combined with the results of the resistive tests to provide a complete picture of the probable structures involved and the severity of injury.
- Special tests are used to confirm *or rule out* particular structures. This is generally the last step of objective formation gathering, and results must be considered in context with the rest of the subjective and objective information.

Table 12-7 summarizes the steps of the evaluation process and the key findings related to that particular step.

TABLE 12-6	Thoracic Outlet Special Tests
Special Test	**Site of Impairment**
Adson's	Between anterior and middle scalenes
Costoclavicular test	Between the first rib (or cervical rib) and the clavicle
Hyper*abduction* + flexion (pectoralis minor test)	Between the pectoralis minor and the first two pair of ribs

Positive response indicates the probable site of impairment.

TABLE 12-7	Matching Each Step of the Evaluation Process with the Key Information It Provides				
	History/Mechanism of Injury	Postural Assessment	Inspection	Functional Tests	Special Tests
Stage of healing	Key information about stage comes from history and mechanism of injury		Key information about stage comes from inspection	Key information about stage comes from functional tests	
Structures involved		In chronic conditions, key information about structures come from postural assessment	Key information about structures comes from inspection	Key information about structures comes from functional tests	Key information about structures comes from special tests
Severity of trauma	Key information about severity comes from history and mechanism of injury		Key information about severity comes from inspection	Key information about severity comes from functional tests	

Review Questions

SHORT ANSWERS

1. What are the two general categories of information for the injury assessment process?

2. Define the terms acute and chronic.

3. What are the three key pieces of information therapists need to determine from the evaluation to establish treatment goals and plan?

4. List all the steps of objective information gathering in the recommended sequence.

5. Explain the meaning of the mnemonic: Locate F.I.D.D.O.

MULTIPLE CHOICE

6. Which of the following is considered a *symptom* of injury?
   a. Description of pain as aching
   b. Measuring a restricted active range of motion
   c. Palpating a tender area
   d. Visible swelling and discoloration

7. Which of these structures in the likely cause of a firm end-feel before the end of a joint flexion?
   a. Tight extensor muscle
   b. Joint capsule
   c. Inflamed bursa
   d. Tight flexor retinaculum

8. Which of these pieces of objective information is considered the key indicator for severity of acute injuries?
   a. Description of pain as sharp
   b. Measurable loss of function
   c. Visible swelling
   d. Presence of heat and discoloration in the tissue

9. What do you suspect is the pathology when active range of motion and passive range of motion are full but painful and isometric resistives tests are strong and pain free?
   a. Moderate strain
   b. Mild nerve impairment
   c. Mild sprain
   d. Moderate sprain

10. Which of the movements should have a normal hard end-feel?
    a. Elbow flexion
    b. Dorsiflexion
    c. Knee extension
    d. Elbow extension

11. What type of end-feel occurs when soft tissue compression stops the movement?
    a. Hard
    b. Firm
    c. Soft
    d. Springy

12. What is the most common type of end-feel in the human body?
    a. Hard
    b. Firm
    c. Soft
    d. Springy

13. What is the strength rating if the athlete can only resist or hold against an isometric pressure?
    a. Normal
    b. Average
    c. Good
    d. Poor

14. The two most important questions to ask when a movement is indicated as painful are "where is the pain" and _____
    a. "how long has it been hurting you?"
    b. "how would you describe it?"
    c. "which part of the movement is painful?"
    d. "does the pain bother you at night?"

15. What is the level of severity of a chronic injury that is painful only during the activity when the activity is not limited?
    a. Mild
    b. Moderate
    c. Moderate plus
    d. Severe

16. Which of these signs of injury is the best indicator of the severity of an acute injury?
    a. Level of pain
    b. Amount of swelling
    c. Description of pain as sharp and stabbing
    d. A decrease or loss of function

17. What are the two components of a loss of function?
    a. Pain and swelling
    b. Tissue discoloration and heat
    c. Strength and range of motion
    d. Crepitus and paresthesia

18. Which of these signs is the best indicator of possible neurologic involvement in the injury?
    a. Aching pain
    b. Shooting pain
    c. Palpable heat and swelling over the spinal column
    d. Throbbing pain with movement

19. Which of these would be considered a *true neurologic* response?
    a. Positive Adson's test
    b. Negative straight-leg raising
    c. Positive Kernig's sign
    d. Negative Tinel's sign

20. If the athlete experiences a radiating pain down the posterior thigh at the 45-degree mark of a straight-leg raising test, what does it indicate?
    a. Possible neurologic trauma at the nerve roots or spinal segment
    b. Pseudo-sciatica
    c. True sciatica
    d. A ruptured disk

REFERENCES

1. Booher JM, Thibodeau GA. Athletic Injury Assessment, 3rd ed. St. Louis: Mosby, 1994.
2. Magee DJ. Orthopedic Physical Assessment. Philadelphia: WB Saunders, 1987.
3. Arnheim DD, Prentice WE. Principles of Athletic Training, 8th ed. St. Louis: Mosby, 1993.
4. Hunter-Griffin LY, Chairman of editorial board. Athletic Training and Sports Medicine, 2nd ed. Park Ridge, IL: American Academy of Orthopaedic Surgeons, 1991.
5. Hoppenfeld S. Physical Examination of the Spine and Extremities, 3rd ed. East Norwalk, CT: Appleton-Century-Crofts, 1982.
6. Rattray F, Ludwig L. Clinical Massage Therapy: Understanding, Assessing and Treating over 70 Common Conditions. Toronto: Talus, Inc, 2000.

Treatment Massage

After completing this chapter, the reader will be able to:

- Define and construct appropriate massage goals and plans for a wide variety of common athletic injuries.
- Estimate appropriate frequency and duration of massage treatments according to the type of injury.
- List at least three generic treatment goals for each stage of healing, and name the types of massage that are most appropriate for use in each stage.
- Explain what distinguishes a sprain from a strain.
- Describe the common factors between acute sprains and strains, tendonitis and chronic strain, and severe hematoma and acute bursitis.
- Describe a good combination of therapeutic massage techniques and a general sequence of application for each stage of healing for:
  a. Acute sprains and strains
  b. Chronic sprains and strains
  c. Hematoma and acute bursitis
  d. Neurovascular compression–tension syndromes
- Explain the probable mechanisms behind a "stitch in the side" and "crick in the neck," and successfully address both of these with therapeutic massage.
- Distinguish between treatment and rehabilitation, and describe a generic sequence of rehabilitation priorities.

When an athlete has suffered a specific injury that causes him or her to stop or significantly alter activity, the therapist can choose from a wide variety of treatment modalities to assist the athlete in the healing process. One choice—treatment massage—includes specific combinations of massage techniques designed to enhance healing of soft tissues and return the athlete to full activity. Because most injuries that occur in athletics are soft tissue traumas, it is logical to include treatment massage as an integral part of total care for the athlete.

Just as maintenance massage requires the therapist to have a solid foundation in sport training techniques and biomechanics, treatment massage demands a clear understanding of the physiology of healing and the general characteristics and treatment protocols for a number of common sport injuries. This chapter outlines general treatment **goals** (what the therapist hopes to achieve) and massage **plans** (how the modalities are combined to achieve the goals) for each stage of the healing cycle. In addition, several sample treatment plans are offered to illustrate appropriate stroke combinations and sequences, and the integration of therapeutic massage into the common treatment protocols used by other sports health care professionals. These are simply examples that help readers clarify their understanding of the general treatment concepts and are not intended to be a step-by-step formula for all cases.

Just as good cooks alter the recipes in their favorite cookbooks, experienced therapists are expected to add their own particular flavor and variations to these example treatment protocols.

Treatment massage is best administered in a clinical environment and focuses on the specific site of trauma as well as the full myofascial chains associated with the injury. This comprehensive approach to treatment is beneficial for all athletes, but of particular importance to those who suffer from chronic injury and persistent pain syndromes. All lymphatic, myofascial, and neuromuscular techniques incorporated in treatment massage must be carefully matched to the condition to be treated. The physiologic changes each technique produces must support the ongoing processes for the current stage of healing and the goals for rehabilitation. The duration and intensity of each session are dependent on the type of injury, stage of healing, severity of injury, and other modalities being used in the treatment of the athlete. In general, acute traumas should be treated more frequently and for shorter periods of time than chronic injuries and conditions (Table 13-1).

> ## From the Field
>
> "Utilizing massage within the practice of athletic training has tremendously improved my palpation and evaluation skills. Massage has been a great benefit for travel, too, minimizing the amount of modalities that I must pack; my hands have become one of my greatest resources!"
>
> Heather Vonasek,
> MS, ATC, NCTMB
> Assistant Athletic Trainer
> University of Vermont

Treatment Massage Goals and Plans

Basically, treatment massage must address the problems identified in the evaluation. More specifically, the *goals* are to decrease the pain, swelling, and limitations to range of motion and function associated with a trauma. The massage *plan* incorporates the lymphatic and deep Swedish techniques to address pain, edema, and circulatory impairment, whereas neuromuscular and myofascial techniques are used to address pain as well as improve functional and range of motion limitations. Treatment massage is distinguished from the event and preventive categories by the liberal use of deep transverse friction (described in Chapter 9) and lymphatic facilitation (Chapter 7). Although both of these massage techniques have limited use in the event and/or preventive categories, they are the foundational components of treatment massage. Basically, the key to the effective use for any of the therapeutic massage techniques is to match the physiologic changes created by the technique to the stage of healing and goals of the treatment/rehabilitation (Table 13-2).

ACUTE STAGE

The treatment goals for the acute stage of healing are to control the amount of hemorrhage and edema, to interrupt the pain and spasm cycle, and to facilitate the formation of the hematoma. Therefore, the massage plan should include lymphatic facilitation to reduce the edema and decrease pain, and neuromuscular techniques in antagonists and synergists to avoid excess muscle spasm that may lead to compensatory motions. Because some muscle splinting is necessary in the acute stage to protect and stabilize the traumatized area, therapists must keep this in mind and apply the neuromuscular techniques with caution. For example, in cases of severe sprain, muscle tension around the injured joint is valuable because the joint has lost its ligament stability. However, muscles farther up and down the myofascial chain should be evaluated and addressed as needed. This is especially true for athletes who are using canes, crutches, braces, and walking casts/boots.

TABLE 13-1	Frequency and Duration of Treatment Massage	
	Frequency	Duration of Session
Acute injury	Daily	10–20 minutes
Chronic injury	Weekly	30–60 minutes

Modified from Archer P, Vaughn B. Therapeutic massage for performance and rehabilitation. Seminar workbook, Indianapolis, 2000.

TABLE 13-2	Treatment Massage According to Stage of Healing	
Key Physiologic Events in Healing Cycle	Treatment Goals/Focus	Clinical Massage Techniques
Acute: Hemorrhage/inflammation Secondary edema Hematoma organization Pain–spasm cycle	Stimulate edema uptake to control secondary edema ↓ Pain ↓ Or prevent secondary muscle spasms	Lymphatic facilitation: Clear the neck and appropriate catchments (start the syphon) Neuromuscular release in antagonists and synergists
Subacute: Resorption of exudate Granulation tissue forms Decreased pain–spasm cycle	↓ Edema and spasm Facilitate formation of flexible and well aligned repair ↑ Range of motion	Continue lymphatic facilitation: Progress toward area of edema Continue neuromuscular release where needed to limit compensatory movement Begin deep transverse friction when swelling is gone
Maturation: Collagen remodeling	Prevent adhesions Facilitate collagen remodeling Return full flexibility/range of motion/strength to area	Continued deep transverse friction over the lesion Myofascial to full fascial chain(s) Neuromuscular release as needed

SUBACUTE STAGE

In the subacute stage, healing actually begins with the laying down of granulation tissue. This regenerative phase of healing is marked by reduction of edema and pain, plus improvements in function and range of motion. Continuing the lymphatic techniques well into the later stage of the subacute phase is important to support these processes. Myofascial techniques, specifically deep transverse friction, will be introduced when swelling has been alleviated. The standard deep transverse friction protocol finishes with ice to prevent irritating the area and pushing an injury backward along the healing continuum. To further this preventive measure, the addition of lymphatic techniques after icing is beneficial as well. Whenever both lymphatic techniques and ice are being used, the proper order of treatment is ice first, then lymphatics because lymph flow is diminished by cold applications.

MATURATION STAGE

The primary goals of the maturation stage include developing a well-organized and flexible scar and improving general flexibility and strength of the injured area. The lymphatic techniques are no longer necessary in most acute injury cases, but may be used instead of ice after deep transverse friction in chronic conditions. All the myofascial, neuromuscular, and basic sports massage techniques are used in this stage of the healing cycle. The specific combination and sequence of techniques are the choice of each therapist, keeping in mind the unique contribution of each method of massage. That is, neuromuscular release reduces muscle tension, myofascial work loosens and softens the connective tissue components of joints and muscles, and lymphatic facilitation reduces swelling and pain. It is in the maturation stage of healing that it is most important to evaluate and treat the full myofascial chain(s) involved in the specific injury to ensure full recovery and decrease the risk of re-injury. This is especially important in the treatment of chronic injuries.

Acute Sprains and Strains

Acute sprains and strains occur when a body part is suddenly forced beyond the normal range of motion, resulting in stretching and tearing of tissue. A **strain** is when only fascia, tendons, and muscles are involved in the injury, and a **sprain** is when ligaments and/or joint capsules have been stretched and/or torn. Depending on the severity of these injuries, they are characterized by rapid swelling, pain, and functional limitations. These clear-cut initial signs and symptoms make it easy to track the progress of acute injuries through the healing cycle with regular evaluation.

COMMON FACTORS

The swelling that occurs in all acute sprains and strains is treated with the same lymphatic sequences (for the upper or

A starting guard for one of the teams in the 1996 NBA Championships suffered a strain to his soleus muscle, which an MRI showed to be about a 50% tear. Everyone believed the guard would not be able to play in the championship series. However, the head athletic trainer and team physician conferred with the team massage therapist to establish a combined treatment plan that included lymphatic facilitation massage: 20-minute sessions two to three times a day. The player also wore a special lymph compression pad and wrap at all times, including during practices, games and at night. He was able to play and perform effectively in all games through the six-game series. The day after the season ended, another MRI was done, and to the amazement of all, the doctors could not find any evidence of the tear. The massage therapist stated that until then the athletic trainer believed that the lymphatic facilitation was a helpful adjunct to his standard treatments, but never saw it as essential and often did not allow massage treatment during the acute stage. After this case, he *and* the athletes became true believers, and lymphatic facilitation was incorporated as a standard part of acute-stage treatment protocols for as long as the therapist was with the team.

lower extremity) throughout the acute and subacute stages because the lymphotomes, watersheds, and catchments are the same regardless of which muscle or joint is involved. For injuries in the upper extremity, most edema must be moved through the axillary catchment to reduce swelling. However, swelling in the acromial region may be moved directly from the acromion over the clavicular watershed line to flow directly into the terminus by-passing the axillary nodes completely (see Fig. 7-17). In the lower extremity, sprains and strains at or distal to the knee can utilize both the anterior pathway to the inguinal catchment and the deep lymphotomes from the popliteal catchment that carries edema from the popliteal directly to the deep nodes in the inguinal catchment (see Fig. 7-12). By using these express lanes from popliteal to the deep inguinals and cisterna chyli, edema removal in the knee, leg, and ankle is much more efficient than when only the anterior lymphotomes are used.

■ TREATMENT GOALS AND PLAN

The treatment goals for each stage of the healing cycle for acute sprains and strains are exactly as outlined in Table 13-2, the priority being increased edema uptake and lymph flow. In the acute stage of these injuries a minimum of 20 minutes of lymphatic facilitation added *after* the standard treatment protocol of R.I.C.E. (rest, ice, compression, elevation) is the most effective combination of modalities. Remember that the proteins in exudate that cause secondary edema cannot be reabsorbed into the capillaries and must be removed through the lymphatic system. Therefore, lymphatic facilitation in the acute stage of healing is an essential element for meeting the treatment goals. Athletes should be taught the opening protocol for lymphatic facilitation (neck; see Fig. 7-9) and encouraged to self-treat each hour or as often as possible while at home. Appropriate massage treatment plans for common acute sprain(s) and strain(s) in the upper and lower extremity are described in Boxes 13-1 and 13-2.

Chronic Sprains and Strains

After three or more acute injury episodes to a specific muscle, tendon, or ligament, the injury is considered a chronic strain or sprain. The term chronic strain also applies to the gradual build-up of **microtrauma** in a muscle, tendon, and/or fascia due to repetitive stressful motion. This second definition makes it clear that chronic strain and tendonitis are essentially the same condition, and both can be treated with the same general goals and plan. As described in Chapter 6, these conditions generally have only mild S.H.A.R.P. (**s**welling, **h**eat, **a**symmetry or a loss of function, **r**edness, **p**ain) indicators and are most often brought to the therapist's attention while in the subacute stage of healing. Therefore, the focus of the massage is less on edema removal and more on reduction of excess muscle and fascial tension and proper healing and alignment of repair fibers.

■ COMMON FACTORS

In both chronic strain and sprain, there has been a proliferation of repair tissue into otherwise healthy areas, and athletes often develop functional adaptations that create complex syndromes of pain, muscle tension, and weakness. Therefore, a key treatment concept for these chronic conditions is that all restrictions that could be adding *stress* to the repetitive motion must be identified and addressed. This requires therapists to fully investigate the myofascial

BOX 13-1 MASSAGE TREATMENT PLAN FOR ACUTE ANKLE SPRAIN

Mechanism of injury: Forced inversion or eversion of the foot and ankle
Commonly seen in: All weight-bearing sports
Massage plan by stage

Acute Stage
Duration 15–20 minutes
1. Lymphatic facilitation: *after* R.I.C.E. (**r**est, **i**ce, **c**ompression, **e**levation) or intermittent compression when used.
   a. Open neck: 15–20 stationary circles at lateral neck + 15–20 stationary circles at terminus
   b. Breathing to empty cisterna chyli
   c. Inguinals: 15–20 stationary circles
   d. Anterior thigh: 10 long strokes
   e. Anterior leg: 10 long strokes
   f. Popliteal: 15–20 stationary circles
   g. Posterior leg: 10 long strokes
   h. Return to step 1 in reverse order. Finish with terminus; no lateral neck
Note: Athlete is taught the self-treatment opening neck protocol and exhale–crunch for home care. Generally, the ankle is supported throughout the acute stage with a brace and/or horseshoe pad and elastic bandage. The use of a short-stretch wrap designed specifically for the management of edema and an edema compression pad constitute a recommended alternative to this standard practice (Chapter 14).
2. Neuromuscular release: Posterior compartment of the leg only; thigh musculature if needed.

Subacute Stage
Duration 15–20 minutes
1. Continue lymphatic facilitation as in the acute stage with the following adjustments:

- Use only 5 exhale–crunches to empty cisterna chyli (step 1b).
- Skip step 1d.
- Step 1h begins the site-specific work with stationary circles as needed at edge of secondary edema. Direct the ankle edema *under the malleoli to the posterior watershed,* and move the edema of the *foot and anterior ankle to the anterior watershed* of the leg.
- Gradually, as edema is reduced, the site-specific work becomes more direct to the damaged ligament(s), and the bulk of the time is spent there (7–10 minutes).
2. Neuromuscular release: Add the lateral and anterior compartment muscles of the leg.
3. Begin massage with deep transverse friction. This should not occur until toward the end of the subacute stage when swelling is sufficiently reduced, and there is no discoloration of tissue over the damaged ligament(s). At this point, therapists may choose to end the session with ice or lymphatic facilitation, or both.

Maturation Stage
Duration approximately 15 minutes
1. Deep transverse friction according to formula in Chapter 9: Administered after any heat modality. When **cryokinetics** are used (Chapter 14), deep transverse friction should *precede* the ice and exercise.
2. Neuromuscular release and lymphatic facilitation as necessary. Be sure to investigate all major muscle groups in the lower extremity for trigger/tender points.

chains related to the injured structures and include a number of general and site-specific myofascial techniques, as well as thorough neuromuscular release in their treatments. A good deal of the treatment session is focused on tissue away from the site of the trauma. As with acute sprains and strains, the basic outline of treatment procedures is the same for all chronic conditions in the upper or lower extremity because the same myofascial chains are involved.

Each treatment plan is individualized according to that athlete's medical history, past injuries, and the demands of the sport and/or position. For example, two athletes with bicipital tendonitis will both be treated with thorough myofascial work in the full arm line. However, the athlete with a history of an elbow dislocation is likely to receive more site-specific work around the elbow than the athlete without such a history. In addition, if one of these athletes is a pitcher in baseball and the other a member of the rowing team, treatments vary according to the difference in the demands of their sport; that is, the superficial back and front lines are of more concern for the rower, and the spiral line plays a larger role for the pitcher.

When chronic strains and sprains have thick and matted scar tissue, or the condition is clearly in the maturation stage of healing, heat packs directly over this tissue may be necessary to soften the collagen and enhance the effectiveness of the myofascial techniques. However, it is recommended that

BOX 13-2 MASSAGE TREATMENT PLAN FOR ACUTE STRAIN OF SUPRASPINATUS

Mechanism of injury: Sudden ↑ intensity in shoulder *ab*duction

Common injury in: Weight lifting, rowing, baseball/softball

Massage plan by stage

Acute Stage
Duration 15–20 minutes
1. Lymphatic facilitation: *after* R.I.C.E. (**r**est, **i**ce, **c**ompression, **e**levation) or intermittent compression when used.
   a. Open neck: 15–20 stationary circles at lateral neck + 1520 stationary circles at terminus.
   b. Axillary catchment: 15–20 stationary circles.
   c. 20–25 Bilateral stationary circles over deltoid watershed (see Fig. 7-17).
   d. Repeat axilla and terminus.
Note: Athlete is taught the self-treatment opening neck protocol for home care, and the appropriate compression and support wraps are applied.
2. Neuromuscular release: Focus on neck, back, and chest musculature.

Subacute Stage
Duration 15–20 minutes
1. Continue lymphatic facilitation: Gradually, as edema is reduced and range of motion improves, *add site-*

specific stationary circles directly over the insertion of the supraspinatus as in step 1d of acute-stage treatment. At that point, the bulk of treatment time (8–10 minutes) is spent alternating between the site-specific stationary circles and clearing the axilla-deltoid. Finish as in acute phase.
2. Toward the end of the subacute stage, *begin massage with deep transverse friction, and end with lymphatic facilitation.*
3. Continue neuromuscular release as needed.

Maturation Stage
Duration approximately 15 minutes
1. Deep transverse friction over supraspinous (Fig. 9-8) according to formula in Chapter 9.
2. Neuromuscular release and lymphatic facilitation as necessary. Be sure to investigate levator scapulae, upper trapezius, infraspinatus, latissimus dorsi/teres major, and pectoralis major/minor for trigger/tender points.
3. Traditional massage to both arms and back if time allows. (This would extend the treatment time an additional 10–15 minutes).

the duration of this heat application is no more than 10 to 15 minutes. The hyperemia that occurs with a longer heat application can make the tissue feel too spongy under the therapist's hands, making landmarks and restrictions difficult to palpate. Moreover, the hyperemia may make it difficult to apply sufficient stretch to the connective tissue to actually break the cross-links and separate the fibers.

■ GOALS AND PLANS

The first treatment priority for chronic strains and sprains is to facilitate appropriate healing and fiber alignment at the site of the tissue damage. Second, muscles in spasm in the myofascial chain must be returned to normal tonus and any fibrous restrictions removed. Deep transverse friction over the affected tendon or ligament accomplishes the first goal, and the evaluation helps the therapist determine the most necessary and appropriate combination of other myofascial and neuromuscular techniques to achieve the second goal. Chronic strains and sprains are also characterized by a low-grade inflammatory response that causes dull pain during or

after activity, depending on severity. Therefore, lymphatic facilitation may be beneficial and should be considered as a standard follow-up to the deep transverse friction treatments.

The massage plan may begin with the direct work at the site of **lesion** or indirect work elsewhere in the myofascial chain. Several variables must be considered in making this choice. Generally, the first treatment priority should be to address the damaged tissue at the site of microtrauma. Therefore, it makes good sense to begin the treatment with site-specific work. However, the general work of reducing muscle tension and fascial restrictions in other areas may provide significant relief of pain and limitation in the affected tendon/ligament, making direct work less intense. Doing the indirect myofascial chain work first also allows therapists to apply hot or cold packs to the affected area in preparation for direct massage. Ultimately, the decision of beginning with direct or indirect work may be dictated by the amount of time available for the treatment massage. Limited time means that the first treatment priority must be addressed and the site-specific work should be done at the beginning of the session. All the necessary indirect work must then be addressed over time with successive treatment sessions.

From the Field

"From my experience as an athlete, coach, and sports massage therapist, I've found that the most important elements of athletic performance revolve around maintaining or improving muscle and joint flexibility, reducing general muscle soreness, and giving athletes lots of positive feedback. I combine several different forms of massage, mostly myofascial, neuromuscular, and Swedish massage techniques to help athletes maintain their desired activity level. Whether it is for general fitness, a weekend work-out, or an elite competition, my experiences and observations along with countless testimonials from the athletes make it clear that massage is one of the most beneficial and important therapies that athletes can invest in."

Sylvia Burns,
LMP, BS, MEd, and Clinical
Sports Massage Specialist
Roosevelt Exercise Training Center,
University of Washington Medical Center
Seattle, WA

Although it is essential that treatment plans for chronic conditions incorporate *both* myofascial techniques for reducing fascial restrictions and neuromuscular release to decrease muscle tension, it does not really matter which of these techniques is applied first in an area. Often the evaluation process may clarify whether the problem is more fascial or neuromuscular in nature, and so that technique is then used first. If the evaluation does not point to one type of restriction over the other, it may be helpful to first use a general neuromuscular technique such as contract–relax to help distinguish the amount of fascial restriction from the neuromuscular tension. For example, if passive range of motion improves dramatically with a contract–relax technique, the amount of fascial restriction is limited because reducing the neuromuscular tension has improved the range of motion. Site-specific myofascial techniques such as reverse-J, and S stroke can be used to relieve restrictions at any point along the myofascial chain as well as directly over the involved structure. When direct work over the lesion and the indirect work throughout the myofascial chain are completed, the treatment can be finished with general Swedish massage if time allows. Finishing with the soothing and gentler Swedish provides the athlete with a sense of reconnection to the whole body with all its healthy parts, deemphasizing the injured area.

Boxes 13-3 and 13-4 show treatment plans for common tendonitis and chronic strain conditions. Figure 13-2 illustrates a specific lymphatic facilitation technique for intra-articular edema or any traumatic edema in and around the knee joint.

Hematomas and Acute Bursitis

Both severe hematomas and acute bursitis are compression traumas of the soft tissue that result in extreme hemorrhage, inflammation, pain, muscle spasm, and disability for the athlete. Perhaps the most common of these are **hip and shoulder pointers**, which are severe hematomas that occur

CASE STUDY 13-2

A 21-year-old male swimmer had been in a shoulder immobilizer for 6 weeks after a SLAP (superior labral anteroposterior) lesion repair. Approximately 4 to 5 weeks into the rehabilitation program, the therapist encountered a peculiar finding; the patient's passive range of motion with external rotation and *ab*duction caused posterior shoulder pain, but there was no restricted end-feel in either of the movements. A little research led the therapist to believe that the pain might be associated with a trigger point in the subscapularis muscle. A thorough soft tissue evaluation confirmed multiple myofascial trigger points in the muscle that accurately reproduced the athlete's pain when palpated. Ten minutes of myofascial and neuromuscular therapy focused on trigger point techniques relieved the pain and increased the athlete's external rotation by 15 degrees (Fig. 13-1; Box 13-3). The increased pain-free range of motion brought the athlete's external rotation to 60 degrees, and the appropriate capsular end-feel could now be assessed to guide the rehabilitation process.

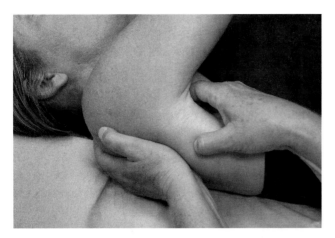

FIGURE 13-1 Subscapularis release. In this position, both neuromuscular and myofascial techniques can be used.

as a result of a sharp blow over the unprotected iliac crest or greater trochanter (hip pointer) and the acromiodeltoid area (shoulder pointer). The mechanism of injury for hip and shoulder pointers is most often a collision or fall that occurs in sports such as soccer, field hockey, rugby, football, basketball, and baseball/softball when the participants do not wear specific padding over these bony prominences. Another compression injury, commonly called a **charley horse**, is a severe hematoma and muscle spasm caused by a sharp blow to the quadriceps or occasionally the hamstrings. This injury is most debilitating when the blow is delivered to the muscle while it is contracted, as when a basketball player is crouched for a rebound and another athlete's knee bangs into their thigh.

Acute bursitis is the sudden inflammation of a bursa caused by either a sudden sharp blow or a sudden increase

---

BOX 13-3 MASSAGE TREATMENT PLAN FOR CHRONIC ROTATOR CUFF STRAIN: SUBSCAPULARIS

Mechanism of injury: Repetitive stressful throwing motion
Commonly seen in: Baseball/softball, racket sports, rowing, swimming, weight lifting
Massage plan by stage

Acute Stage
Chronic injuries rarely present with acute-stage signs and symptoms. However, some heat and very light swelling may be found in the anterior shoulder with this chronic rotator cuff strain. In this case, follow the acute-stage treatment plan outlined previously for an acute strain of the supraspinatus.

Subacute Stage
Duration 15–20 minutes
1. Locate and release any neuromuscular points with specific focus on the following:
   - Subscapularis (see Fig. 13-1) and infraspinatus–teres minor
   - Biceps and triceps brachii
   - Pectoralis major and minor
   - Levator scapulae and upper trapezius
   - Middle trapezius/rhomboids
   - Sternocostal points
2. Deep transverse friction to the subscapularis insertion (see Fig. 9-7) according to formula in Chapter 9.
   - Duration from 1 to 5 minutes

Maturation Stage
Duration 15–20 minutes
1. Continue deep transverse friction according to formula in Chapter 9.

- May be preceded by heat therapy.
- Actual deep transverse friction over the insertion should be approximately 5–7 minutes in duration at this point.
2. Broad plane and site-specific myofascial techniques for full chain; these may include:
   - Anterior neck broad plane pin-and-stretch
   - Anterior shoulder broad plane pin-and-stretch
   - Braced-fingers friction over deltopectoral junction
   - Site-specific pin-and-stretch through the fascial septa of biceps and triceps brachii
   - Braced-thumb friction over the long head of the triceps tendon
   - Muscle rolling of biceps and triceps brachii, sternocleidomastoid, and the anterior and posterior muscles of axilla
3. Traditional massage to arms, back, and chest if time allows (additional 10–15 minutes). Some neuromuscular release (detailed in step 1 of the subacute stage) may be incorporated here rather than being a separate step. The active-assistive techniques should include the following:
   - Deltoid
   - Biceps and triceps brachii
   - Pectoralis major

BOX 13-4 MASSAGE TREATMENT PLAN FOR PATELLAR TENDONITIS (PATELLOFEMORAL SYNDROMES)

Mechanism of injury: Repetitive stressful knee flexion and extension; predisposing factors: excessive Q-angle, muscle weakness, and/or imbalance in the quadriceps
Commonly seen in: Running and jumping sports
Massage plan by stage

Acute Stage
Chronic injuries rarely present with acute-stage signs and symptoms. However, some heat and very light (palpable only) swelling may be found in the anterior knee. In this case, follow the acute-stage treatment plan outlined previously. An overhand/underhand position for lymphatic facilitation at the knee joint is used to address swelling/inflammation in the patellar tendon (see Fig. 13-2).

Subacute and Maturation Stage
Duration 15–20 minutes
1. Locate and release any neuromuscular points with specific focus on the following:
   - Hamstrings and quadriceps
   - Gluteals and hip flexors

- *Adductors*
- Iliotibial band
2. Broad plane and site-specific myofascial work for lower extremity to include the following:
   - Skin rolling to lumbosacral aponeurosis, iliotibial band, and all three compartments of the leg. If the rolling is easy and without restriction, move on to next area.
   - Braced-fingers friction around greater trochanter to insertions of iliotibial band and hamstrings, common origin of hamstrings, and over the hip flexor tendons and inguinal ligament.
   - Site-specific frictions to retinacula of the knee.
   - Muscle rolling to iliotibial band, gastrocnemius, and lateral compartment of the leg.
3. Deep transverse friction to the patellar tendon (see Fig. 9-10) according to formula in Chapter 9.
4. Traditional massage of full lower extremity (include active-assistive releases) and back if time allows. (This would extend the treatment time an additional 10–15 minutes.)

in the intensity of compression stress over the bursa by the tendon/ligament it is protecting. If the mechanism of injury is not a sudden sharp blow, it must be presumed that the increased muscle and fascial tension over the bursa is related to a sudden change in the normal movement demands on that area. It occurs most often in the bursae around the elbows and knees and occasionally in the trochanteric bursa because these are the most vulnerable to external compression trauma. If a sufficient amount of force is delivered, the

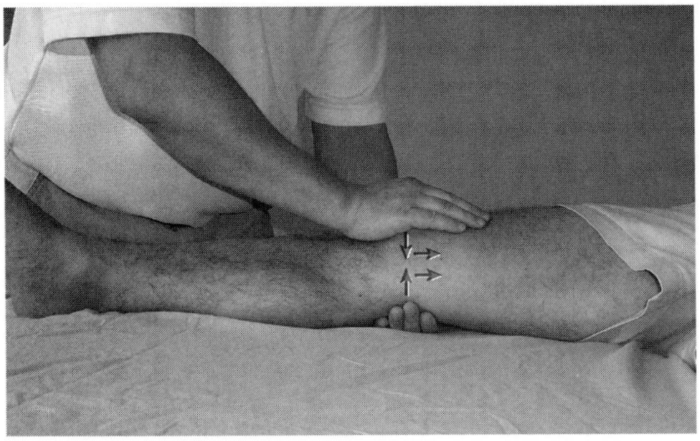

FIGURE 13-2 With anterior or intracapsular swelling in the knee, this overhand and underhand position for lymphatic stationary circles is a very effective method of edema removal.

bursa can rupture, which is immediately apparent from the large pouch of fluid spilled into the area.

■ COMMON FACTORS

Both hematomas and an acute bursitis are characterized by extreme swelling, pain, and muscle spasm, which makes the treatment goals for both very similar to that for acute sprains/strains. Other common factors are that these conditions are localized to a specific area or structure and have a sudden onset, making their progression through the healing cycle similar and easy to monitor. The major distinction between the two conditions is that bursae are encapsulated structures and the swelling is exacerbated by increased fluid production from the synovial lining of the bursa. Therefore, it is not easily reabsorbed by either the cardiovascular or lymphatic system, making the resolution of the swelling in acute bursitis much slower. Regardless of this difficulty, treatment of both acute bursitis and severe hematomas is enhanced by the addition of lymphatic facilitation. In addition, the cause of the tension stress irritating the bursa must be determined and changed for complete resolution of acute bursitis. To do this, the athlete's equipment, exercise/ training programs, work and leisure activities all must be evaluated and adjusted as necessary.

It is important to note that mismanagement of severe hematomas may lead to a separate pathology known as **myositis ossificans** (Fig. 13-3). In this condition, exacerbation of the original hematoma—either from re-injury or overly aggressive attempts at edema removal—causes more hemorrhage, which interferes with the resorption of the primary edema. Eventually, the body simply calcifies the exudate as a speedy way to repair the damaged tissue. This bone deposit in the middle of a muscle can irritate the surrounding tissue with every movement and can be extremely sensitive to pressure.

■ GOALS AND PLAN

The priority treatment massage goal for both hematomas and acute bursitis is to reduce swelling and pain and to protect the area from further trauma. The combination of general massage proximal to the swelling followed by the appropriate lymphatic facilitation sequence is the most effective treatment massage plan for the acute stage (Boxes 13-5 and 13-6). The muscle spasms and trigger/tender points in the surrounding muscle groups are definitely a secondary priority and should not be addressed with neuromuscular release until the pain and swelling of the acute stage have subsided. Myofascial techniques, especially the site-specific strokes, are contraindicated until the maturation stage in these two conditions because of the fragile nature of the edematous tissue. Therapists are reminded that lymphatic facilitation work directly at the site of edema begins at the periphery of the secondary edema, as described in Chapter 7.

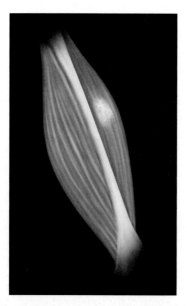

FIGURE 13-3 Myositis ossificans, calcium deposits formed within a muscle, can occur when a severe hematoma is re-aggravated and the healing process disrupted.

From the Field

"In my opinion, therapeutic massage is a vital component of training for optimal athletic performance. Event massage (on-site preparation for and recovery from athletic performance) and clinical sport massage (for restoration and maintenance of healthy muscle function) serve to enhance the physical and mental preparation of athletes at all levels of participation. At the elite levels of performance such as professional athletics, or with world class amateur and collegiate athletes, a sports medicine team would be incomplete without a licensed and skilled sports massage therapist."

Robyn Wilson, LMT, ATC

President, University Sports Massage, Inc
Performance Consultant (Massage Therapy),
University of Florida Athletic Association

Neurovascular Compression or Tension Syndromes

Several neurovascular compression–tension syndromes can commonly develop in active people. In each of these syndromes, muscle spasm and/or fascial restrictions lead to tension, causing strain or compression of a specific nerve and/or blood vessel (Boxes 13-7 and 13-8). The athlete's complaint is of an aching and/or tingling pain that often radiates into distal body regions. Chapter 12 details the distinguishing signs and symptoms of these syndromes (see Table 12-5) and describes some special tests that should be used in the evaluation of these complaints.

■ COMMON FACTORS

Neurovascular compression–tension syndromes are categorized as chronic conditions, but these pathologies rarely have tissue tearing or stretching. Therefore, they do not

BOX 13-5 MASSAGE TREATMENT PLAN FOR HIP POINTER

Mechanism: Sharp blow to unprotected iliac crest and/or greater trochanter
Commonly seen in: Soccer, volleyball, rugby, football, field hockey, basketball, baseball/softball
Massage plan by stage

Acute Stage
Duration 20–25 minutes
1. Lymphatic facilitation full body on affected side. These steps are depicted in Figure 7-16.
   a. Open the neck with 15–20 stationary circles to lateral neck and terminus.
   b. Empty axilla with 15–20 stationary circles.
   c. Clear the lymphotomes on the torso from the umbilical watershed to the axilla with as many long strokes as needed. *Note:* Severe edema and ecchymosis may require edema to be moved across the sagittal watershed to flow into the opposite axilla and/or inguinal catchments.
   d. Empty cisterna chyli and iliac trunks: 5 resisted breaths at cisterna → 5 at right iliac trunk → 5 at cisterna → 5 at left iliac trunk → 5 at cisterna (substitute 5 exhale–crunches if time is a factor).
   e. Empty inguinals with 15–20 stationary circles.
   f. Repeat 5 resisted breaths over cisterna chyli.
   g. Repeat 15–20 stationary circles over inguinals.
   h. Finish by repeating c, then b, then a.
Note: Neuromuscular and myofascial techniques are contraindicated in the acute stage with this type of severe hematoma because of the fragile nature of the edematous tissue.

Subacute Stage
Duration 20–25 minutes
1. Repeat acute-stage lymphatic facilitation through step e. Then add:
   a. Site-specific edema removal at periphery of secondary edema with stationary circles as needed (20–30 strokes).
   b. Empty the inguinals and cisterna again.
   c. Repeat steps c through a in reverse order.
Note: The edema-specific work in step 1 should be repeated at several points along the periphery of the edema, especially if the bruising and swelling extend over a watershed. For efficient edema removal of a bruise that begins at the greater trochanter and extends up the athlete's side to the mid-lateral rib cage, superficial lymph flow must be directed bilaterally toward both the affected and unaffected axilla and the inguinal catchments, as well as across the sagittal, umbilical, and/or inguinal watershed lines.

Maturation Stage
Duration 20–25 minutes
1. Continue the lymphatic facilitation as outlined in the subacute stage.
2. Relieve and release trigger and tender points in surrounding musculature with the appropriate neuromuscular release technique.

BOX 13-6 MASSAGE TREATMENT PLAN FOR ACUTE SUBACROMIAL BURSITIS

Mechanism: Sudden increase of intensity and/or duration of shoulder motion, or a change in biomechanics of the motion (see Fig. 12-7)
Commonly seen in: Any sport or activity with overhead arm motion, such as baseball, tennis, swimming
Massage plan by stage

Acute Stage
Duration 10–15 minutes, using the same treatment plan as outlined previously for treatment of an acute strain of the supraspinatus

Subacute Stage
Duration 15 minutes
1. Continue lymphatic facilitation: Gradually, as edema is reduced and range of motion improves, *add site-specific stationary circles* at the periphery of the swelling.
2. Continue neuromuscular release as needed with focus on rotator cuff, pectoralis major and minor, latissimus dorsi and teres major, and biceps brachii.

Maturation Stage
Duration approximately 15 minutes
1. Continue neuromuscular release and lymphatic facilitation as necessary.
2. Traditional massage to arms, chest-neck, and back as time allows. Some neuromuscular release (detailed in step 2 of the subacute stage) may be incorporated here rather than being a separate step.

have a specific healing cycle and do not present with the standard signs and symptoms such as swelling, heat, discoloration, and asymmetry. The specific pathology in these conditions is generally a combination of muscle spasms, fascial tension, and anatomic anomalies such as cervical ribs that compress or overstretch specific nerves and/or blood vessels. Compression of the neurovascular bundle between muscles in spasm, such as compression of the brachial plexus between the middle and anterior scalenes, is a *direct* compression. Muscle spasms and fascial restrictions that create excessive tension and compress or pull on the nerve/blood vessel when the body part is in a particu-

---

BOX 13-7 MASSAGE TREATMENT PLAN FOR PIRIFORMIS SYNDROME/SCIATICA

Mechanism of injury: No clear mechanism; hypertonicity and/or spasms of the piriformis muscle compress the sciatic nerve

Commonly seen in: Any athlete; most common predisposing factors are postural or functional (sport-specific) adaptation of excessive hip rotation—either internal or external

Massage plan

1. Locate and release any neuromuscular points. At a minimum, the trigger/tender points in the following muscles must be addressed:
   - Piriformis; gluteus medius, minimus, and maximus; and the sacral junctions
   - Hamstrings and *add*uctors
   - Iliotibial band and tensor fasciae latae
2. Broad plane and site-specific myofascial work for the full lower extremity. At a minimum, include these myofascial techniques:

- Skin rolling to lumbosacral aponeurosis and iliotibial band if possible.
- Linear shift to lumbosacral aponeurosis, iliotibial band, and hamstrings.
- Braced-fingers friction around greater trochanter and common origin of hamstrings and over the hip flexor tendons and inguinal ligament.

3. Traditional massage to legs and back. The traditional massage should include the following:
   - Linear friction through the fascial septa of the posterior thigh
   - Contract–relax neuromuscular release as needed (only needed if tension points remain from step 1)
   - Active-assistive release of hamstrings and quadriceps
   - Hip lift–compress and tracing of the ilium

BOX 13-8 MASSAGE TREATMENT PLAN FOR THORACIC OUTLET SYNDROME

Mechanism of injury: Chronic strain of neck and/or shoulder; often a secondary pathology that develops after a fractured clavicle, whiplash, or shoulder dislocation

Commonly seen in: Collision/impact sports such as football, hockey, wrestling, soccer, and throwing sports

Massage plan

Duration 20–30 minutes

1. Broad plane and site-specific myofascial release that includes the following:
   - Skin rolling from lumbosacral aponeurosis up paraspinals to neck
   - Broad plane pin-and-stretch to anterior shoulder and neck
   - General friction and site-specific pin-and-stretch to scalenes
   - Lift and unwind pectoralis major
   - Muscle rolling to upper trapezius and levator, pectoralis muscles, posterior neck, and latissimus-teres major junction

2. Locate and release any neuromuscular points. Some points may be released in conjunction with the myofascial work in step 1, and others may be included in the traditional massage outlined in step 3. Specific focus should be given to the following:
   - Sternocleidomastoid and scalenes
   - Pectoralis minor and subclavius
   - Levator scapulae and upper trapezius
   - Middle trapezius/rhomboids and sternocostal points

3. Traditional massage to arms, chest, neck, and back which should include neuromuscular release for any remaining trigger/tender points and active-assistive release of:
   - scalenes (Fig. 13-4A, B)
   - deltoid
   - pectoralis major (see Fig. 11-18; Fig. 13-5A and B)

lar position, are considered *indirect*. A good example of an indirect compression–tension syndrome is hypertonicity of the pectoralis minor and subclavius, compressing and pulling the brachial plexus and/or subclavian artery against the first two pair of ribs. In both direct and indirect compression–tension syndromes, therapists must address the site of compression, as well as the full myofascial chain.

GOALS AND PLAN

The treatment priority for neurovascular compression–tension syndromes is to reduce muscle tension and fascial restrictions that are irritating the neurovascular bundle. The treatment plan is heavy on neuromuscular and myofascial techniques, which should then be followed by traditional massage to help reduce the general ischemic condition of the tissue. In some neurovascular compression cases, a significant part of the compression is due to low-grade inflammation and edema. For example, light to moderate levels of edema can occur around the finger flexor tendons in severe cases of carpal tunnel syndrome (Fig. 13-6; Box 13-9). In chronic compartment syndromes, there is typically as much edema as there is muscle tension causing the compression. In these cases, edema removal via lymphatic facilitation is an important element of the treatment plan; perhaps as important as reduction of muscular tension and fascial restrictions.

Miscellaneous: Stitches and Cricks

Many athletes have regularly occurring problems that are not thought of as specific injuries because no spe-

cific tissue damage occurs. Two common examples are waking up with a "crick in the neck," or getting a "stitch in the side" while running. Even though no tissue has been traumatized and no clear cause has ever been described for either of these conditions, an athlete's ability to perform can be significantly reduced by either of these. Both conditions are of an acute nature without the traditional S.H.A.R.P. signs and symptoms of injury, and they both go away in a few hours or days even if nothing is done. Because athletes cannot wait for things to go away, therapists must be able to intervene, and soft tissue manipulation is the key to relief of both of these conditions.

There are several theories on what causes a stitch in the side, including spasms of the intercostals and/or diaphragm, fascial restrictions, indigestion or gas, and any combination of these. For relief of the stitch, a myofascial lift over the full abdomen and lower thoracic tissue is generally the most successful method of relief (Fig. 13-7) and may be all that is required. Therapists should begin the lift directly over the affected area first and proceed through the entire region. Be sure to lift from the bottom portion of the role of tissue to avoid a pinching pain. Therapist and athlete should "feel" a release of the fascia, and, depending on how severe the restriction is, a clear click or pop may also be heard. If there is no sense of release with this lift, several additional steps can be used in any sequence: (1) horizontal plane diaphragm release (see Fig. 9-23), (2) tracing the diaphragm (see Fig. 11-19), or (3) positional release for intercostals tender points (Fig. 13-8).

The muscle spasm that is called "crick in the neck" is most likely due to a false stretch reflex signal from the muscle spindle related to gamma gain. During sleep, we rarely are able to keep all the neck muscles in neutral tension, leading to gamma gain in those that are held in shortened

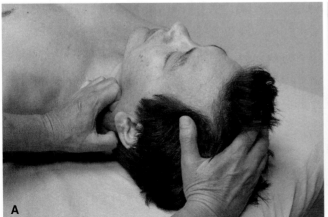
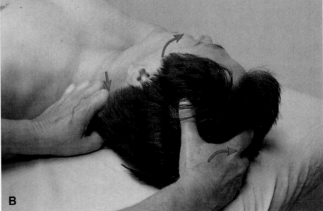

FIGURE 13-4 Active release of the sternocleidomastoid and scalenes. (A) Begin by hooking the anterior edge of the sternocleidomastoid muscle with your knuckles and applying a light downward pressure. **(B)** While maintaining this downward tension in the tissue, assist the athlete in a slow rotation of the head to the opposite side.

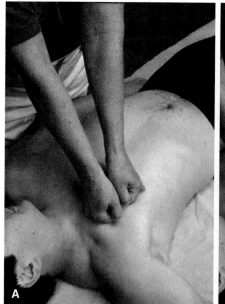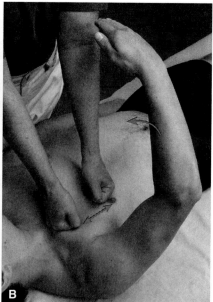

FIGURE 13-5 Active-assistive broadening. Another method of active-assistive broadening for the pectoralis major uses two hands to stroking across the fibers as the athlete carries out a slow horizontal adduction of the shoulder.

positions. When we toss and turn or get startled awake by the alarm, the sudden lengthening of these muscles causes protective spasms that lock the posterior-lateral muscles into tensile stressed and painful positions. Therefore, relief can generally be accomplished through positional release and general massage. Often, this condition has been exacerbated by the athlete's repeated attempts to stretch his or her stiff neck, meaning that the general massage may be the most appropriate first step. The relaxation from general massage may be needed before specific treatment is applied, and the positional release is easily incorporated into the

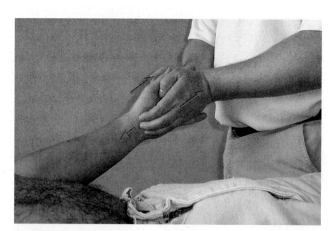

FIGURE 13-6 Lymphatic facilitation stroke for carpal tunnel syndrome. A specific lymphatic facilitation stroke helps reduce compression and irritation in the carpal tunnel. Squeeze the athlete's hand between both of yours so the fingertips rest over the joint line and lean back to apply slight traction to the wrist. Opening the joint with the traction improves the effectiveness of the stationary circles applied bilaterally with the fingertips.

neck, back, and chest massage. Figure 13-9 depicts tender point/positional release for the posterior neck, and therapists must not forget to find and release the offending spasms and tender points in the anterior and lateral muscles around the neck.

Treatment and Rehabilitation: Two Different Processes

In addition to matching the choice of massage techniques to the physiology of healing, therapists must also have a clear understanding of the overall treatment and rehabilitation goals used in sports medicine. Without this overview of the entire process, it is difficult to work well with and support the other members of the sports health care team, and athletes may get mixed information that can negatively affect their compliance with the treatment plans. There are several different ways to state the different phases of injury treatment and rehabilitation, but the two overriding concepts are to first support tissue healing and repair, or **treatment**, and then to focus on return of function, or **rehabilitation**. All the preceding examples of massage plans are based on matching the physiologic effects of the massage technique to the stage of healing to facilitate and enhance the process, which makes them *treatment* plans. Just like the healing cycle, rehabilitation (the return to full function) is an ongoing and overlapping process that cannot truly be separated from healing. However, by dividing rehabilitation into stages or phases, both athletes and ther-

BOX 13-9 MASSAGE TREATMENT PLAN FOR CARPAL TUNNEL SYNDROME

Mechanism of injury: Repetitive stressful wrist and finger flexion or secondary pathology with acute wrist sprain or strain

Commonly seen in: Racket and implement sports such as tennis, javelin, and shot-put or sports such as gymnastics that require acute impact and chronic strain on the wrists

Massage plan

Duration 20–30 minutes

1. Broad plane and site-specific myofascial release that includes the following:
   - Skin rolling to anterior and posterior forearm.
   - Site-specific pin-and-stretch to anterior and posterior forearm.
   - Muscle rolling to the flexor (medial) and extensor (lateral) muscle groups at the elbow, biceps and triceps brachii, and pectoralis major/minor.

   - Site-specific friction (double-thumb or braced-fingers) to broaden the flexor retinaculi and transverse carpal ligament. If swelling is evident or questionable, this direct friction is *contraindicated*.
2. Locate and release any neuromuscular points. Some points may be released in conjunction with the myofascial work in step 1.
   - Subscapularis and pectoralis minor
   - Wrist and finger flexors (anterior forearm)
   - Wrist and finger extensors (posterior forearm)
   - Sternocostal points
   - Thenar and hypothenar eminence
3. Finish with lymphatic facilitation for upper extremity that includes the special carpal tunnel stroke depicted in Figure 13-6 and, if time allows, traditional massage to arms, chest, neck, and back that includes active-assistive releases to anterior and posterior forearm.

apists have a better understanding of the intermediate steps that need to be taken to achieve the return to full function. Short-term goals can be established, and progress more easily measured by breaking the process into a few stages. The most generic representation of the sequence of rehabilitation priorities is:

1. Range of motion
2. Strength
3. Coordination
4. Endurance

As is true for the entire process, there is much overlap between each of these stages. Each stage has its own levels

of progression, and different members of the sports health care team make their primary contributions in different stages. Massage therapists play a primary role in the first step in rehabilitation—healing and returning pain-free range of motion—and continue to focus on this while other members of the health care team carry out the remaining stages of rehabilitation. Of course, as range of motion

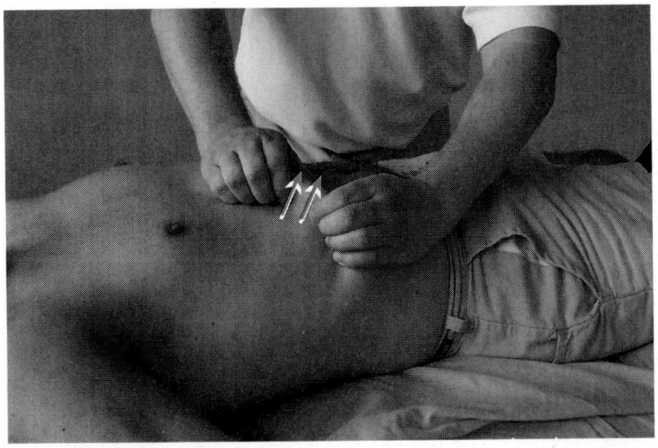

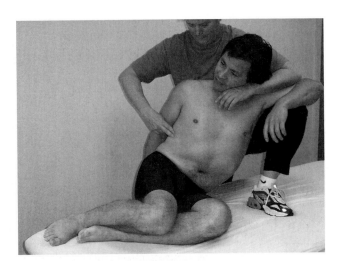

FIGURE 13-8 Positional release for tender points in the ribs/intercostals. The athlete is supported with the arm on the opposite side of the point draped over the therapist's knee/thigh. As the athlete leans away from the point, the therapist applies slight posterior rotation of the torso and full rotation of the head toward the side with the point.

FIGURE 13-7 A firm lift of the abdominal fascia can be very effective at relieving a stitch in the side.

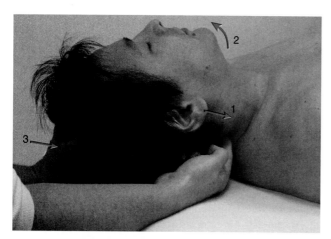

FIGURE 13-9 Positional release for tender points in the deep paraspinal muscles of the neck (transverse–spinalis group) requires three different maneuvers: (1) lateral flexion of the head toward the point, (2) slight rotation of the head/neck to the opposite side, and (3) compression to the cervical spine on the exhale of a deep breath to fully shorten the muscles. The therapist must maintain a monitoring pressure over the point, feel for tissue softening with each movement, and make sure that the chin is still in relative alignment with the sternum before adding the compression.

exercises progress from passive to active, strength and coordination are also being developed to a small degree. However, massage therapists should not consider returning to full strength, coordination, or endurance as their rehabilitation goals.

SUMMARY

- It is important to know what specific tissue changes you hope to accomplish (treatment goals) and which massage techniques are best at doing that (treatment plan) before beginning the massage.
- In general, acute-onset injuries should be treated more frequently, especially in the acute and subacute stages, than chronic-onset conditions.
- The treatment goals for each stage of the healing cycle can be briefly summarized as follows: acute—stabilize and control; subacute—enhance and improve; maturation—prevent adhesions and return to full function.
- In the acute stage of healing, the most important therapeutic massage technique is lymphatic facilitation. Neuromuscular and myofascial techniques become more important during the late subacute and maturation stages.
- Chronic injuries generally present in the subacute and/or maturation stages, making the myofascial and neuromuscular techniques more appropriate choices for soft tissue treatments.
- When both ice and lymphatic facilitation are used to help control swelling, ice should precede the lymphatic techniques.
- Regardless of the location, all sprains and strains have the same treatment goals and follow the same basic plan. There are also common goals and basic treatment plans between chronic strains and tendonitis, severe hematoma and bursitis, and all neurovascular compression–tension syndromes (Table 13-3).

TABLE 13-3	Treatment Massage Priorities and Techniques for Common Injury Categories	
Injury/Condition	**Treatment Massage Priorities**	**Massage Techniques**
Acute sprains and strains	1. Improve edema uptake and lymph flow 2. Facilitate proper fiber alignment in repair tissue	1. Lymphatic facilitation 2. Deep transverse friction in subacute and maturation stages
Chronic strains and sprains	1. Facilitate proper fiber alignment in repair tissue 2. ↓ Fibrous adhesions and neuromuscular restrictions in full myofascial chain	1. Deep transverse friction over site of lesion 2. Myofascial and neuromuscular release in full myofascial chain 3. Follow deep transverse friction and myofascial release with lymphatic facilitation
Hematoma and acute bursitis	1. Improve edema uptake and lymph flow 2. ↓ Secondary muscle spasms	1. Lymphatic facilitation 2. Neuromuscular release in subacute and maturation stages
Neurovascular compression–tension syndromes	1. ↓ Muscle spasm over compressed nerve/blood vessel 2. ↓ Fibrous adhesions in full myofascial chain	1. Neuromuscular and myofascial release over site and full myofascial chain

Review Questions

SHORT ANSWERS

1. What are the two most unique massage components of treatment massage?

2. List the primary treatment goals for any acute injury in the subacute stage of healing.

3. Describe the recommended treatment frequency and duration ratios for acute and chronic injuries.

4. Describe the appropriate use of neuromuscular techniques during the acute stage of healing.

5. Define myositis ossificans, and explain how the condition develops.

MULTIPLE CHOICE

6. Which combination of treatment massage techniques is most appropriate for chronic strain syndromes?
   a. Lymphatic facilitation and trigger point
   b. Deep transverse friction and broad myofascial release
   c. Contract–relax and positional release
   d. Linear shift and lymphatic facilitation

7. What is the treatment priority for the acute stage of a hip pointer?
   a. Reduce muscle tension throughout the chain.
   b. Increase circulation.
   c. Improve edema uptake.
   d. Reduce myofascial restrictions throughout the chain.

8. At what stage of healing would it be appropriate to first use the stationary circles of lymphatic facilitation directly at the site of edema?
   a. Acute
   b. Subacute
   c. Maturation
   d. Never directly at the site of edema

9. Although acute tendonitis and acute bursitis are treated with a similar treatment plan, which stroke is contraindicated for the bursitis, even in the later stages of healing?
   a. Trigger point release
   b. Lymphatic stationary circles
   c. Linear shift in the myofascial chain
   d. Deep transverse friction

10. Lymphatic facilitation should direct swelling associated with an acute rotator cuff strain toward the axillary catchment and _____.
    a. over the acromion and clavicular watershed to the terminus.
    b. across the umbilical watershed to the inguinal catchment.
    c. down to the cubital catchment via medial arm watershed.
    d. across the anterior sagittal watershed to the opposite axilla.

11. The full myofascial chain releases are most necessary in which of these injury categories?
    a. All injuries in the subacute stage
    b. Acute sprains and strains
    c. Neurovascular compression syndromes
    d. Severe hematoma

12. Massage treatment sessions for acute injuries should have a _____ frequency and a _____ duration.
    a. high and short
    b. short and high
    c. high and long
    d. short and long

13. When neuromuscular release is used in the acute-stage treatment plan, it should be applied in _____.
    a. the injured muscle
    b. antagonists and synergists
    c. in the area of swelling
    d. only to muscles that are distal to the site of injury

14. What is the suggested minimum amount of time for treatment of an acute injury?
    a. 5 minutes
    b. 20 minutes
    c. 10 minutes
    d. 30 minutes

15. What is the suggested minimum amount of time for treatment of a chronic injury?
    a. 5 minutes
    b. 20 minutes
    c. 10 minutes
    d. 30 minutes

16. What is the recommended duration of heat application over a deeply matted scar before site-specific friction?
    a. 5–7 minutes
    b. 10–15 minutes
    c. 15–20 minutes
    d. 20–30 minutes

17. What is the treatment priority in syndromes such as sciatica?
    a. Decrease tension and restrictions.
    b. decrease inflammation and swelling.
    c. Increase circulation and range of motion.
    d. Increase strength and endurance.

18. In thoracic outlet syndrome, what muscles are considered priorities for treatment?
    a. Iliopsoas, piriformis, quadratus lumborum
    b. Sternocleidomastoid, sternalis, pectoralis major
    c. Scalenes, pectoralis minor, subclavius
    d. Serratus anterior, levator scapulae, rhomboids

19. In carpal tunnel syndrome, what muscles are considered priorities for treatment?
    a. Pectoralis major and minor
    b. Latissimus dorsi and teres major
    c. Wrist and elbow extensors
    d. Finger and wrist flexors

20. What does it indicate when a contract–relax technique does *not* create any improvement in the restricted movement?
    a. There are probably tender points that need to be released.
    b. The restricted range of motion may be from fascia or joint capsule.
    c. Reciprocal inhibition must be used to release the antagonist.
    d. The muscle is in contracture and cannot be released.

SUGGESTED READING

1. Houglum PA. Concepts in rehabilitation of patellofemoral pain syndrome. Athletic Therapy Today 2004;9(3):66–71.
2. Simons DG, Travell JG, Simons LS. Myofascial Pain and Dysfunction: The Trigger Point Manual, 2nd ed. vol. 1: Upper Half of Body. Philadelphia: Lippincott Williams & Wilkins, 1999.
3. Arnheim DD, Prentice WE. Principles of Athletic Training, 8th ed. St. Louis: Mosby, 1993.
4. Hunter-Griffin LY, Chairman of editorial board. Athletic Training and Sports Medicine, 2nd ed. Park Ridge, IL: American Academy of Orthopaedic Surgeons, 1991.
5. Rattray F, Ludwig L. Clinical massage therapy: Understanding, assessing and treating over 70 conditions. Toronto; Talus Inc, 2000.
6. Hendrickson T. Orthopedic Massage. Baltimore: Lippincott Williams & Wilkins, 2002.
7. Cook JL et al. Overuse tendinosis, not tendonitis. Part 2: Applying the new approach to patellar tendinopathy. The Physician and Sports Medicine 2000;28:31.
8. Gazzillo LM, Middlemas DA. Therapeutic massage techniques for three common injuries. Athletic Therapy Today 2001;6(3):5–9.
9. Prentice WE. Therapeutic Modalities for Physical Therapists, 2nd ed. New York: McGraw-Hill, 2002.

Common Therapeutic Modalities in Sports Health Care

OBJECTIVES

After completing this chapter, the reader will be able to:

- Define and distinguish between the terms hydrotherapy, thermotherapy, cryotherapy, and contrast therapy.
- Explain the physiologic effects of heat and cold applications.
- Name several methods of heat and cold applications, and explain the advantages, disadvantages, and common use for each.
- Name the indications and contraindications for various heat and cold applications.
- Compare and contrast standard elastic wraps with short-stretch wraps used for edema control.
- Understand how to integrate therapeutic massage with several other common sports health care modalities.

Each time therapeutic massage is added to a treatment protocol, therapists must make decisions about how to integrate the soft tissue techniques with all of the other elements in the athlete's care without disrupting the healing, overworking the tissue, or extending the total treatment time to an unreasonable level. Although each situation must be evaluated when it comes along, a few simple guidelines can help direct this decision making. First, therapists must recognize what modalities fall under their specific scope of practice according to their credentials. In most states, only manual range-of-motion exercises and perhaps hydrotherapy are within the scope of practice for a massage therapist. Second, a general understanding of several common modalities used within sports health care helps therapists make well-informed decisions about how to integrate therapeutic massage with these modalities. For example, both ice and lymphatic facilitation are used to help reduce traumatic edema. However, because cold decreases lymph flow, it is important to use ice before lymphatic facilitation to gain the full benefit of both modalities. When all members of the health care team understand the basic indications, contraindications, and effects of all modalities being used, athletes are more likely to receive the comprehensive and well coordinated treatment needed to return them to full activity as soon as possible.

Hydrotherapy

Hydrotherapy is the use of water in any form—fluid, solid, or vapor—for therapeutic purposes. This is a very broad definition that brings several different modalities such as whirlpools, steam baths, and ice massage under one umbrella even though some hydrotherapies are cold applications and others are heat. There are two general schools of thought regarding hydrotherapy. The orthopedic perspective is directed toward supporting the healing cycle, whereas the naturopathic viewpoint is more focused on stimulating body-wide systemic functions. Because therapeutic massage in athletics has the main goal of supporting the healing cycle, it seems more appropriate to discuss hydrotherapy from the orthopedic perspective.

Therapists must keep in mind that all forms of hydrotherapy—whether hot or cold applications—have some cautions and contraindications that are generally the same as for classic massage[1-6]:

- Never use hydrotherapy over open wounds or rashes.
- Never use hydrotherapy in individuals with malignancy, lymphedema, or undiagnosed conditions.

- Never use hydrotherapy when there is a possibility of internal hemorrhage.
- Use great caution with all hydrotherapy during pregnancy. Only small local applications are advised to avoid any possibility of exposing the fetus to extreme temperatures.
- Always monitor the athlete and the tissue being treated during treatment.

In addition to these general contraindications, hydrotherapy should not be used if there is compromised circulation or sensation. Because the primary homeostatic mechanism for adjusting to changes in temperature occurs in the circulatory system—that is, heat is dissipated via peripheral vasodilation and increased circulation to the skin and conserved via peripheral vasoconstriction and shifting blood volumes to internal organs—hydrotherapy applications can create a dangerous level of tissue and/or cardiovascular distress for those with significantly impaired circulation. If there is decreased sensory input in an area, such as in paralysis or temporary neural compression syndrome, the risk of tissue damage is high owing to the athlete's inability to perceive and report pain. In addition, hydrotherapy packs, and heat therapies in particular, *should be placed on the athlete* rather than the athlete sitting or lying on the pack. This decreases the risk of tissue damage because superficial vessels have been compressed and circulation compromised. Additional cautions and contraindications that are specific to cold or heat are discussed in the sections that follow.

■ CRYOTHERAPY

The therapeutic use of cold is called cryotherapy. The application of cold to injured tissue is a general depressant to normal metabolic activities. Whenever cryotherapy is used, the athlete experiences a sensory progression that begins with first recognizing the sensation of cold. Within 4 or 5 minutes, the area of application begins to burn and then a deep aching sensation closely follows. Seven to 10 minutes into the cold treatment, the area feels numb to the athlete. The numb sensation is interpreted to mean that the physiologic effects of cold are fully engaged in the tissue being treated. At that point, therapists may choose to end the cryotherapy, or sustain and deepen the physiologic benefits by extending the cryotherapy for another 5 to 10 minutes, or do some light stretching and/or movement exercises. As a general rule, cryotherapy over thin tissue areas such as the wrist/hand/fingers should have a duration of 5 to 10 minutes, whereas a 15- to 20-minute duration is more appropriate when cold is applied over thicker tissue such as the hamstrings or quadriceps. Cryotherapy treatments should never exceed 30 minutes in duration for a single application because of the risk of frostbite. Following are the specific physiologic effects of cold in the area of application[1-6]:

- Vasoconstriction that limits local blood flow
- Decreased pain (analgesic effect)
- Decreased muscle spasm
- Decreased lymph flow

When these effects are considered, it is easy to see why cryotherapy is the preferred modality during the acute stage of the healing cycle. Cryotherapy accomplishes the treatment goals in the acute stage by creating vasoconstriction to help control hemorrhage and diminish primary edema, and the pain-spasm cycle is effectively interrupted because both pain and spasm are diminished by cold. Pain is decreased via the gate control theory and slowed nerve impulses.[1-5] Because nerve impulses are slower, the signal for muscle contraction is also slowed. This method of reducing spasm is better described as *raising the muscle threshold*. By reducing pain and raising the muscle threshold to reduce spasm, the muscle spindle/stretch reflex is also quieted, and pain-free active range of motion is improved. This allows active movement to be initiated during the acute stage of healing. The most important benefit of active movement during the acute stage of healing is the reduction of edema that occurs from muscle contraction facilitating venous and lymphatic flow. During the subacute stage of healing, active movement is essential for creating well-organized granulation tissue. **Cryokinetics**, a specific modality that combines ice and movement, can be used throughout the healing cycle rather than switching to a heat modality during the subacute and maturation stages. The use of cryokinetics has been demonstrated to be as effective, or more effective, than heat modalities at returning athletes to activity after acute injuries.[1,5]

There are several different methods of applying cryotherapy, and each has a few advantages and disadvantages. Table 14-1 describes the most common methods of cryotherapy, lists the advantages and disadvantages, and gives the suggested use in conjunction with therapeutic massage. For the most part, massage therapists use ice packs and ice massage more than any of the other methods of cold application.

Cryotherapy is clearly indicated during the acute stage of the healing cycle and any time there are signs and symptoms of inflammation and/or hemorrhage. A specific contraindication for cryotherapy is **Raynaud's syndrome.** In this condition, the arterioles in the extremities, usually hands and feet, respond to cold with severe vasoconstriction. This severe vasoconstriction is first recognized by changes in tissue color of the fingers or toes, that is, a blanched and/or cyanotic appearance. In addition, athletes may experience sharp pain, dizziness, and sometimes nausea during cryotherapy. Until athletes have this type of reaction, they may not know they have the condition, requiring therapists to perform thorough intakes and always monitor athletes closely during all cryotherapy applications. Some indicators that an athlete may have Raynaud's phenomenon include awareness that they are easily

TABLE 14-1	Comparison of Cryotherapy Methods		
Method	**Advantages**	**Disadvantages**	**Integration with Massage**
Spray coolants	Contained, easily and precisely applied	Only superficial effect Require special training	Used only in spray and stretch in trigger point therapy
Ice bag	Therapeutic effect at muscular level Inexpensive and readily available Compression and elevation can also be used	Uneven cooling; air pockets create areas of poor cooling Can be messy	After deep transverse friction After cramp management To reduce pain and spasm before manual exercise
Gel or chemical cold pack	Easy for at-home treatment Therapeutic effect at muscular level	Loses cold quickly Develops frost on outside surface that can freeze tissue	Same as with ice pack
Immersion (cold whirlpool)	Even and thorough cooling especially around joints Therapeutic effect at muscular level	Not readily available in all settings Cannot use compression, elevation, or massage in other areas at same time Messy	Same as with ice pack
Ice massage	Isolates precise area for treatment Easy for at-home treatment Therapeutic effect at muscular level	Messy Therapist unable to continue work in another area during ice massage	Before and/or after deep transverse friction May substitute for spray in spray and stretch

chilled, always having cold hands or feet, or having an episode of frostbite in their history. When an athlete has Raynaud's syndrome, the immersion and ice-bag forms of cryotherapy *must* be avoided. If the therapist believes cryotherapy is still a necessary part of this athlete's treatment (eg, after the first session of deep transverse friction), the intensity of the application must be decreased by using a cool compress rather than an ice bag and by shortening the duration of the treatment to 5 minutes or less.[2,6]

■ THERMOTHERAPY

The therapeutic use of heat is called thermotherapy. The application of heat to injured tissue is a general stimulant to normal metabolic activities. Similar to cryotherapy, the physiologic effects of thermotherapy are fully engaged approximately 10 minutes into the treatment, and a standard duration of treatment is 15 to 20 minutes, depending on the tissue being treated and the method of thermotherapy. The local physiologic effects of heat are:

- Vasodilation and hyperemia (improved local blood flow)
- Decreased pain
- Increased nerve impulse conduction (facilitated pathways)
- Improved pliability/extensibility of collagen
- Improved lymph flow

Because of these effects, thermotherapy can be indicated in the subacute and maturation stages of healing, but are definitely contraindicated in the acute stage. An important distinction between heat and cold therapy is that heat does not *directly* decrease muscle spasm the way cold does. Because nerve impulse conduction is increased with heat, the muscle threshold is lowered or facilitated, making the muscle spindle/stretch reflex a little more sensitive to sudden lengthening. However, because pain is reduced via the gate control theory and the general soothing sensation of heat on the nervous system as a whole, muscle relaxation is considered a *secondary or indirect* effect of thermotherapy.

Because it is difficult to be sure how far into the subacute stage an injury may be, heat should be used with great caution or not used at all (consider cryokinetics instead) in this stage of healing. During the maturation stage of an acute injury or when treating chronic injuries with thick matted repair tissue, the improved local circulation and collagen pliability created by heat are very helpful in achieving full range of motion. Other specific contraindications to heat include *thrombophlebitis, severe arterio- or atherosclerosis, and uncontrolled hypertension.*[1-3,6] Although individuals with Raynaud's phenomenon may also be somewhat sensitive to extreme heat, it is not a specific contraindication.

Common methods of heat application are outlined in Table 14-2, with the advantages and disadvantages of each listed along with suggestions for integration with mas-

TABLE 14-2	Comparison of Thermotherapy Methods		
Method	**Advantages**	**Disadvantages**	**Integration with Massage**
Hydrocollator pack (moist heat pack)	Immediate transfer of heat. Always available and easy to store. Easy to work in other tissue during application	Requires separate protective covering. Frequent cleaning of heating unit. Not easy to use in small or bony areas	Before general massage, myofascial applications, and stretching. After extensive myofascial work in chronic conditions
Heating pad (dry heat)	Easy for at-home treatments. Easy to work in other areas during application	Heat remains superficial. Slower transfer of heat (must heat up)	Not recommended
Thermophore (moist heating pad)	Affects deeper tissue than heating pad does. Always available and easy to store. Easy to work in other areas during application	Slower transfer of heat (must heat up). Not easy to use is small or boney areas	Before general massage, specific myofascial work, and stretching
Whirlpools	Immediate transfer of heat. Molds to area; good for bony areas. Even and thorough heating	Wet and messy. Not readily available in all settings. Cannot perform massage at same time. Frequent cleaning	Before general massage, specific myofascial work and stretching
Steam/sauna	Immediate transfer of heat. Full body; internal and external effects	Only available in spa or clinical setting. Full-body treatment	Before general massage. After extensive myofascial work

sage. In general, moist heat applications do a better job of transferring heat to the body than dry heat applications, creating physiologic changes at a deeper level in the tissue. The "heat rub" creams and lotions are not included in this table because they do not actually increase the temperature of tissue to any significant level. However, these topical analgesics can be beneficial to athletes because the superficial sensation of heat can be very soothing and can help with general relaxation.

Two additional thermotherapy modalities outside the scope of practice for massage therapists are ultrasound and diathermy. Ultrasound projects high-frequency sound waves through tissue to increase tissue temperature, whereas diathermy projects a high-frequency electrical impulse to generate heat in the tissue. Because they are both forms of thermotherapy, they should generally be applied before therapeutic massage.

■ CONTRAST THERAPY

In sports health care, contrast therapy is the alternating application of heat and cold over the injured tissue area for therapeutic effect. The intention of contrast therapy is to cre-

ate an alternating vasoconstriction and vasodilation, sometimes called a vascular pump or flush, to help reduce edema during the subacute stage of healing.[1-3] However, this effect has not been well established in research. Because the cardiovascular system is *not* the primary system for edema removal, cryokinetics and lymphatic facilitation, which are proven methods of edema reduction, are a better choice.

Compression Pumps and Short-Stretch Wraps

With the advent of intermittent compression pumps, the use of compression to control edema formation in the acute stage of injury has extended to using it for reducing edema during the subacute stage. Compression pumps completely surround an injured area with pressure by using a sleeve that is slipped over the extremities and pressurized with air—often cold air. The compression pumps used in sports medicine usually have three or four individual chambers, and the distal chambers are filled with more pressure than the proximal ones. For an upper extremity, the standard compression levels from distal to proximal is usually 60-30-15 mmHg, and pressure is applied intermittently at a 30-seconds-on and 30-seconds-off ratio for a total treatment time of approximately 20 minutes.[7–9] The suggested compression range for lower extremity edema is slightly higher, ranging from 40 to 80 mmHg.[7] Several empirical and clinical trials using circumference measurements of an edematous area before and after the use of a compression pump have confirmed that circumference is decreased by this method of treatment. However, very little research has been done using total fluid volume measurements with these treatment parameters, which makes it difficult to say with any degree of certainty that improved edema uptake and lymph flow are the reason for the decreased circumference. Without measuring a change in fluid volumes in the tissue, the decreased circumference could simply be due to pushing the fluid into adjacent areas.

In contrast to the intermittent compression pumps commonly used in sports medicine, lymphedema specialists use sequential pneumatic sleeves that have more chambers along their length—usually five or six—and inflate the chambers with much less pressure than the compression pumps.[8,10,11] In the 1980 *British Journal of Surgery*, Lawrence and Kakkar reported that a compression formula of 18 mmHg in the distal chamber progressing to 14, then 12, 10, and finally 8 mmHg in the proximal chamber created a significant improvement in venous return without adverse effects on subcutaneous blood or lymph flow. When pressures were increased to 30-26-18-14 and 12 mmHg, the venous return improved even more, but the initial lymphatic and subcutaneous blood flow were significantly reduced.[8] Theoretically, edema uptake and lymph flow may be inhibited by compression of 30 mmHg or more,[8–12] suggesting that therapists may want to try lower levels of compression with their intermittent compression pumps to avoid possible occlusion of the superficial lymphatic vessels that might impede edema uptake. In addition, the use of lymphatic facilitation, specifically clearing the neck and all appropriate catchments, before the application of compression pumps may also improve their effectiveness.

The value of maintaining compression while the athlete is away from the clinic is universally recognized. At this time, the standard practice is to use elastic bandages or neoprene sleeves over the region of edema. Sometimes, felt pads or inserts are used to increase compression in a specific location of edema, that is, a felt horseshoe placed around the malleolus for treatment of an ankle sprain. These wraps/bandages are used because they supply high compression during rest and provide little resistance to muscle contraction, thus allowing the athlete to move comfortably. In other words, the standard elastic wrap has a high *resting pressure* (compression of the tissue when the limb is at rest), and a low *working pressure* (compression of the tissue during movement/muscle contraction). However, this does not help stimulate edema uptake or lymph flow, because

From the Field

"As a certified lymphatic therapist I was first introduced to short-stretch wraps as a key part of comprehensive lymphedema treatments. When I was working as a massage therapist for an NBA team, I convinced the athletic trainer to try them for management of the swelling that occurred with athletic injuries. The results were pretty dramatic. The athletes who went home with the short-stretch wraps wore them all night long, and when we took the wraps off for treatment, the swelling did not return as quickly. The athletic trainer was convinced and wanted to buy a bunch, but couldn't find them anywhere in his standard supply catalogues. I directed him to the company that sells lymphedema treatment supplies, where he found them listed as lymphedema bandages."

Dale Perry, LMT, CLT
Albany, NY

some resistance to expansion during contraction is necessary to propel lymph through their vessels. Moreover, the high resting pressure can cause pain during periods of inactivity, such as at night, which often causes athletes to loosen or remove the compression wrap. In treatment of lymphedema, a compression wrap that has very little elasticity, a **short-stretch wrap**, has been demonstrated to be more effective. Compared with standard elastic bandages, these short-stretch wraps have a *low* resting pressure and a *high* working pressure (Fig. 14-1). Low resting pressure creates compression without discomfort during periods of inactivity, and high working pressure of the bandage resists expansion during muscle contraction to squeeze the superficial lymph vessels, thus facilitating lymph flow.[8,10,11] Although

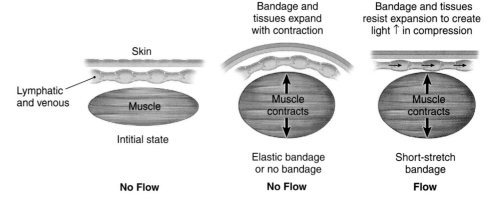

FIGURE 14-1 Elastic wrap versus short-stretch wrap. An elastic wrap expands with the muscle contraction and loses compression, whereas a short-stretch wrap resists full expansion to squeeze lymph vessels and veins to stimulate flow.

these shorts stretch wraps have traditionally been used only in treatment of lymphedema, they are now effectively being utilized for the treatment of traumatic edema as well.

SUMMARY

- When using multiple modalities, it is important to consider the indications, contraindications, and benefits of each to integrate them appropriately.
- Sports health care therapists may use only those modalities that fall within their specific scope of practice and must communicate effectively with all members of the health care team regarding their inclusion of these modalities.
- Cryotherapy is used to decrease pain and muscle spasm and to control primary edema. Therefore, it is best suited

for treatment during the acute and subacute stages of healing.
- Thermotherapy is used to decrease pain, to enhance muscle relaxation, increase local circulation, and to enhance collagen flexibility. Therefore, it is best suited for treatment during the maturation stage of healing.
- As a general guideline, cryotherapy should be administered after intense soft tissue manipulation such as deep transverse friction, but before lymphatic facilitation.
- As a general guideline, thermotherapy should be administered before most therapeutic massages and may also be beneficial after comprehensive myofascial sessions.
- Short-stretch wraps are a better method of compression bandaging than the standard elastic wrap for control and reduction of traumatic edema.

Review Questions

SHORT ANSWERS

1. Define cryotherapy and list the primary physiologic effects of this type of treatment.

2. Define thermotherapy and list the primary physiologic effects of this type of treatment.

3. Name the most appropriate kind of hydrotherapy for each stage in the healing cycle.

MULTIPLE CHOICE

4. How does cold reduce muscle spasm?
   a. By reducing circulation via vasoconstriction
   b. By raising the muscle threshold
   c. By lowering the muscle threshold
   d. Via increased metabolism

5. Both heat and cold reduce pain via what mechanism?
   a. Raising muscle threshold
   b. Loosening the collagen
   c. Decreasing metabolic activity
   d. Gate control method

6. Contraindications to all forms of hydrotherapy include breaks in the skin or rashes, malignancy, lymphedema, and _____.
   a. asthma
   b. Raynaud's syndrome
   c. areas with a circulatory or sensory deficit
   d. fibromyalgia

7. Ultrasound and diathermy are common sports health care modalities that are classified as _____.
   a. cryotherapy
   b. thermotherapy
   c. hydrotherapy
   d. compression therapy

8. What is the primary intention of contrast therapy?
   a. To decease metabolism
   b. To reduce muscle spasm
   c. To reduce swelling
   d. To improve collagen flexibility

9. Additional contraindications for thermotherapies include uncontrolled hypertension, arteriosclerosis, and _____.
   a. thrombophlebitis
   b. dehydration
   c. fibromyalgia
   d. neurologic compression–tension syndromes

10. Short-stretch wraps are a better choice than standard elastic wraps because they have _____.
    a. high resting pressure and low working pressure
    b. higher overall compression ratio
    c. lower overall compression ratio
    d. low resting pressure and high working pressure

REFERENCES

1. Prentice WE. Therapeutic Modalities for Physical Therapists, 2nd ed. New York: McGraw-Hill, 2002.
2. Prentice WE. Therapeutic Modalities for Allied Health Professions. New York and St. Louis: McGraw-Hill, 1998.
3. Drez D, ed. Therapeutic Modalities for Sports Injuries. Chicago: Year Book Medical Publishers, 1989.
4. Knight K. Cryotherapy: Theory, technique, and physiology. 1985, Chatanooga Corporation.
5. Knight KL. Cryotherapy in sports medicine. In: Scribner K, Burke W, eds. Relevant Topics in Athletic Training, 1978.
6. Werner R. A Massage Therapist's Guide to Pathology, 3rd ed. Baltimore: Lippincott Williams & Wilkins, 2005.
7. Hooker DN. Intermittent compression devices. In: Prentice WE, ed. Therapeutic Modalities for Physical Therapists, 2nd ed. New York: McGraw-Hill, 2002.
8. Casley-Smith JR. Modern Treatment of Lymphoedema. Adelaide, Australia: Henry Thomas Laboratory, Lymphoedema Association of Australia, 1994.
9. Johansson K, Lie E et al. A randomized study comparing manual lymph drainage with sequential pneumatic compression for treatment of postoperative arm lymphedema. Lymphology 1998;31:56–64.
10. Perry, DE, Hanlon H. Lymphatic Techniques for Injury Rehabilitation, vol. 1: Upper Extremities; Course Workbook. Koru Seminars, 2000.
11. Perry DE, Hanlon H. Lymphatic Techniques for Injury Rehabilitation, vol. 2: Lower Body; Course Workbook. Koru Seminars, 2000.
12. Eliska O, Eliskova M. Are peripheral lymphatics damaged by high pressure manual massage? Lymphology 1995;28:21–30.

Massage Categories and Common Brand Names

Category	Description	Common Names
Swedish massage	Use of lubricant for sliding–gliding style of work; full-body focus for general relaxation and health maintenance.	Combines "standard strokes" of effleurage, pétrissage, friction, vibration, passive range of motion, and tapotement
Myofascial/deep tissue	Any technique focused on stretching and broadening of fascia and other connective tissues; usually without lubricant. Intention is to improve structural alignment and range of motion, and decrease pain and ischemia.	Hellerwork®, Rolfing®, myofascial release (MFR), structural integration, Aston Patterning®, craniosacral, active releasing technique (ART™), soft tissue release, muscle energy technique (MET™)
Neuromuscular (trigger point/tender point)	Any technique that reduces resting muscle tension. Intention is to normalize muscle tension and decrease pain that limits range of motion.	Neuromuscular technique (NMT), trigger point, Strain Counterstrain®, tender point, positional release, muscle energy technique (MET)®, myotherapy
Lymphatic	Any system of light to moderate depth strokes based on anatomy and physiology of the lymphatic system. Intention is to stimulate edema uptake and other lymphatic processes.	Manual Lymphatic Drainage (MLD)®, lymphatic massage, lymphedema techniques
Movement therapies	Focused, patterned, conscious movement designed to decrease muscle tension, improve pain-free movement, and balance emotions.	Feldenkries®, Alexander technique, Rosenwork, Trager®, Hakomi, Qui gong, Tai Chi
Reflexive/zone therapies	Stimulation of defined energy zones, dermatomes, chakras, or points with light or deep pressure to improve systemic functions and decrease pain.	Shiatsu, foot reflexology, bindegewebs (CTM), Therapeutic Touch®, chakra balancing, acupuncture, acupressure
Energy techniques	Touching/holding/stroking (often without physical contact) of defined energy zones, chakras, or points with intention to balance the energy flow.	Polarity®, Reiki®, Qui gong, Therapeutic Touch®, touch for health, chakra balancing

Muscle Focus for Massage by Sport

SPORTS THAT EMPHASIZE LOWER BODY

- Basketball
- Field or ice hockey
- Lacrosse
- Downhill skiing
- Soccer
- Track

MUSCLE FOCUS FOR LOWER BODY SPORTS

Focus includes the following major muscle groups and their fascial zones/tendons:

- Lumbar muscles
- Gluteals
- Hamstrings
- Gastrocnemius/soleus
- Quadriceps
- Iliopsoas/hip flexors
- *Add*uctors
- Anterior and lateral compartments of the leg

Sport		Expanded Focus for Maintenance Massage
Basketball		• Full back • Shoulders
Field or ice hockey		• Full back • Shoulders
Lacrosse		• Full back • Shoulders
Downhill skiing		• Full back
Soccer		• Abdominals • Neck
Track	Sprints/hurdles	• Diaphragm • Chest/neck
	Long jump/high jump	• Abdominals • Chest/neck
	Distance/cross-country	• Full back • Chest/neck

SPORTS THAT EMPHASIZE UPPER BODY

- Baseball/softball
- Golf
- Kayak/paddling
- Pole vault
- Swimming
- Tennis/racket sports

MUSCLE FOCUS FOR UPPER BODY SPORTS

Focus includes the following major muscle groups and their fascial zones/tendons:

- Full back and posterior neck
- Shoulder (deltoid and rotator cuff)
- Pectoralis major and minor
- Biceps brachii
- Triceps brachii
- Iliopsoas and abdominals
- Anterior and posterior forearm
- Palm of hand

Sport	Expanded Focus for Maintenance Massage
Baseball/softball	• Gluteals • Hamstrings • Quadriceps and knees
Golf	• Back (focus is mostly lumbar) • Knees • Feet
Kayak/paddling	• Gluteals • Hamstrings
Pole vault	• Gluteals • Hamstrings • Quadriceps
Swimming	• Gluteals • Hamstrings • Quadriceps and knees (especially for breast-strokers)
Tennis/racket sports	• Gluteals • Hamstrings • Quadriceps and knees

SPORTS THAT REQUIRE FULL BODY FOCUS

- Crew/rowing
- Cross-country skiing
- Cycling
- Field events
- Gymnastics
- Volleyball
- Wrestling

FULL BODY FOCUS

The event massage focus for athletes in sports that demand use of major muscle groups from both the upper and lower body begins by attending to any tight or sore areas identified by the athlete. After that, work through each muscle group listed as thoroughly as time allows.

Sport	Massage Should Include These Regions and/or Muscles
Crew/rowing	• Full lower body (decreased focus anterior/lateral compartments) • Full back • Chest • Forearms
Cross-country skiing	• Full lower body (decreased focus anterior/lateral compartments) • Full back • Chest • Shoulders
Cycling	• Quadriceps and hip flexors • Hamstrings and gluteals • Upper back • Chest and neck

Field events
  • Javelin
  • Shot put
  • Hammer
	• Full lower body (decreased focus anterior/lateral compartments)
	• Full back
	• Chest
	• Shoulders
	• Triceps and biceps

Gymnastics	• Focus varies with event
Volleyball	• Full lower body (decreased focus anterior/lateral compartments) • Low back • Chest and neck • Shoulders
Wrestling	• Full back • Abdominals • Hamstrings • Quadriceps • Gastrocnemius/soleus

A Quick Reference for Distinguishing Sign and Symptoms by Body Region

Foot/Ankle Evaluation

Athlete's Complaint	History and Mechanism	PA and Tissue Inspection	Functional Tests	Probable Condition
Numbing or burning pain in foot				
• Forefoot	*Chronic:* Repetitive activity on ball of foot; poor arch support; shoes too narrow in toe box.	Morton's toe; fallen metatarsal arch; callus build-up under 2nd–4th metatarsal heads; webbed tissue between 2nd and 3rd toes.	Deep pincer pressure between 3rd and 4th metatarsal heads recreates pain; metatarsal squeeze test recreates pain.	Morton's neuroma
• Whole foot/ankle	As above, plus history of ankle sprain or fracture; ankle "gives out."	Pronation and/or pes planus; thick fibrous tissue around malleolus.	Positive Tinel's test; possible ↓ in pulse.	Tarsal tunnel syndrome
Aching pain in foot and/or heel	*Chronic:* Poor arch support; running, jumping, walking.	Burning or sharp pain in arch at distal edge of calcaneus; first step in AM excruciating; point tender at medial distal heel on plantar surface; plus any or all of these: pronation; pes cavus; Morton's toe.	Forced dorsiflexion with toe extension may reproduce pain + reveals pronounced medial cord in plantar fascia.	Plantar fasciitis
		Pain in heel; point tender at middle or posterior calcaneus; Achilles tendon thick and gritty.	Crepitus and/or pain in Achilles during active dorsiflexion and plantar flexion.	Achilles tendonitis
Ankle pain and swelling	*Acute:* Forced inversion or eversion of ankle.	PA not relevant in acute injury; overt swelling at medial or lateral malleolus; ecchymosis.	Weak and painful inversion and/or eversion; + anterior drawer or other ligament laxity test.	Ankle sprain
	Chronic: Repetitive stressful motion.	Little or no swelling; gritty; thick feel to tendons. Swelling and redness at tendons.	Crepitus at peroneal tendon during AROM (eversion); possible weak eversion. Crepitus and pain in anterior tendons during AROM. Possible crepitus, pain, and/or weakness as above.	Peroneal tendonitis. Extensor tendonitis Tenosynovitis

Leg/Knee Evaluation

Athlete's Complaint	History and Mechanism	PA and Tissue Inspection	Functional Tests	Probable Condition
Anterior leg pain	*Chronic:* Repetitive stressful movement; change in running surface (hard to soft or vice versa); aching pain along anteromedial or posterolateral crest of tibia that increases with activity.	Possible pronation or pes planus; little or no heat and swelling; palpable bumps over tibial crest with point tenderness.	Weak and painful inversion and dorsiflexion, or . . . Weak and painful inversion and plantarflexion.	"Shin splints," either Anterior tibial stress syndrome or . . . Posterior tibial stress syndrome
	Chronic: As above, except pain is point specific on the tibia.	As above, except specific point tenderness on bone.	Tapping proximal or distal to point-tender location yields tingle or buzz at the tender site.	Stress fracture
	Chronic: As above, or . . . *Acute:* Due to traumatic compression (kick, fall, blow); describes "full" and/or "tight" pain over entire anterior compartment.	Full anterior compartment tight, swollen, and tender; skin appears taut and shiny; possible redness or ecchymosis.	↓ or absent pedal pulse; weak or absent dorsiflexion and inversion	*Acute or chronic anterior compartment syndrome
Posterior leg pain	*Acute:* Forceful plantar flexion with knee extended; pop or tearing sensation in proximal posterior leg.	Swelling and ecchymosis of medial calf; point tender at medial head of gastrocnemius; palpable defect in gastrocnemius contour.	Weak and painful plantar flexion when weight bearing; noticeable change in Thompson's test.	Tennis leg (strained/torn medial gastrocnemius)
	Acute: Forced dorsiflexion (heel drops) during plantar flexion contraction, ie, stopping momentum by putting foot up on wall.	Same as above without the palpable muscle defect.	Negative Thompson's test; painful but strong plantar flexion with weight bearing.	Ruptured plantaris
Medial knee pain	*Chronic:* Runner with possible history of tight hamstrings; aching/burning pain at medial joint line and/or medial proximal shaft of tibia.	Pronated feet and/or knock-kneed; palpable swelling and thick-boggy tissue over pes anserine bursa.	Painful but full knee flexion; full strength but ↑ pain with resistives; negative MCL stress test.	Pes anserine bursitis
	Acute: valgus force + medial rotation while knee is flexed; sharp pain and "pop" reported at time of injury.	Intra-articular swelling; heat; point tenderness at medial joint line.	Pain and/or laxity (loss of firm end feel) with valgus stress to MCL.	Sprained/torn MCL
			Knee locks in flexion and/or "gives out" when weight bearing; crepitus or crunching sensation to athlete during AROM; + Apley's compression test.	Torn medial meniscus

*Although rare, the same complaints in the lateral or posterior leg indicate possible compartment syndromes in those areas.

Region	Symptoms	Signs	Special Tests	Diagnosis
Posterior knee pain	*Chronic:* Aching in popliteal space that ↑ with activity; swelling that comes and goes in popliteal space.	Soft pocket of swelling in popliteal space; *not* point tender.	Nothing remarkable	Popliteal/Baker's cyst
	Chronic: Aching in posterolateral knee; history of running downhill.	Tender along posterolateral knee; *not* tender over hamstring tendon; crepitus with AROM.	Nothing remarkable	Popliteus tendonitis
	Chronic: Forceful extension during hamstring contraction, i.e., sprinters start out of blocks; pain at hamstring tendon(s); aching or pulling pain.	Little or no swelling or heat; palpable tension in hamstrings; possible TPs.	Strong but painful resisted knee flexion; crepitus with AROM.	Chronic hamstring tendon strain (tendonitis)
	Acute: As above, except sharp pop/tear when injured.	Palpable defect in tendon contour; possible swelling.	Weak and painful resisted knee flexion.	Acute hamstring tendon strain
Lateral knee pain	*Chronic:* Most common in female runners and jumpers; aching pain along lateral joint line and/or femoral condyle.	Little or no swelling; possible heat along lateral knee; point tenderness at lateral joint line and/or femoral condyle.	Lateral drift of thigh during iliopsoas tension test; + Noble compression test; + Ober's test	Iliotibial band syndrome
	Chronic: Forceful extension during hamstring contraction; Aching pain over biceps femoris tendon.	Little or no swelling or heat; palpable tension in hamstrings; possible TPs.	Strong but painful resisted knee flexion; crepitus with AROM.	Chronic hamstring tendon strain (tendonitis)
	Acute: As above, except sharp pop/tear when injured.	Palpable defect in tendon contour; possible swelling.	Weak and painful resisted knee flexion.	Acute hamstring tendon strain
	Acute: Varus force and rotation of the knee; felt pop or tear in joint at time of injury.	Diffuse extra-articular swelling and ecchymosis over lateral knee; point tender over lateral joint line and/or head of fibula.	Pain and/or laxity (loss of firm end-feel) with varus stress to LCL.	Sprained/torn LCL
	Acute: As above, and reports that knee tends to lock or get stuck.	As above	Positive Apley's compression test	Torn lateral meniscus
Anterior knee pain	*Chronic:* Runners and jumpers, especially after lots of stairs or downhill workouts; aching pain over the top of the patella that ↑ with activity.	Little or no swelling; point tenderness at inferior pole or superior medial pole of patella.	Crepitus over patella with AROM; pain or ↑ discomfort with resisted knee flexion.	Patellar tendonitis
	Chronic: As above, except pain located under the patella; grinding during activity; aching after activity.	As above, except point tender along medial and/or lateral borders of patella; ↑ Q-angle and/or poor VMO development.	+ Clarke's sign	Chondromalacia (patellofemoral syndrome)
	Chronic: Adolescent athlete; excessive knee extension stress.	Enlarged tibial tuberosity; point tender at tibial tuberosity.	Nothing remarkable	Osgood-Schlatter's
	Acute: Knee buckled or gave out during external rotation of slightly flexed knee; sudden sharp pain at patella; possible direct blow to side of patella.	Point tender along borders of patella; possible ↑ Q-angle and/or poor VMO development.	+ Patellar apprehension test	Patellar subluxation

AROM, active range of motion; LCL, lateral collateral ligament; MCL, medial collateral ligament; TP, trigger point; VMO, vastus medial oblique.

Thigh/Hip/Low Back Evaluation

Athlete's Complaint	History and Mechanism	PA and Tissue Inspection	Functional Tests	Probable Condition
Lateral hip pain	*Acute:* Traumatic compression to lateral hip and/or torso.	Moderate to severe swelling and ecchymosis over iliac crest or ranging from mid torso through mid thigh; point tenderness.	Painful AROM, with probable decrease in pain-free range.	Hip pointer (severe contusion)*
	Acute: Same as above but to greater trochanter; sharp and/or burning pain over trochanter.	Moderate to severe swelling over greater trochanter; point. tender over greater trochanter.	As above	Acute trochanteric bursitis
	Chronic: Running and jumping activities, especially downhill or stairs; sharp and/or burning pain over trochanter.	As above, plus gritty thick tissue at greater trochanter; possible TPs in TFL, quadriceps and/or gluteals.	+ Ober's test; painful resisted hip *abduction*	Chronic trochanteric bursitis
	Chronic: As above; tight, tense and aching full lateral hip.	Taut, tender and gritty iliotibial band; no swelling, heat, or ecchymosis; probable TPs in TFL and/or gluteals; possible point tenderness at lateral joint line of knee.	As above	Iliotibial band syndrome
Groin pain	*Chronic:* Cycling, horseback riding, gymnastics and downhill running; deep groin pain across pubic bone that ↑ with activity; possible abdominal discomfort.	Point tender over pubic symphysis; palpable misalignment or increased gap; spasm and tension in adductors; possible mild swelling and heat.	Pain and weakness with resisted bilateral hip *adduction* and/or stretch of adductors.	Pubic symphysitis
	Acute: Forced *abduction* of hip; sudden sharp pain; pop or tearing sensation at time of injury.	Tenderness and possible palpable muscle defect in adductors.	Pulling pain with stretch of adductors; painful and/or weak resisted adduction.	Acute adductor strain

*Any severe contusion can progress to myositis ossificans if retraumatized or improperly treated.

Radiating/burning pain in posterior hip and/or thigh	*Chronic:* Repetitive stressful lifting and twisting activities; crew, power lifting; history of tight hamstrings and/or gluteals.	General muscle tension of low back, gluteals, and hamstrings; TP at mid-gluteal; externally rotated hips.	SLR causes radiating pain at approx. 75–85° of hip flexion, relieved with passive external rotation of hip; symptoms occur with resisted external rotation of hip.	Sciatica from piriformis compression
	Chronic: As above, or with excessive sitting on hard surfaces.	Pain reproduced with firm palpation over ischial bursa; mild swelling or thick, fibrous tissue at ischial tuberosity.	Pain at end point of passive straight-legged hip flexion; painful resisted hip extension.	Ischial bursitis
	Chronic: Low back strain.	See below	SLR causes radiating pain at approx. 35–70° of hip flexion.	Lumbosacral nerve root strain and/or compression
	Acute: Low back strain.	See below	As above, plus possible change in bowel or bladder function, and + Valsalva test.	As above
Low back pain	*Chronic:* Low intensity and repetitive bending, lifting, and twisting activities; general aching, muscle soreness, and stiffness; no radiating pain.	Widespread muscle tension of low back and hips; various TPs; no heat and/or swelling; any or all of these: high ilium, anterior or posterior pelvic tilt, point tender over sacroiliac joint.	Pain, stiffness, and/or limited AROM of trunk and hip; negative SLR; possible + Ober's test or iliopsoas tension test.	Chronic soft tissue strain of low back
	Acute: High intensity bending, lifting, and twisting activities; pop and sudden sharp pain followed by rush of warmth across low back; may or may not have continued activity depending on severity.	As above, except with possibility of heat and/or swelling in low back; possible point tenderness over spinous processes or interspinous spaces.	As above, plus possible weak and painful resisted torso rotation and/or extension.	Acute soft tissue strain of low back

SLR, straight-leg raising; TFL, tensor fasciae latae; TP, trigger point.

Neck/Shoulder Evaluation

Athlete's Complaint	History and Mechanism	PA and Tissue Inspection	Functional Tests	Probable Condition
Anterior shoulder pain	*Chronic:* Swimming, throwing, crew, etc.; aching pain over anterior shoulder that ↑ with activity; worst at beginning and end of activity.	Little or no swelling; point tender over bicipital groove.	Crepitus at biceps tendon with AROM; light stretch pain in anterior shoulder with passive shoulder extension with elbow extension; weak and painful resisted shoulder flexion; +Spee's test; no painful arc.	Bicipital tendonitis (chronic strain)
		As above, except with swelling along bicipital groove.	As above	Tenosynovitis
	Chronic: As above, but pain may be a constant ache both during and after activity.	Little or no swelling; point tender at greater tubercle of humerus and/or at anterolateral edge of acromion.	Painful arc; negative Spee's test; +impingement test; painful and weak resisted *abduction.*	Chronic strain of supraspinatus
		Swelling and/or heat at anterior lip of acromion; thick tissue and point tenderness in same region.	Pain with active flexion and external rotation plus painful arc; pain at end point of passive hyperextension and horizontal *abduction;* negative Spee's test; +impingement test; pain with resisted external rotation and horizontal *abduction.*	Subacromial bursitis
	Acute: Lifting especially deltoid flys; sudden sharp pain; pop or tearing sensation when injured.	Mild swelling and/or heat; point tender over greater tubercle of humerus and/or at anterolateral edge of acromion.	Painful arc; weak and painful *abduction;* negative Spee's test.	Acute rotator cuff strain (supraspinatus)
	Acute: Throwing or freestyle swimming; sudden sharp pain; pop or tearing sensation when injured.	Mild swelling and/or heat; point tender at lesser tubercle of humerus.	No painful arc; weak and painful resisted internal rotation; negative Spee's test.	Acute rotator cuff strain (subscapularis)

Posterior shoulder pain	*Chronic:* Swimming especially backstroke, throwing, racket sports; aching pain that ↑ with activity.	Little or no swelling and heat; point tender posterior greater tubercle; tissue gritty and taut.	Weak and painful external rotation and horizontal *abduction*.	Chronic rotator cuff strain (infraspinatus or teres minor)
	Acute: As above; sudden sharp pain; pop or tearing sensation at time of injury.	Swelling and/or heat; point tender posterior greater tubercle.	As above	Acute rotator cuff strain (infraspinatus or teres minor)
Radiating, numbness, and/or tingling shoulder to elbow	*Chronic:* Aching and numbing in shoulder at night; arm heavy and/or weak; possibly history of clavicular fracture.	Protracted and medially rotated shoulders; forward head; no swelling, heat, or point tenderness; general muscle tension of neck and shoulders.	One or all of these: + Roos test + Adson's test + Pectoralis minor test + Wright's or military test Loss or diminished strength of upper extremity.	Thoracic outlet syndrome Scalene compression Pectoralis minor Compression Costoclavicular compression Burner/stinger (brachial plexus strain)
	Acute: Shoulder compression with lateral neck flexion to opposite side; sharp burning radiating pain followed by numbness and loss of arm function.	Nothing remarkable		
	Acute: Whiplash or neck compression injury; sharp pain; pop or tearing sensation at time of injury; possible radiating pain with sneezing and coughing.	Often point-tender spinous processes and/or interspinous spaces; general muscle spasm in neck and shoulders.	+ Compression-Distraction test; + Kernig's test; loss or diminished function of myotome and/or dermatome; possible changes in speech, vision, or hearing.	Nerve root impingement (possible disc involvement)
Lateral superior shoulder pain	*Acute:* Blow to lateral or superior aspect of shoulder.	Point tender at AC joint; possible ↑ in space at joint; swelling and heat.	+ Acromial squeeze test; painful and limited AROM.	Shoulder separation (AC sprain)
	Acute: As above	Point tender, swelling and ecchymosis over AC.	NA	Shoulder pointer (severe hematoma)

AC, acromioclavicular; AROM, active range of motion.

Elbow/Forearm/Wrist Evaluation

Athlete's Complaint	History and Mechanism	PA and Tissue Inspection	Functional Tests	Probable Condition
Dorsal wrist pain	*Chronic:* Repetitive stressful motion of the wrist; history of wrist sprain.	Observable lump over dorsal joint line; nodule firm, round and point tender; no heat or swelling.	Pain and pinching sensation with forced wrist extension.	Synovial cyst (can occur at anterior or medial wrist)
	Acute: Fall on hand with extended wrist; sharp pain and pop at time of injury.	Observable protrusion at hypothenar eminence; point tender; possible swelling, but no heat.	Painful and limited wrist AROM.	Dislocated carpal
	Acute: Wrist forced beyond normal range of motion; sharp pain; pulling tearing sensation at time of injury.	Swelling, heat and point tenderness at joint line.	As above, + ligament laxity tests.	Wrist sprain
Lateral elbow pain	*Chronic:* Racket sports and activities that require repetitive stressful wrist extension and forearm supination; aching pain during and after activity.	Point tenderness at lateral humeral epicondyle or lateral supracondylar ridge; thick, gritty and fibrous tissue at site; possible tension and TPs in posterior forearm.	Painful and weak wrist extension.	Tennis elbow or lateral humeral epicondylitis (chronic strain of extensor carpi muscles)
	Acute: Forceful varus stress of elbow; sharp pain; pop or tearing sensation at time of injury.	Point tenderness, swelling and heat at lateral joint line.	+ Ligament laxity with varus stress; probable painful and ↓ AROM.	Radial collateral ligament sprain

AROM, active range of motion.

Medial elbow pain	*Chronic:* Racket sports, golf, and baseball pitching; activities that require repetitive stressful wrist flexion and pronation; aching pain during and after activity.	Point tenderness at medial humeral epicondyle or medial supracondylar ridge; thick, gritty and fibrous tissue at site; possible tension and TPs in anterior forearm.	Painful and weak wrist flexion.	Golfer's elbow or medial humeral epicondylitis (chronic strain of flexor carpi muscles)
	Acute: Forceful valgus stress of elbow; sharp pain; pop or tearing sensation at time of injury.	Point tenderness, swelling and heat at medial joint line.	+ Ligament laxity with valgus stress; probable painful and ↓ AROM.	Ulnar collateral ligament sprain
Numbing or tingling to hand and fingers	*Chronic:* History of wrist sprain or fracture; gripping or repetitive wrist flexion or finger flexion activities; numbing, tingling, and/or weakness in thumb, index, and middle fingers; aching at night.	Flat carpal tunnel; tight and tender anterior forearm muscles with probable TPs; swelling unlikely; no heat.	+ Tinel's test; + Phalen's test; weakened grip strength.	Carpal tunnel syndrome
	Chronic: Numbing and tingling as above; no history of sprain or fracture; no aching at night.	Normal over carpal tunnel; general tension and possible TPs of forearm; TP in subscapularis.	Negative Tinel's test; negative Phalen's test.	Subscapularis trigger point
	Chronic: Numbing and tingling pain in little and ring fingers; repetitive throwing, racket, or bat activities.	Tender over track of ulnar nerve and paresthesia with palpation.	+ Tinel's test at elbow; negative Phalen's test; diminished motor function of ring and little fingers.	Ulnar nerve compression or tension
	Acute: As above, but due to traumatic compression of medial elbow.	As above, plus possible swelling	As above	As above

AROM, active range of motion; TP, trigger point.

Selected Special Tests

Foot and Ankle

Test and Indication	Description	Positive Finding	Figure
Metatarsal squeeze: Morton's neuroma	Use thumbs and index fingers to apply a firm pincer grip on either side of the 2nd and 4th metatarsal heads. Squeeze the metatarsal heads together, and maintain this compression while wiggling the metatarsals up and down.	Re-creates pain	
Tinel's test: A generic test used in a variety of locations to evaluate site-specific neurologic tension and/or compression	Firm tapping over the site.	Radiating tingling or shocking sensation	
Ligament laxity	Specific application of pressure in direction the ligament is supposed to limit joint excursion.	Soft end-feel and pain	

Leg and Knee

Test and Indication	Description	Positive Finding	Figure
Thompson's test: Torn Achilles or gastrocnemius	Squeezing the belly of the gastrocnemius to test integrity of Achilles tendon.	↓ or absent plantar flexion	
Apley's compression: Meniscal tears	Athlete prone with knee flexed just short of 90 degrees. Apply firm compression of the joint and simultaneous medial then lateral rotation of the tibia. Modifying the amount of knee flexion can also improve findings.	Crunch, grind, or pain	
Clarke's sign: Chondromalacia	Athlete is supine with knee extended. Therapist passively slides patella inferiorly and maintains this position by cupping the hand over the superior edge of the patella. Athlete is instructed to contract quadriceps to pull patella up under the hand of the therapist.	Crunch, clunk, and pain	
Patella apprehension: Patellar subluxation	Athlete lies supine with knee resting over a low bolster. Therapist applies lateral excursion pressure to the patella as the knee is passively lifted into full extension.	Athlete apprehensive, anxious and may stop the exam.	

(continued)

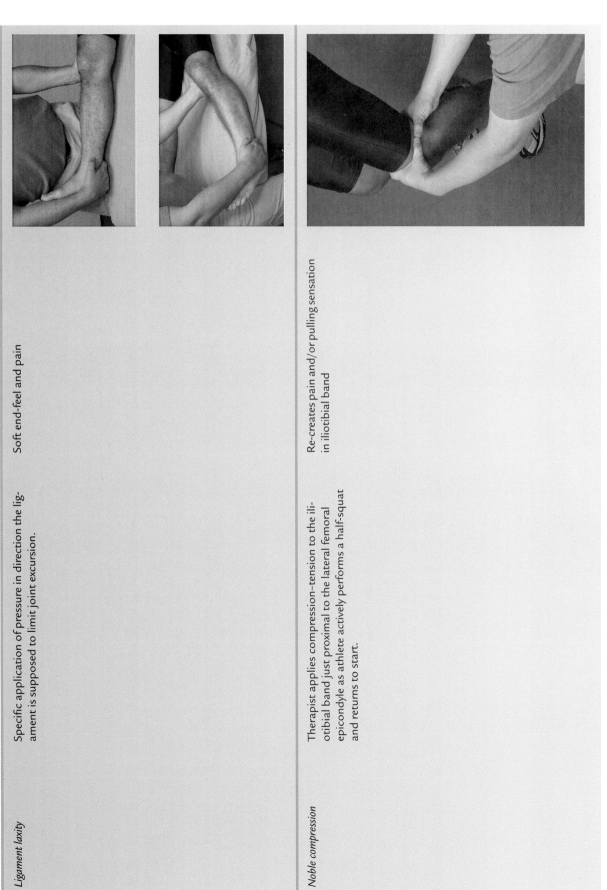

Ligament laxity

Specific application of pressure in direction the ligament is supposed to limit joint excursion.

Soft end-feel and pain

Noble compression

Therapist applies compression–tension to the iliotibial band just proximal to the lateral femoral
epicondyle as athlete actively performs a half-squat
and returns to start.

Re-creates pain and/or pulling sensation
in iliotibial band

Leg and Knee (Continued)

Test and Indication	Description	Positive Finding	Figure
Ober's test: Iliotibial band tension/ restriction	Tests for tension and fascial restriction in iliotibial band and full lateral thigh and low back. Athlete is side-lying with both knees partially flexed. Therapist passively moves top leg/thigh to slight hip extension, then lowers it to the table.	Knee cannot be lowered to the level of the bottom leg.	

Thigh, Hip, Low Back

Test and Indication	Description	Positive Finding	Figure
Straight leg raise: Nerve root or spinal segment compression/ tension	Athlete lies supine as therapist passively raises the straight leg into hip flexion. Dorsiflexion of the ankle intensifies a tension syndrome.	Radiating pain in hip and/or lumbo-sacral spine occurs between 35° and 70° hip flexion.	
Straight leg raise: Sciatica/piriformis syndrome	Athlete lies supine as therapist passively raises the straight leg into hip flexion. Then adds external rotation at point of pain.	Radiating pain in hip and/or thigh between 75° and 90° hip flexion that is relieved by external rotation.	Same as above plus external rotation at point of pain.
Iliopsoas tension/length test:	Athlete in supine curl (knees to chest) at the end of table, positioned so the ischial tuberosities are off the edge of the table. Therapist slowly lowers one thigh to its natural resting point.	Thigh does not rest parallel or below the line of the table.	

Neck and Shoulder

Test and Indication	Description	Positive Finding	Figure
Spee's test: Biceps brachii strain (acute and chronic)	Resisted straight arm shoulder flexion with palm up.	Weak and painful	
Impingement test: Supraspinatus strain and/or shoulder bursitis	Shoulder is positioned at 90° flexion and slight *abduction*. Therapist stabilizes at elbow to resist athlete's external shoulder rotation.	Pain and weakness	
Acromion squeeze: Shoulder separation/ acromioclavicular sprain	Therapist grips athlete's shoulder and squeezes anterior and posterior on either side of acromioclavicular joint.	Excess motion at acromioclavicular joint and possible pain	

(continued)

Neck and Shoulder (Continued)

Test and Indication	Description	Positive Finding	Figure
Costoclavicular test: TOS from compression/ tension between *clavicle and 1st and 2nd pair of ribs*	Compresses and posteriorly rotates the athlete's clavicle while checking the radial pulse. Perform the maneuver on athlete's exhale for best results.	Re-creates pain and/or ↓ radial pulse	
Pectoralis minor test: TOS from *pectoralis minor* compression/tension	Athlete's arm is hyperflexed, *abducted*, and externally rotated as therapist check radial pulse.	Re-creates pain and/or ↓ radial pulse	

Test	Description	Positive finding
Roos test: General finding of thoracic outlet syndrome	Athlete holds both arms at 90° *abduction*, elbow and wrist flexion. Athlete performs rapid finger flexion in this position for about 30 seconds.	Re-creates pain and/or ↓ radial pulse
Adson's test: Thoracic outlet syndrome (TOS) from *scalene muscle* compression and/or tension	Athlete's arm is passively *abducted* and extended with palm up. Therapist checks radial pulse as athlete turns head toward and/or away from that side. A common modifier is to have athlete take a deep breath and hold it to further tighten the scalenes.	Re-creates pain and/or ↓ radial pulse
Cervical compression: Nerve root compression in cervical spine	Therapist gently presses the crown of the athlete's head to compress the cervical spine as the athlete slowly exhales a deep breath.	Radiating pain down the spine and/or shoulder, or numbing sensation anywhere in the upper extremity
Kernig's test: Nerve root or spinal segment compression/tension.	Athlete lies supine and actively flexes neck and applies slight overpressure with hands behind head at the end of the movement.	Radiating pain down the spine

Elbow, Forearm, Wrist

Test and Indication	Description	Positive Finding	Figure
Phalen's test: Carpal tunnel syndrome	Athlete presses palms together in "prayer position" and slowly draws hands down to increase intensity of compression. Repeat with posterior side of hands; drawing hands upward to increase intensity of tension.	Re-creates pain	
Varus/valgus test: Ligament laxity	Therapist applies varus and valgus stress to elbow in slightly flexed elbow.	Soft end-feel and possible pain	

Answers to Chapter Review Questions

CHAPTER 1

1. a. Adjustable-height legs with secure locking mechanism. b. Detachable and adjustable face cradle. c. Minimum 2 inches of foam. d. Strong middle cross piece and hinge. e. Strong material for carrying case with shoulder strap, portable tables in the 5- to 15-pound range.
2. a. Multi-plane adjustable face cradle. b. Adjustable chest pad, leg height, and seat, quick and easy set up. c. Carrying case with shoulder strap or wheels.
3. Support the spine in a relaxed neutral position, avoids compression over soft tissues like stomach and breasts, provides the most comfortable and stable side-lying support for athletes, and is lightweight and easy to use in any environment.
4. a. O, b. C, c. L/G, d. C, e. O.
5. a
6. b
7. c
8. b
9. d
10. b
11. d
12. c
13. a
14. c
15. c
16. d

CHAPTER 2

1. Basic sports massage is scientific and intuitive application of massage, movement, and stretching to physically active people.
2. Effleurage, pétrissage, friction, vibration, tapotement.
3. a. Inflamed or edematous tissue. b. Varicose veins. c. Open wounds or skin rash/lesions. d. Cysts or tumors. e. Hematomas.

4. b
5. c
6. d
7. a
8. c
9. d
10. c
11. b
12. a
13. c
14. d
15. c
16. a
17. b
18. d
19. b
20. a

CHAPTER 3

1. Fluid return
2. Contraction of the heart and stretch—recoil of arteries.
3. Skeletal muscle contraction and respiratory pump.
4. Initial vessels, collecting capillaries, primary vessels (lymphangia), collecting trunks, deep collecting ducts.
5. a. **Catchment**—the primary lymph node beds
   b. **Watershed**—nonstructural divisions that mark the regional drainage areas of the lymphatic system; the location of the highest number of anastomoses
   c. **Starling forces**—the pressures created by different fluid volume and protein concentrations within and outside the capillary beds, which create and control capillary filtration and reabsorption
   d. **Oncotic pressure**—osmotic pressure created by the concentration of protein on either side of a semipermeable membrane
   e. **Angion**—the working unit of a lymphangia that has autonomic contractions to help propel lymph

through the primary vessels; a segment of the lymphangia marked by one-way valves at both ends

6. b
7. d
8. a
9. c
10. a
11. b
12. c
13. d
14. d
15. a
16. c
17. b
18. d
19. c
20. a

CHAPTER 4

1. **Muscle tone**—the amount of natural firmness of a muscle created by density of tissue and fluid volumes within
   Motor tone—The constant low-grade tension in a muscle related to neuromuscular signals; tonic contraction of several motor units in a muscle to maintain posture
   Tensile stress—The descriptor used to indicate that the "tight" muscle is being held in a long position (eccentric).
   Atrophy—Wasting away of muscle tissue due to disuse
   Hypertrophy—Building up/thickening of muscle fibers due to exercise
   Contractile stress—Descriptor used to indicate that the "tight" muscle is being held in a short position (concentric).
2. (1) Always found in a taut band of tissue; (2) has a distinct nodular feel to it; (3) compression of the point recreates a predicable pattern of pain related to the particular muscle housing the point; (4) muscle is hypersensitive to stretch
3. Tension is applied to the attachments pulling toward the center of the muscle, and the middle of the muscle (belly) bunches up or broadens.
4. Increased mechanical strain, impaired circulation or ischemia, dis-use or prolonged immobility, trauma/local inflammatory response, mental/emotional distress
5. c
6. d
7. b
8. a
9. c
10. d
11. c

12. a
13. d
14. b
15. a
16. c
17. b
18. d
19. a
20. b

CHAPTER 5

1. Macrophages, plasma cells, mast cells, and fibroblasts.
2. The superficial front and back myofascial chains work together to maintain posture.
3. Gluteus maximus, gluteus medius, vastus lateralis, latissimus dorsi.
4. Brow of the frontal bone, occipital ridge, sacrum, ischial tuberosity, femoral condyles, calcaneous, plantar surface of the phalanges.
5. Base of the cranium, thoracic inlet, diaphragm, pelvic floor.
6. a
7. c
8. b
9. d
10. a
11. c
12. d
13. a
14. a
15. b
16. c
17. b
18. d
19. a
20. c

CHAPTER 6

1. Swelling, Heat, A loss of function, Redness, Pain.
2. Sensory perception of pain causes muscles to go into a protective spasm that creates ischemia and further irritate free nerve endings, leading to more pain, which then becomes a self-perpetuating cycle.
3. Primary edema is the amount of hemorrhaged fluid from the damaged tissues and cells. Secondary edema is the additional swelling added to primary edema due to increased interstitial oncotic pressure pulling water out of healthy tissue and cells in an attempt to dilute the high concentration of proteins.
4. c
5. c

6. a
7. d
8. d
9. a
10. c
11. c
12. b
13. b
14. d
15. a
16. b
17. c
18. d
19. a
20. c

CHAPTER 7

1. (1) Raise table height, position athlete closer to side of table, change side of the table frequently, (2) use a step stool or box to rest front foot on during the work, and (3) use slight flexion and extension of the front knee during the application of stationary circles to keep hands relaxed and shoulders down.

2. All use very light pressure and apply slight stretch to the skin; the tissue must be fully released and allowed to snap back to its original position between strokes; strokes are applied in the direction that facilitates normal lymph flow; to be effective strokes must be repeated 15 to 20 times over the same location/tissue.

3. 1) Current infection
   2) Kidney dysfunction
   3) Active tuberculosis
   4) Current thrombosis, embolism, or phlebitis
   5) Congestive heart failure

4. LF improves edema uptake to help manage both primary and secondary edema formation; it helps relieve pain; it stimulates the lymphatic system while the other standard care measures manage edema via the circulatory system.

5. b
6. c
7. a
8. b
9. d
10. c
11. a
12. c
13. c
14. d
15. a
16. b
17. c
18. d

19. b
20. a

CHAPTER 8

1. Examples are post-isometric relaxation, muscle energy technique, Aston patterning, neuromuscular technique, NeuroKinetics, active release technique, myotherapy, strain-counterstrain, positional release, and others.

2. *Trigger point techniques*—use therapeutic compression over a palpable hypersensitive nodule to reduce the contraction knot believed to be the cause of the point.
   Positional release—uses repositioning, usually shortening, of the muscle housing the tender point to relieve the hypersensitivity of the point and to reduce tension in the muscle; based on the theory of gamma gain leading to a false stretch reflex report from the muscle spindle.
   Proprioceptive techniques—manipulates normal muscle reflexes such as reciprocal inhibition and Golgi tendon organ function to reduce muscle tension; uses contract-relax.

3. (1) The point has a nodular feel to it; (2) always occurs in a taut band of tissue; (3) moderate pressure creates exquisite pain; (4) athlete recognizes the pain elicited by the compression; (5) the pain radiates in a predictable pattern into surrounding tissue; and (6) the muscle housing the point has a painful limit to full stretch.

4. (1) Reciprocal inhibition, (2) proprioceptive neuromuscular facilitation specifically contract–relax, (3) muscle energy techniques, (4) post-isometric relaxation.

5. c
6. b
7. c
8. d
9. a
10. c
11. b
12. d
13. c
14. a
15. d
16. b
17. c
18. b
19. c
20. b

CHAPTER 9

1. Any technique with the primary intention of loosening, stretching, and/or broadening connective tissue. Myofascial techniques include Hellerwork, rolfing, struc-

tural integration, deep tissue techniques, myofascial release, muscle release technique, matrix repatterning, and others.

2. (1) Postural assessment, (2) general palpation that includes skin rolling and fascial excursion, (3) passive range of motion, (4) contract–relax techniques.

3. Direct myofascial technique is directed over the restriction and/or in the direction of restricted movement. Indirect myofascial technique focuses on areas other than the site of specific tissue restriction and/or in a direction that feeds slack into the restricted tissue.

4. (1) Severe hematoma, (2) local infection, (3) traumatic edema, (4) open wounds or fractures, (5) degenerative joint disease.

5. Deep transverse friction (DTF) must be preceded by thorough warming/preparation of the tissue, applied without an emollient, applied with a broad enough stroke to stretch the tissue. Muscles and tendons are short/soft during DTF and sheathed tendons on stretch; stroke is perpendicular to the fiber run of the muscle. DTF is applied frequently enough to effect long-term change.

6. c
7. b
8. a
9. d
10. b
11. d
12. b
13. c
14. b
15. d
16. a
17. c
18. b
19. a
20. c

CHAPTER 10

1. Soften and loosen fascia and other connective tissue; decrease excess muscle tension; enhance the hyperemia response in the muscles used in the activity; and provide kinesthetic feedback that helps create a positive state of mind.

2. Return muscles to resting tone and length; assist venous return to support metabolic recovery; deactivate trigger/tender points that may have developed during activity; reduce risk of delayed-onset muscle soreness.

3. Post-event is done at a slower pace and rhythm than pre-event, and the depth of strokes is moderated as needed.

4. (1) position the outside hand at the hip with fingers up and the inside hand on the medial side of the knee (ath-

lete's knee is bent and resting over therapist's forearm; (2) lift/push the hip up slightly and slide the knee into adduction as you supinate the hand to create external rotation of the hip; (3) unwind the quadriceps and apply light traction to release the sacroiliac joint. Indicators that the position should not be used include elevation of the hip, inability to keep the bent leg and ankle on the table, and the athlete's feeling uncomfortable.

5. Rhythmic compressions, pétrissage, friction.
6. d
7. a
8. c
9. b
10. c
11. d
12. a
13. a
14. c
15. b
16. a
17. d
18. c
19. a
20. b

CHAPTER 11

1. Maintenance massage (1) can identify restrictions and limitations in the pre-season physical to begin remedial work at the start of training; (2) can enhance the warm-up and cool-down processes; (3) can enhance general flexibility and ability to relax; (4) can help identify and remove soreness related to training before an injury occurs as a result of regular and thorough assessment of the muscles, tendons, and fascia.

2. Specific muscle release is any method that reduces muscle tension and/or fibrous adhesions in a muscle.

3. Goals are (1) to reduce general muscle hypertonicity/spasm; (2) to stretch, broaden, and loosen connective tissue; and (3) to enhance general flexibility; decrease the likelihood and impact of delayed-onset muscle soreness.

4. Upper body sports: baseball/softball, kayak/paddling, tennis and racket sports, golf, swimming.

5. Lower body sports: track/cross-country running, cycling, basketball, soccer, ice/field hockey, lacrosse, downhill skiing.

6. c
7. a
8. a
9. d
10. a
11. b
12. c

13. d
14. b
15. c
16. a
17. c
18. d
19. b
20. c

CHAPTER 12

1. Subjective and Objective.
2. Acute = sudden onset and easily measured progression through the healing cycle (short duration). Chronic = gradual onset and difficult to measure progression through healing (long/undetermined duration).
3. Stage of healing; Structures Involved; Severity.
4. Postural assessment, tissue inspection (visual and palpation), range of motion assessment (active then passive); strength tests, special tests.
5. Location, Frequency, Intensity, Description, Duration, and onset of pain/problem.
6. a
7. a
8. b
9. c
10. d
11. c
12. b
13. a
14. b
15. a
16. d
17. c
18. b
19. c
20. a

CHAPTER 13

1. Deep transverse friction and lymphatic facilitation.
2. Reduce edema, improve circulation, return range of motion, begin facilitation of flexible organized scar, continue to decrease pain-spasm cycle.

3. Acute—high frequency and low duration; chronic—low frequency and high duration.
4. In antagonists and synergists away from the site of trauma in the myofascial chain.
5. Myositis ossificans is bone/calcium formation within a muscle; it develops when a hematoma is repeatedly traumatized.
6. b
7. c
8. b
9. d
10. a
11. c
12. a
13. b
14. c
15. d
16. b
17. a
18. c
19. d
20. b

CHAPTER 14

1. Cryotherapy is the therapeutic use of cold. Primary physiologic effects are vasoconstriction that decreases local circulation, decreased metabolism, rise muscle threshold, reduction of spasm, decrease in pain.
2. Thermotherapy is the therapeutic use of heat. Primary physiologic effects are vasodilation that increases local circulation, increased metabolism, decreased pain, general muscle relaxation, softening and improved pliability of collagen.
3. Acute stage—cryotherapy; subacute stage—contrast or cryokinetics; maturation stage—thermotherapy or cryokinetics.
4. b
5. d
6. c
7. b
8. c
9. a
10. d

Glossary

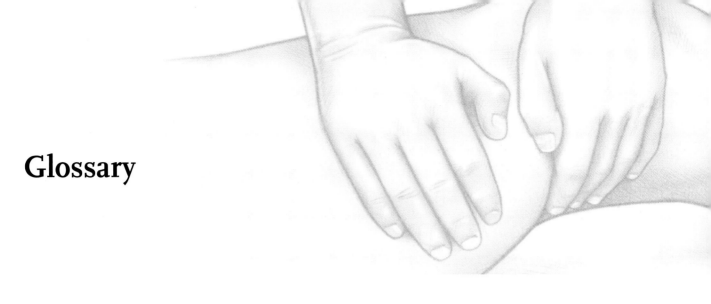

Acute—Term used to indicate an injury of sudden onset and short duration (an easily measured progression through the healing cycle).

Acute bursitis—The sudden inflammation of a bursa caused by either a sharp blow or a sudden increase in the intensity of the compression stress over the bursa by the tendon/ligament it is protecting.

Adhesion—A sticking together of connective tissue due to the diminished capacity of group substance caused by dehydration or injury.

Anastomosis—The end-to-end arrangement of multiple lymphatic collecting capillaries, similar to a capillary network in the cardiovascular system. Lymph flow can go in either direction across an anastomosis.

Anchor filaments—Microscopic fiber that extends from an initial lymphatic vessel into the interstitial tissue.

Angulus venosus—The junction between the lymphatic and cardiovascular division of circulation. Also referred to as the *terminus*.

Anthropometric—A measurement of the human body, including craniometry, osteometry, skin-fold evaluation for subcutaneous fat estimation, and height and weight measurement.

Aponeurosis—The broad flat sheet of fibrous connective tissue or tendon that connects skeletal muscles to bone.

Arthrokinematics—The normal and necessary joint play that allows free movement of the articular surfaces of the bones within a joint.

Available range of motion—The range of movement of a joint measured with passive range of motion.

Basic sports massage—A combination of deep Swedish massage and a few strokes specific to sports massage such as rhythmic compression, pin-and-stretch, and active release.

Capillary exchange—The process of fluid exchange that occurs between the blood and tissue.

Capillary filtration—Movement of fluid and dissolved substances from the blood to the interstitium.

Capillary fluid pressure (CFP)—The hydrostatic pressure created by the water content in the blood in capillaries.

One of four Starling forces that regulates fluid movement in the body.

Capillary reabsorption—The movement of fluid and dissolved substances back into the blood.

Catchment—An area in which several lymph nodes are clustered together, forming a bed of lymph nodes.

Charley-horse—A severe hematoma and muscle spasm caused by a sharp blow to the quadriceps, or occasionally to the hamstrings.

Chemical activation—The action that occurs when chemicals are released by damaged cells or secreted by surrounding tissues in response to the injury. Chemicals such as kinins, prostaglandins, serotonin, and histamine become part of the exudate. Each plays a role in the acute stage of healing by creating vasodilation, calling in macrophages and fibroblasts, and/or increasing the permeability of the vessels and tissues in the injured area.

Chronic injury—A gradual-onset trauma or damage to some part of the body.

Circulatory edema—Edema caused by dysfunction or disease in the cardiovascular system.

Cisterna chyli—A small bulge located at the base of the thoracic duct approximately at the level of the second vertebrae. It serves as a passive collecting well for lymph from the lower extremities and also gives an extra boost to lymph flow into and through the thoracic duct in response to deep breathing.

Collagen fibers—A bundle of thinner protein fibrils in parallel arrangement, similar in structure to the muscle fibers, which are tough and resistant to stretch because of the structure of the fibers.

Collecting capillary—A vessel that collects lymph from several initial lymphatic vessels.

Collecting trunk—A larger lymphatic vessel where primary lymph vessels converge after exiting catchment areas.

Colloidal osmotic pressure—A pressure differential two colloidal fluids (water and protein) separated by a membrane that creates movement of water toward the higher concentration of proteins to establish equilibrium between the substances.

Compressive pétrissage—A pétrissage stroke that presses the superficial tissue away from the underlying structures. The two types are kneading and lift and press (fulling).

Contractile—The ability to contract or shorten.

Contract–relax—The technique in which the tight muscle, or target muscle, is engaged in an isometric contraction and then relaxed.

Contrast therapy—A hydrotherapy treatment that uses alternating applications of heat and cold to help reduce traumatic edema.

Cryotherapy—The use of cold and/or ice applications for therapeutic purposes.

Deep collecting ducts—The right lymphatic and thoracic ducts of the lymphatic system. These deep ducts receive lymph from the collecting ducts and return it to cardiovascular circulation.

Dense connective tissue—Tissue that contains thicker more densely packed collagen fibers, less ground substance, and a low number of cells, making it strong and resistant to tensile stresses.

Diffusion—A passive transport mechanism based on the tendency of molecules of a substance to move from a region of high concentration to one of lower concentration.

Direct techniques—Myofascial techniques that are applied in the area of complaint and in line with the direction of restriction.

Edema—A local or generalized condition in which the interstitial spaces contain an excessive amount of tissue fluid.

Edema uptake—The movement of interstitial fluid into the initial lymphatic vessels.

Effleurage—A classic/Swedish massage stroke in which the hands glide or slide over the superficial tissue.

Elastic—A description used to describe a substance that can be stretched and then returns to its original state.

Elastic fiber—One of three types of connective tissue fibers; made up of a protein called elastin, which makes the fiber more "stretchy" than either collagen or reticular fibers.

End-feel—The distinct feeling palpated by therapists and/or sensed by the athlete at the end of the range of movement of a joint due to anatomic and physiologic restrictions that stop the motion.

Endomysium—A layer of connective tissue that covers the outside of each individual muscle fiber or cell.

Epimysium—The most superficial layer of connective tissue that surrounds a skeletal muscle.

Extensibility—A functional characteristic of some tissues and fibers in the body to lengthen or expand when force is applied. Extensibility implies that the tissue cannot snap back to its original length like an elastic tissue does.

Extravasate—The escape of blood, intracellular, and interstitial fluids from damaged cells, vessels and tissues into the surrounding tissues when strain, sprain, and/or compression trauma occurs.

Exudate—The accumulated fluid in tissue due to the collective escape of blood and intracellular and interstitial fluids.

Fibroblasts—A specialized connective tissue cell that secretes protein substances and that makes up both ground substance and the fibers in the matrix of connective tissue; the primary "repair cells" for the healing cycle.

Fibrous connective tissues—A connective tissue that contains thicker and more densely packed collagen fibers, less ground substance, and a low number of cells, making it strong and resistant to tensile stresses.

Filtration—A passive transport mechanism based on differences in pressure. Filtration moves substances from an area of high pressure to an area of lower pressure.

Firm end-feel—An end-feel that indicates that tension in the soft tissue is stopping the movement.

Friction—Any stroke that applies compression and stretch to tissue.

Frostbite—A condition in which prolonged exposure to cold has caused tissue to freeze.

Frostnip—First-degree or superficial frostbite.

Fulling—One form of compressive pétrissage in which the tissue is first lifted, or gathered into the middle of the tissue mass, then pressed down into the bone while the hands glide out across the fibers, pulling the tissue away from the middle.

Functional range of motion—The usable range of movement for a joint that is associated with active movement.

Goals—The desired outcome that therapists hope to achieve with massage.

Granulation tissue—Fragile threadlike fibers that begin the repair of damaged tissue in the subacute stage of healing.

Ground substance—The intercellular fluid in all connective tissues, mostly made of water, but also containing a unique protein and a polysaccharide chain that serve as water magnets for the ground substance.

Hard end-feel—An end-feel that indicates that bone has run into bone to stop the passive movement.

Heat exhaustion—A physiologic stress condition that occurs when the body has a combination of dehydration, excess loss of electrolytes, and depletion of energy.

Heat stress syndromes—Overheating conditions, such as heat stroke and heat exhaustion.

Heat stroke—A severe physiologic stress condition in which the core temperature of the body has increased to a life-threatening level. The condition is due to some combination of dehydration, prolonged physical exertion, and environmental conditions of high heat and/or high humidity.

Hematoma—A bruise.

Hematoma organization—The last step in the acute stage of the healing cycle, when fibroblasts begin to move to the perimeter of the exudates and establish a loose-knit net around the exudate.

Hemorrhage—An abnormal internal or external discharge of blood.

Hip or shoulder pointers—Severe hematomas that occur as a result of a sharp blow over the unprotected iliac crest and greater trochanter or the acromiodeltoid area.

Histamine—A chemical substance released by specialized connective tissue cells called *mast cells* when tissue is damaged or stressed. Histamine causes an increase in capillary permeability and blood vessel vasodilation in the area of its release.

Hydrotherapy—The use of water in any form for therapeutic purposes.

Hyperemia—An increase in the quantity of blood in capillary network. Hyperemia is generally indicated by external reddening of the tissue.

Hypothermia—A condition brought on by an excess loss of heat, which is most likely to occur with a combination of cool temperature, wind, and wet clothing.

Indirect myofascial techniques—Techniques that are applied outside the area of the area of complaint or in the opposite direction of the restriction.

Inert tissues—Tissues that do not contract; includes bone, articular cartilage, menisci, ligaments, bursae, and joint capsules.

Inflammation—The basic immune response that occurs in reaction to any type of bodily injury.

Initial vessel—The first capillary in the lymphatic vascular network.

Interstitial fluid pressure (IFP)—The hydrostatic pressure created by the water content in the interstitial spaces. One of four Starling forces that regulates fluid movement in the body.

Interstitial oncotic pressure (IOP)—The osmotic pressure created in the interstitial spaces by the protein content of the interstitial fluid. One of four Starling forces that regulates fluid movement in the body.

Intralymph valves—One-way valves located throughout the primary lymphatic vessels (lymphangia) and at the junction between collecting capillaries and the primary lymph vessels. These valves prevent lymph backflow and create a slight propulsion pressure within the lymph vessel when they close.

Jump response—The action of pulling away or flinching in response to moderate compression palpation over a tender point.

Kinetics—The therapeutic practice of combining cold and movement to facilitate the healing cycle and begin rehabilitation of an injury. First, cold is applied to reduce pain and muscle spasm; the active movement through the pain-free range of motion is then used.

Lesion—An injury or wound; stretching, compression, or tearing of tissue.

Ligament laxity test—Structural stress tests used to test the integrity of ligaments in synovial joints throughout the body.

Local twitch response—A visible or palpable transient contraction of fibers within the taut muscle band associated with myofascial trigger points.

Long stroke (L/S)—A lymphatic facilitation stroke applied by lightly engaging the superficial tissue in slight stretch, then sliding full hands or flat fingers over the surface of the skin.

Lumen—Inside diameter of a vessel.

Lymph—The interstitial fluid once it enters the initial lymphatic vessels.

Lymphangia—Another term for a primary lymph vessel.

Lymphatic facilitation (LF)—A unique style of massage specifically directed at reducing traumatic edema.

Lymphatic obligatory load—The volume of fluid from capillary filtrate that remains in the interstitium after capillary reabsorption—approximately 10%—which must be picked up by the lymphatic system for return to general circulation. Many metabolic by-products, proteins, and other cellular substances are carried in the fluid of the obligatory load.

Lymphatic terminus—The junction between the lymphatic and cardiovascular division of circulation. Also called the *angulus venosus*.

Lymphedema—An abnormal accumulation of tissue fluid in the interstitial spaces due to dysfunction or failure in the lymphatic system.

Lymphotome—The anatomic connection between a specific group of initial vessels, collecting capillaries, and lymphangia that forms a single pathway for lymph flow.

Mast cells—Cells that are distributed throughout all types of connective tissue and that produce histamine and heparin, two chemicals that play important roles in the healing cycle.

Matrix—The background substance of cells, comprising ground substance and fibers.

Mechanism of injury—The description of the how an injury occurred.

Microtrauma—Microscopic irritation and/or tearing of tissue related chronic injuries.

Modality—A method or application of any therapeutic agent used to affect physical and/or physiologic changes.

Movement barriers—Conditions that restrict movement, such as muscle tension, fascial restrictions, the structural integrity of joints, edema, or pain; the point at which therapist or athlete sense resistance to a movement.

Muscle cramp—A short-term temporary muscle contraction that creates dysfunction and pain that affects a single training session or competition. Common causes include muscle fatigue, dehydration, and excessive loss of metabolites.

Muscle splinting—The pain signal to the brain that initiates a protective motor response causing a reflex contraction of the muscles surrounding the injured area.

Musculotendinous junction—The area in which muscle makes the transition to the fibrous connective tissue of the tendon.

Myofascial pain syndrome—A regional pain condition in which nonmuscular trigger points can occur in cutaneous, ligamentous, fascial, and periosteal tissue.

Myofascial techniques—Any method used to stretch, broaden, and soften fascia and other connective tissue elements.

Myositis ossificans—A condition in which there is growth of a bony deposit within the muscle and/or surrounding soft tissue. It usually follows trauma that involves significant hemorrhage that may have been mismanaged.

Neuromuscular release (NMR):—Any massage technique that is directed at reducing abnormal muscle tension and spasm.

Oncotic pressure—An osmotic pressure caused by high levels of protein molecules.

Osmosis—A specialized form of diffusion in which the solvent, usually water, passes through a semi-permeable membrane from a region of lower concentration of solute to that of a higher concentration.

Osmotic pressure—The pressure that develops when water is drawn into tissue in an attempt to balance different concentration gradients.

Osteokinematics—A measurement of the movement of a bone when it swings through a range of motion around the axis in a joint, such as flexion, extension, abduction, adduction, or rotation.

Paresthesia—A sensation of pins and needles, tingling, or burning and aching described with neurologic or circulatory impairments.

Perimysium—A connective tissue layer that divides the muscle into several different internal components by wrapping around a bundle of several muscles fibers to make a fascicle.

Periosteum—Tough connective tissue that is the outer covering of bone.

Pétrissage—Massage stroke in which superficial tissues are separated from the underlying surfaces with a grasping, lifting motion of the hands.

Plans—The combination of modalities used to achieve the desired treatment goals and the projected time frame for therapy.

Plasma—The fluid portion of blood.

Plasma oncotic pressure (POP)—Osmotic pressure created inside the cardiovascular capillary by the protein content of the blood.

Position of ease—A position of comfort or decreased tension used in positional release to release tender points. It is generally a shortened position for the muscle housing the tender point.

Prelymphatic channels—The unorganized and unstructured pathway in the interstitium that fluid flows through before reaching initial lymphatic vessels.

Primary edema—The amount of hemorrhaged fluids from the damaged tissues and cells in strain, sprain, and/or compression trauma.

Primary lymphedema—A congenital or genetic defect in the development or function of the lymphatic system resulting in an insufficient fluid return function of the system.

Raynaud's syndrome—Circulatory conditions in which arterioles in the extremities respond to cold with severe vasoconstriction.

Respiratory pump—Changes in cavity pressure caused by the contraction of the diaphragm that facilitates venous and lymphatic fluid flow.

Reticular fibers—Connective tissue fibers similar to collagen in structure and function but thinner and more delicate. They form the network of connective tissue that surrounds and gives support to smooth and skeletal muscle cells, nerve fibers, and the connective tissue framework for organs.

Right lymphatic duct—The deep collecting duct of the lymphatic system that collects fluid from the upper right quadrant of the body and carries it back to the cardiovascular system at the junction of the right jugular and subclavian veins.

Secondary edema—The amount of traumatic edema that continues to form during the acute stage of healing after the initial hemorrhage has been stopped. The increased interstitial oncotic pressure after injury is the primary cause of secondary edema.

Secondary lymphedema—Lymphatic system pathology; a gross regional edema that occurs when lymph nodes or vessels are damaged or destroyed, such as in radiation therapy, surgery, or chemotherapy.

Signs—The measurable and quantifiable or objective information about a particular injury or condition.

Site-specific technique—A myofascial technique that applies compression and stretch of tissue over a specific structure or small region of muscle or fascia.

Skin rolling—A specific type of myofascial assessment and treatment in which the therapist applies a loose pincer grip to the skin, causing a roll of tissue to pop up and be rolled between thumb and fingers.

Soft end-feel—An end-feel that occurs when a mass of soft tissue stops the movement.

Solutes—The solid substances of a solution.

Spasms—A sustained muscle contraction that is commonly the result of chronic low-grade strains or functional adaptations to a repeated position or pattern of movement.

Specific muscle release—Any neuromuscular or myofascial method/stroke that reduces muscle tension and/or fibrous adhesion in muscle.

Sprain—An injury in which ligaments and/or joint capsules have been stretched or torn.

Starling forces—Four distinct forces acknowledged as the regulatory mechanisms for capillary exchange of fluid. The four forces are capillary fluid pressure, interstitial fluid pressure, plasma oncotic pressure, and interstitial oncotic pressure.

Stationary circle (S/C)—A stroke in which the superficial tissue is engaged in a light stretch and carried through an "L" pattern of movement, then released and allowed to snap back into place while the therapist's hand circles back to re-engage the tissue at the starting point of the stroke. Stationary circles stretch tissue in two vectors: first across the line of lymph flow and then in-line with lymph flow.

Strain—An injury where only fascia, tendons, and muscles are involved.

Structural effects—Changes in muscle and connective tissue created by massage.

Symptoms—The subjective information or what the athlete tells you about an injury or trauma to any part of the body.

Systemic effects—The cellular, circulatory, and/or nervous system changes created by massage.

Target muscle—Tight muscle that is the target of the proprioceptive neuromuscular facilitation (PNF) techniques.

Technique—A specific type of massage that has strokes sharing the same general intentions and methods of application.

Tendon—The fibrous connective tissue cord formed by the extension and melding of epi-, peri-, and endomysium to connect muscles to bone.

Tendonopathies—A generic term that describes any form of irritation, stretching, or tearing of tendons that create pain and dysfunction. Inflammation may or may not be a part of this condition.

Tenoperiosteal junction—The point at which the fibrous connective tissue of the tendons weaves into the periosteum.

Tensegrity—A term that describes a structure that maintains structural integrity via a system of guidewires and tension cords between solid structures; compression or tension in any one area is reflected throughout the system.

Therapeutic pressure—Amount of pressure applied to a trigger point to deactivate the point.

Thermotherapy—The application of heat for therapeutic purposes.

Thixotropic—The ability of ground substance in connective tissue to change between the gel (more solid) and sol (more soluble or fluid) state in response to temperature change and movement.

Thoracic duct—The deep collecting duct of the lymphatic system that is situated in the central thoracic and abdominopelvic cavities. It is responsible for the collection of lymph from the other three fourths of the body and returns it to cardiovascular system at the left terminus.

Thoracic outlet syndrome (TOS)—A compression–tension syndrome of the neurovascular bundle that passes through the posterior triangle of the neck out to the upper extremity.

Tissue excursion—The amount of slide–glide allowed by superficial fascia before it resists further movement. This type of palpation is used to access the mobility of broad areas of superficial fascia such as the lumbosacral aponeurosis and iliotibial band.

Traumatic edema—The localized and temporary swelling of tissue associated with soft tissue injury and/or the exertion of exercise, including the acute or chronic sprains, strains, and hematomas common to sports and exercise.

Vasoconstriction—Narrowing of the artery lumen that generally restricts blood flow.

Vasodilation—A widening of the artery lumen that reduces resistance to blood flow.

Viscoelastic—A unique quality of fascia to extend owing to the unwinding of collagen fibers and thixotropic changes in ground substance.

Watershed—A thin area of tissue that gives regional organization to the multiple lymphotomes into the body. The highest percentage of anastomoses are located at the watersheds, allowing lymph flow to be directed into different lymphotomes and catchments.

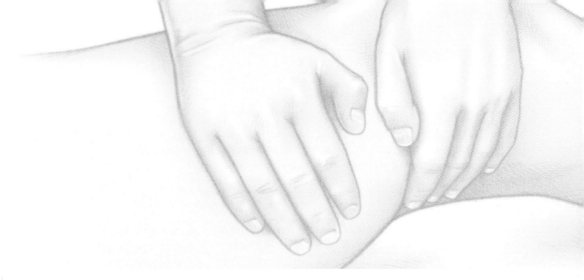

Index

Note: Page numbers followed by t and f indicate tables and figures, respectively. Those followed by b indicate boxed material.